Practical UROLOGY
(Instruments, Pathology, Radiology)
A Comprehensive Guide

Practical UROLOGY
(Instruments, Pathology, Radiology)
A Comprehensive Guide

SECOND EDITION

Editors

Ravindra B Sabnis MS MCh
Chairman
Department of Urology
Muljibhai Patel Urological Hospital
Nadiad, Gujarat, India

Arvind P Ganpule MS DNB MNAMS
Vice-Chairman
Department of Urology
Muljibhai Patel Urological Hospital
Nadiad, Gujarat, India

Sujata K Patwardhan MS MCh
Professor and Head
Department of Urology
Seth GS Medical College and KEM Hospital
Mumbai, Maharashtra, India

Assistant Editors

Abhishek G Singh MS MCh DNB
Fellow in Endourology and Laparo-robotic Urology
Consultant Urologist
Muljibhai Patel Urological Hospital
Nadiad, Gujarat, India

Abhijit P Patil MS MCh DNB
Consultant Urologist
Muljibhai Patel Urological Hospital
Nadiad, Gujarat, India

Rohan S Batra MS DNB
Consultant Urologist
Muljibhai Patel Urological Hospital
Nadiad, Gujarat, India

Forewords
P Venugopal
Mahesh R Desai
Prokar Dasgupta FKC
Thomas RW Herrmann

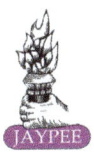

JAYPEE BROTHERS MEDICAL PUBLISHERS
The Health Sciences Publisher
New Delhi | London

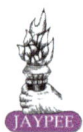 **Jaypee Brothers Medical Publishers (P) Ltd**

Headquarters
EMCA House
23/23-B, Ansari Road, Daryaganj
New Delhi 110 002, India
Landline: +91-11-23272143, +91-11-23272703
+91-11-23282021, +91-11-23245672
E-mail: jaypee@jaypeebrothers.com

Corporate Office
Jaypee Brothers Medical Publishers (P) Ltd.
4838/24, Ansari Road, Daryaganj
New Delhi 110 002, India
Phone: +91-11-43574357
Fax: +91-11-43574314
E-mail: jaypee@jaypeebrothers.com

Overseas Office
JP Medical Ltd.
83, Victoria Street, London
SW1H 0HW (UK)
Phone: +44-20 3170 8910
Fax: +44(0)20 3008 6180
E-mail: info@jpmedpub.com

Website: www.jaypeebrothers.com
Website: www.jaypeedigital.com

© 2022, Jaypee Brothers Medical Publishers

The views and opinions expressed in this book are solely those of the original contributor(s)/author(s) and do not necessarily represent those of editor(s) of the book.

All rights reserved by the author. No part of this publication may be reproduced, stored or transmitted in any form or by any means, electronic, mechanical, photocopying, recording or otherwise, without the prior permission in writing of the publishers.

All brand names and product names used in this book are trade names, service marks, trademarks or registered trademarks of their respective owners. The publisher is not associated with any product or vendor mentioned in this book.

Medical knowledge and practice change constantly. This book is designed to provide accurate, authoritative information about the subject matter in question. However, readers are advised to check the most current information available on procedures included and check information from the manufacturer of each product to be administered, to verify the recommended dose, formula, method and duration of administration, adverse effects and contraindications. It is the responsibility of the practitioner to take all appropriate safety precautions. Neither the publisher nor the author(s)/editor(s) assume any liability for any injury and/or damage to persons or property arising from or related to use of material in this book.

This book is sold on the understanding that the publisher is not engaged in providing professional medical services. If such advice or services are required, the services of a competent medical professional should be sought.

Every effort has been made where necessary to contact holders of copyright to obtain permission to reproduce copyright material. If any have been inadvertently overlooked, the publisher will be pleased to make the necessary arrangements at the first opportunity. The **CD/DVD-ROM** (if any) provided in the sealed envelope with this book is complimentary and free of cost. **It is Not meant for sale.**

Inquiries for bulk sales may be solicited at: jaypee@jaypeebrothers.com

Practical Urology (Instruments, Pathology, Radiology): A Comprehensive Guide / Ravindra B Sabnis, Arvind P Ganpule, Sujata K Patwardhan

First Edition: 2016

Second Edition: **2022**

ISBN: 978-93-90595-66-2

Contributors

Abhijit P Patil MS MCh DNB
Consultant Urologist
Muljibhai Patel Urological Hospital
Nadiad, Gujarat, India

Abhishek B Ladhha MS DNB
Fellow in Uro-oncology
Amrita Institute of Medical Science
Kochi, Kerala, India

Abhishek G Singh MS MCh DNB
Fellow in Endourology and Laparo-robotic Urology
Consultant Urologist
Muljibhai Patel Urological Hospital
Nadiad, Gujarat, India

Amit Jojera MD
Consultant Pathologist
Muljibhai Patel Urological Hospital
Nadiad, Gujarat, India

Amit S Bhattu MS DNB
Clinical Fellow in Urological Oncology and Robotic Surgery
University of Miami, Miller School of Medicine
Miami, Florida, USA

Arvind P Ganpule MS DNB MNAMS
Vice-Chairman
Department of Urology
Muljibhai Patel Urological Hospital
Nadiad, Gujarat, India

Gopal Tak MS DNB
Consultant Urologist
Asian Institute of Nephrology and Urology (AINU)
Hyderabad, Telangana, India

Jigish B Vyas MS DNB
Consultant Urologist and Transplant Surgeon
Zydus Hospital
Pramukhswami Medical College and Shree Krishna Hospital
Anand, Gujarat, India

Jitendra V Jagtap MS DNB
Fellow in Endourology and Laparo-robotic Urology
Consultant Urologist
Global Hospital
Mumbai, Maharashtra, India

Mahesh R Desai MS FRCS
Managing Trustee
Muljibhai Patel Urological Hospital
Past President, Urological Society of India (USI)
Past President, Endourology Society Inc
Past President, Societe Internationale de Urologie (SIU)
Nadiad, Gujarat, India

Nitiraj B Shete MSc Statistics
PhD pursuing
Biostatistician
Muljibhai Patel Urological Hospital
Nadiad, Gujarat, India

Raghuram Ganesamoni MS MRCS
MCh
Fellow in Endourology and Laparo-robotic Urology
Consultant Urologist
Ganesamoni Hospital
Nagercoil, Tamil Nadu, India

Rahul A Chrimade MS MCh
Consultant Urologist
Department of Urology
RR Hospital
Nashik, Maharashtra, India

Ravindra B Sabnis MS MCh
Chairman
Department of Urology
Muljibhai Patel Urological Hospital
Nadiad, Gujarat, India

Rohan S Batra MS DNB
Consultant Urologist
Muljibhai Patel Urological Hospital
Nadiad, Gujarat, India

Sanika A Ganpule MBBS DMRE
Consultant Radiologist
Muljibhai Patel Urological Hospital
Nadiad, Gujarat, India

Shailesh Soni MD
Head, Department of Pathology
Muljibhai Patel Urological Hospital
Nadiad, Gujarat, India

Shashikant K Mishra MS DNB
Fellow in Endourology and
Laparo-robotic Urology
Consultant Urologist
Precision Urology Hospital
Lucknow, Uttar Pradesh, India

Sujata K Patwardhan MS MCh
Professor and Head
Department of Urology
Seth GS Medical College and KEM Hospital
Mumbai, Maharashtra, India

Foreword

I deem it a great honour to be invited again to write a forward for the Second Edition of the book by Ravindra B Sabnis, Sujata K Patwardhan and Arvind P Ganpule on 'Urology Instrumentation A Comprehensive Guide' now renamed as 'Practical Urology (Instruments, Pathology, Radiology) A Comprehensive Guide'. This has added contributors of young minds in Indian Urology who are fast making a name for themselves in the field of Urology. The earlier book on 'Instrumentation' became a grand success and soon became a near bible for all those taking exit exams in Urology. As rightly mentioned in the preface of second edition, there were many who felt that a book addressing most aspects of practical exam was indeed necessary and that included I as well.

In the practical exam in Urology, time is a real worrying aspect and the candidate is expected to answer the questions posed without much delay and in few sentences. As an Examiner who has conducted many exams, I found that for many who are taking the exit exam, answering at times become a nightmare and many a time the answers are found inadequate. This is where this edition of the book is going to be a boon for all who are taking up the exit exams in urology, be it MCh (urology) or DipNB (Urology).

This book is not only valuable to the trainees as mentioned but is a good recipe for those who are examiners or are probably being considered as an examiner. Good questions asked is a necessity for examiners. They should be to the point with clarity.

Apart from updating the Section on 'Instruments', the book has additional sections on 'Uropathology', Uroradiology' apart from a section on 'Chemotherapy schedules for Urological Malignancies' which will be of considerable use for all. It has also details of 'operative procedures' commonly asked in exit exams. Overall I find this book will become a must for all practicing Urology and a boon for those in training and planning to take up the exam.

The Editors and Contributors need a special mention in making it possible for bringing out such an 'all inclusive book' on practical aspects of Urology. Their efforts and perseverance need to be lauded. I am sure this edition will be in considerable demand as the earlier one. With the popularity this book will gain, I am sure that I may have the privilege to write forwards for subsequent editions soon to follow.

P Venugopal
Prof (Emeritus) Urology,
Kasturba Medical College (KMC)
Mangaluru, Karnataka

Foreword

I am delighted to pen this foreword for this new form of old book on Instrument.

I must compliment and congratulate Drs Sabnis, Patwardhan, and Ganpule for the hard work they have put in to make sure that this volume sees the light of the day.

When students appear for the practical examination, they are well read, know everything but have to revise what they have read, and need information which is concise, to the point, and in the manner that is required in a practical exam. For a long time, such books were lacking. The editors had come out with the first edition, which gave all information about instruments. Because contents were of practical relevance, it quickly became popular and in no time became a "bestseller".

In the second edition, several new sections have been added, which I feel is huge value addition. I have read a few chapters in details and what I have realized, that the format is very reader friendly, and the flow of information is as if a student is actually appearing for exam, especially pathology and radiology sections. The colored photographs and diagrammatic explanation of photos, flowcharts, and tables appear quite attractive, and are likely to leave an everlasting impression in the reader's mind. Compiling chemotherapy regimens was a great idea as this aspect is often difficult to remember and quickly forgotten. These new chapters would serve as a one-stop reference for all postgraduates appearing for their exit examinations.

I feel this book will be useful not only to students appearing for exam but also to all Urologists, be it junior or senior.

I am particularly pleased to see that majority of the contributors of this book are past students of the Muljibhai Patel Urological Hospital. It gives me an immense sense of satisfaction and pride. I have no doubt that this book will also become the "Best of bestsellers".

I wish to congratulate once again all those who contributed.

Mahesh R Desai
Managing Trustee and Chief Consultant Urologist
Muljibhai Patel Urological Hospital, Nadiad, Gujarat, India
Past President, Urological Society of India
Societe Internationale de Urologie and Endourology Society

Foreword

It is a pleasure to write a foreword to this excellent book by Dr Ravindra B Sabnis, Arvind P Ganpule and Sujata K Patwardhan, now in its second edition. The text itself has evolved significantly from the first edition which focussed on urological instrumentation and is now arranged in four neat sections. This is clearly to bring it up-to-date with our ever-progressive specialty where numerous recent advances have occurred to directly improve the care of our patients.

I enjoyed reading every section and wish I had such a succinct text myself when preparing for my exit exams. The Questions/Answers format is particularly useful for trainees in the sub-continent preparing for their MCh or DNB exams. The text could also potentially be of considerable help to candidates preparing for similar exams elsewhere in the world such as the FRCS(Urol) or FEBU. Urology is after all a global specialty.

This is a modern book that covers everything from the basics of cystoscopy to the recent developments in miniaturization of instrumentation for PCNL. It avoids obvious pitfalls and bias by objectively comparing the outcomes of open, laparoscopic and robot-assisted radical prostatectomy. It covers the latest Grade Grouping for prostate cancer which the editor of every major journal has been trying to promote since it superseded the Gleason scoring system. And finally, it is right up-to-date with current chemotherapy and immunotherapy for urological cancers. It entices students to learn about biostatistics and trial design, so that they can not only appraise the scientific literature critically but perhaps even contribute to it in the future.

The contributors read like a "who is who" in Indian urology, from the stars of the future to the most experienced surgeons. It is well illustrated, easy to read and the ideal revision text to impress your examiners.

This is a must read and I would happily have it in my library, either as a traditional printed version or in an electronic format for a kindle!

Prokar Dasgupta FKC
King's Health Partners Foundation Professor of Surgery
Editor in Chief, BJUI 2012-20

Foreword

It is my distinct pleasure and honor to contribute a foreword to the second edition of "Practical Urology – Comprehensive Guide", formerly known in first edition as "Urology Instrumentation – A Comprehensive Guide" by editors Drs Ravindra B Sabnis, Sujata K Patwardhan, and Arvind P Ganpule.

In the light of PubMed, YouTube, and Google, one could ask: What is the need for textbooks today? as Dr YouTube and Dr Google seem to be the most accomplished forums to study and learn the friends and foes of contemporary urology. I presume that the internet (in front of the paywall) probably takes you to your next "like" on Twitter, Instagram, or LinkedIn but surely does not make you fulfil the requirements for passing your exit exams in urology for either MCh or DipNB.

Although having stood all my exams in Europe, I still can confirm the above as an eyewitness (and fortunately not as an examinee) of the Saturday's "Improvement hours" during my time as a fellow at the Muljibhai Patel Urological Hospital in 2003. The motto of the European Space Agency (ESA) "per aspera ad astra" gained real reference at that time to me. My formidable colleagues in residency, who had passed the selection process to enter the residency program at this institution, by showing their knowledge in urology beforehand in a non–multiple choice written exam with Campbell's urology, as the examination subjects were put to the acid test to guarantee good performance at their exit exams, for the sake of themselves, their patients, and last but not the least the honor of the institution. I can therefore confirm that the first edition would already have been very useful in those days, in 2003 and for sure from the beginning, as it structured and distilled the essence out of urology and made it "practically available".

This enhanced version of the first edition with added sections such as Uropathology, Uroradiology and Uro-oncology has evolved into a true Vademecum not only for the future examinee who is eager to pass the exam with flying colors but also for the practicing urologist as well.

The channels on which we receive information today are so diverse that it has become a challenge itself to select and display the relevant facts. Therefore, I would like to thank the editors and contributors for their honorable efforts in providing such a fine book. Your efforts will pay off for residents, for urologists, and last but not the least for examiners inside the urological universe.

Thomas RW Herrmann MD PhD MSc FEBU
Director of Urology Spital Thurgau AG
Head of Department of Urology Kantonspital Frauenfeld
Chairman German Working Group for Endourology – AK Endourologie
Member German Working Group for Operative Techniques –
AK Operative Techniken
Member of ESUT
Member of European Guideline Panel for Non-neurogenic Male LUTS
Associate Editor World J Urology
Associate Editor SIU Journal

Preface to the Second Edition

We are happy to release this second edition of "Urology Instrumentation A Comprehensive Guide".

After overwhelming success of first edition, for long time, we were contemplating to come out with second edition. After release of first edition, we got feedback from many. Most students were happy to about the content which they found very useful during exam. We got lot of suggestions to add many more sections. Hence we decided that when we come out with second edition, we will not restrict to instruments but add many other sections which are useful for students when they appear for exam.

So this book is now, no longer restricted only to instruments in urology. Apart from revamping Instruments section other 3 sections area added. In Instruments section, we have added many new chapters which will be useful to practicing urologists also. Section on Uropathology covers all specimens and specimen related questions and answers to them. Similarly in Uroradiology, we have included all typical and common X-rays, CT scans…etc. Each imaging study has details of what questions can be asked and how those can be answered. Last Miscellaneous section, we have added chapter on Biostatistics which is now not only important aspect in practical, but this chapter elaborates many common statistical methods in simplified manner. If someone has conduct a study and analyze it, then this chapter will be very helpful. Lastly various important and landmark trials and common chemotherapy regimes are given. This will give readymade information at one glance.

Thus this book is now named as "Practical Urology (Instruments, Pathology, Radiology) A Comprehensive Guide". Because of all new added sections, we feel, this book will not only be useful to Trainees of MCh or DNB courses but also be useful to practicing urologists, who wish to remain updated with latest information. Biggest benefit is, all this information is available in a comprehensive manner in one book. This book will also be useful to urology trainee abroad who have similar exit exam pattern.

It would be unfair if we fail to acknowledge that hard work of our assistant editors and contributors towards completion of this book. We thank Dr P Venugopal, Dr MR Desai, Dr Prokar Dasgupta, and Dr Thomas Herman for going through the book and writing forward. We also thank M/s Jaypee Brothers Medical publications (P) Ltd, New Delhi, India to have accepted the project and come out with his book.

Ravindra B Sabnis
Arvind P Ganpule
Sujata K Patwardhan

Preface to the First Edition

During various National Boards, University and mock examinations as an examiner, we realized that most students become shaky when they appear for instrument viva. This is probably because there is no dedicated book for reading. They go through various atlas/catalogues provided by companies, that contains lots of unnecessary information, and hence, students are under pressure to face this viva.

Over the years, we realized that there is need to have a book on this topic. We decided to write a small booklet to give information about commonly asked instruments in examination. While writing the booklet, suggestions came from many colleagues about not restricting scope of the book only to those examination-going trainees but expand it to give full information about all urological instruments. We accepted suggestions and decided to have this compressive guide of all urological instruments. We also decided to add chapters such as disposables, laparoscopic/robotic instruments, energy sources, sterilization methods, etc. so as to give value to the book.

Urology is rapidly advancing branch and it is more so in urological instrumentations. Within short-time, new instruments come which makes whole armamentarium quite big. In our attempt to provide updated information, we have referred to various catalogues and textbooks, however, as medical facts keep changing, newer things keep adding, some information may be lacking or may be old, hence the book should be viewed keeping this in mind.

We feel, the book will not only be useful to the trainees of MCh or DNB courses but also to all urologists, who wish to remain updated with various instruments in urology. We also feel that the book will be useful abroad especially in countries, where examination pattern is somewhat similar to ours.

It would be unfair, if we fail to acknowledge the hardwork of our assistant editors and contributors towards completion of the project. We thank Glenn M Preminger, Michael YC Wong, Mahesh R Desai, Olivier Traxer, Steeve Doizi, Percy Jal Chibber and P Venugopal for going through the book and writing forewords. We also thank M/s Jaypee Brothers Medical Publishers (P) Ltd, New Delhi, India to have accepted to publish this rather unusual book.

Ravindra B Sabnis
Sujata K Patwardhan
Arvind P Ganpule

Contents

SECTION 1: INSTRUMENTS

1. Cystoscope and its Accessories — 3
Introduction and Brief History   3
The Cystoscope Sheath   4
Bridges   8
Obturators   9
Special Types of Cystourethroscopes and their Uses   10
Flexible Cystourethroscope   13
Meatotomy Scissor   17

2. Visual Internal Urethrotomy, Otis Urethrotome — 21
Sachse's Optical Urethrotomy   21
Blades   22
Otis Maurmyers Urethrotome   23

3. Transurethral Resection of the Prostate Instruments — 25
Introduction and History of Transurethral Resection of
the Prostate Instruments   25
Resectoscope Sheath (Monopolar)   25
What is a Rotating Resectoscope?   27
Working Element   29
Irrigating Fluids in Transurethral Resection of the Prostate   34
Transurethral Resection of the Prostate Syndrome   35
Accessories to Evacuate Prostate Chips   36

4. Bipolar Transurethral Resection of the Prostate — 38
Introduction   38
Irrigation in Bipolar Transurethral Resection of the Prostate   39
Advantages of Bipolar Transurethral Resection of the Prostate   39
Limitations of Bipolar Technology   39
Types   39

5. Cystolithotrity Instruments — 43
History and Brief Introduction   43

6. Percutaneous Nephrolithotomy Instruments — 48
Instruments   48
Access Needles   48
Percutaneous Nephrolithotomy Tract Dilators   50
Nephroscopes   55
Ultramini Percutaneous Nephrolithotomy   60
Energy Sources   66

7. Semirigid Ureteroscopy — 74
Introduction   74
Evolution of Ureteroscopes   74
Classification   75
Karl Storz 7/9.9 Fr Semirigid Ureteroscope   76
Richard Wolf Ureteroscopes   78
Olympus Ureteroscopes   79
Accessories   79
Instruments Used in Retrograde Endopyelotomy   79

8. Flexible Ureteroscope — 81
Evolution of Flexible Ureteroscopes   81
Types of Flexible Ureteroscopes   81
Basic Design of a Flexible Fiberoptic Ureteroscope   82
Optical System   82
Parts of a Conventional Fiberoptic Flexible Ureteroscope   82
Why Dual Deflection has Disappeared?   84
What do you Mean by Active and Passive Deflection?   84
What is Leakage Tester?   84
Accessories   87

9. Laparoscopy and Robotics Instruments — 91
Laparoscopic Instruments   91
Armamentarium   91
Video and Imaging   92
Access Devices   96
Insufflation Devices   97
Trocars   99
Instruments Used for the Retroperitoneal Approach   104
Laparoscopic Scissors   107
Laparoscopic Staplers   113
Miscellaneous Instruments   114
Angle of View   114
Special Laparoscopes   115
Newer Instruments   115
New Platforms for Laparoscopy   117
Robotics Surgery in Urology   117

10. Energy Sources in Open, Laparoscopic, and Robotic Surgery 122
Introduction 122
Definitions 122
Classification 123
Electrosurgical Tissue Effects 125
Advance Bipolar Systems 126
Argon Beam Coagulator 132
Safety Consideration 134

11. Accessories 137
Ureteric Catheter 137
Guidewires 140
Double J Stent 142
Description of Individual Catheters 145
Various Size Parameters and Color Coding of Catheters 147
Baskets and Retropulsion Devices 150
Urethral Balloon Dilators 153
Ureteric Dilator 153
Passive Dilators: Double J Stents 153
Percutaneous Nephrolithotomy Accessories 157

12. Sterilization 160
Definitions 160
Approach to Disinfection and Sterilization 161
Different Methods of Sterilization 161
Aldehyde 165
Formaldehyde 166
Steps of Sterilization and Processing of Surgical Instruments 167

13. Open Urology Instruments 174
Open Surgery Retractors 174
Vascular Instruments 177
Uses of Vascular Instruments 179
Stone Holding Forceps 179
Use 180
Instruments Used in Urethral Surgery 181

14. Pediatric Urology 186
Pediatric Endourology Instruments 186
Deflux 195
Diagnostic and Therapeutic Indications 198
Diagnosis 198
Therapy 198

15. Lasers in Urology — 199
Introduction   199
Classifications of Laser as per its Use in Urology   199
Mechanism of Laser Beam Production in Holmium Laser   201
Neodymium:Yttrium Aluminum Garnet Laser   202
Potassium Titanyl Phosphate Laser   202
Holmium:Yttrium Aluminum Garnet Laser   202
Thulium:Yttrium Aluminum Garnet Laser   203
Thulium Fiber Laser   203
Anatomy of a Laser Fiber   204
Fiber Size   206
Role of Shape Tip and Configuration of the Laser Fiber   206
Newer Technologies that Enhance the Performance of a High Watt Holmium Laser   207
Different Techniques of Laser Lithotripsy   210
Techniques of Enucleation   211

SECTION 2: URORADIOLOGY

16. Stricture Disease — 215
Pan Anterior Urethral Stricture   215
Distal Bulbar Stricture   217
Post Traumatic Posterior Urethral Injuries   218
Proximal Penile Urethral Stricture   223

17. Benign Bladder Diseases — 225
Bladder Diverticulum   225
Neurogenic Bladder   227

18. Pediatric Urology — 229
Bilateral Primary Obstructive Megaureter   229
Posterior Urethral Valves with Reflux   231
Bilateral Posterior Urethral Valves   233

19. Urolithiasis — 237
Bilateral Renal Calculi   237
Staghorn Stone   238
Nephrocalcinosis   243
Bilateral Ureteric Stone   244
Calculus in Ectopic Kidney   246

20. Renal Imaging — 250
Pelvic Ureteric Junction Obstruction   250
Angiomyolipoma   254

Renal Mass   256
Renal Mass with IVC Thrombus   258
Small Renal Mass   260

21. Bladder and Ureteric Imaging 262
Lower Ureteric Mass   262
Transitional Cell Carcinoma   263
Bladder Mass   265
Bladder Mass with Nonfunctioning Kidney   266

22. Adrenal Mass 268
Adrenal Mass   268

23. Miscellaneous 273
Trauma   273
Retrocaval Ureter   279

SECTION 3: UROPATHOLOGY

24. Renal Pathology 283
Specimen 1: Nephrectomy with Upper Ureteric Stones   283
Specimen 2: Xanthogranulomatous Pyelonephritis   284
Specimen 3: Autosomal Dominant Polycystic Kidney Disease   285
Specimen 4: Angiomyolipoma with Hematoma   288
Specimen 5: Large Angiomyolipoma   289
Specimen 6: RCC (Clear Cell)   290
Specimen 7: RCC (Chromophobe)   292
Specimens 8 and 9: Oncocytoma   293
Specimen 10: RCC (Pappilary)   295
Specimen 11: Radical Nephroureterectomy   298
Specimen 12: Wilms' Tumor   300

25. Bladder and Ureter Pathology 304
Specimen 13: Cystectomy   304
Specimen 14: Nephroureterectomy with Cystectomy   306
Specimen 15: Distal Ureteric Tumor   308

26. Penile Mass 310
Specimen 16: Radical Penectomy   310
Specimen 17: Partial Penectomy   311

27. Testicular Mass 314
Specimen 18: Testicular Tumor   314

28. Adrenal Mass — 318
Specimen 19: Adrenal Tumor 318

29. Prostatic Pathology — 321
Specimen 20: Radical Prostatectomy 321

SECTION 4: MISCELLANEOUS

30. Chemotherapy in Urological Malignancies — 327
Introduction 327
Chemotherapy for Bladder Cancer 327
Bacillus Calmette–Guérin (BCG) 328
Chemotherapy for Muscle Invasive Bladder Cancer 330
Immunotherapy for Bladder Cancer 333
Chemotherapy for Carcinoma Prostate 334
Adjuvant Therapy for Renal Cell Carcinoma 336
Chemotherapy in Squamous Cell Carcinoma of Penis 340
Chemotherapy in Testicular Cancers 341
BEP Protocol 341
EP Regimen (Etoposide and Cisplatin) 343
TIP Protocol (Paclitaxel, Ifosfamide, and Cisplatin) 343
VEIP Protocol (Vinblastine, Ifosfamide, and Cisplatin) 345
Chemotherapy for Neuroendocrine Tumors of Genitourinary System 345
Chemotherapy for Adrenocortical Carcinoma 346
Chemotherapy for Wilms' Tumor 347

31. Operative Notes — 350
Hypospadias 350
Distal Hypospadias 350
Proximal Repair 351
Complications 353

Anterior Urethral Strictures 355
Grafts 356
Urethral Strictures 356

Progressive Perineal Urethroplasty 357
Steps 358
Anastomosis 359
Complications 360

Vesicovaginal Fistula Repair 360
Nephrectomy 362
Preoperative Evaluation 362
Indications for Simple Nephrectomy 362
Steps 363

Partial Nephrectomy   363
Complications of Partial Nephrectomy   365
Radical Nephrectomy   366
Steps   366

Pyeloplasty   367
Dismembered Pyeloplasty   367
Complications   368

Surgeries for VUR   369
Principles of Antireflux Surgery   369
Approaches   369

Radical Prostatectomy   369
Surgical Approach   370
Surgical Technique   370
Complications   371

Radical Cystectomy   372
Complications   373

Adrenalectomy   374
Preoperative Preparation for Adrenalectomy   374
Open Adrenalectomy   376
Complications   377

Penile Mass   378
Partial Penectomy   378
Total Penectomy   379

Radical Orchiectomy   380
Partial Orchiectomy   381
Complications   382

Retroperitoneal Lymph Node Dissection   382
Types   382
Preoperative Planning   382
Steps   382
Inferior Vena Cava Thrombectomy   387
Politano–Leadbetter Technique   387
Glenn Anderson Technique   388
Cohen's Cross Trigonal Technique   389
Leich-Gregoir Extravesical Approach   390
Complications   391

32. **Biostatistics**   393
Statistics   393
Biostatistics   393
Kurtosis   399
Types of Error in Analysis   402
Screening and Diagnostics Tests   407

Receiver Operating Characteristic Curves   411
Regression Analysis   413
Survival Analysis Kaplan–Meier Curves   421

33. Research Methodology   422
Study Designs   422
Observational Studies   422
Experimental Studies   426
Systematic Reviews and Meta-analysis   436

Index   **445**

SECTION 1

Instruments

CHAPTER 1

Cystoscope and its Accessories

INTRODUCTION AND BRIEF HISTORY

Maximilian Carl Nitze is credited with the invention of modern cystoscope, which was primarily used for inspection of the bladder. This was publicly demonstrated in 1879. It used an electrically heated platinum wire for illumination, a cooling system which used flowing ice water and telescopic lens for visualization. In 1887, following the invention of the light bulb by Thomas Edison, Nitze constructed a cystoscope that did not require the cooling system.

Cystoscopes are manufactured by various companies namely, Karl Storz, GmbH, Richard Wolf, GmbH, and Olympus Inc. We shall be describing the instruments by Karl Storz GmbH with some technical detailing from other manufacturers wherever necessary.

For many years, Karl Storz™ cystoscopes were utilizing the older nomenclature for sizes of the cystoscopes. In the 1990s, the numbering of cystoscope sheath changed. Although the nomenclature changed, the actual size did not (**Table 1**). For the purpose of uniformity, we will describe the new Storz numbering schema.

The parts of a rigid cystoscope assembly (**Fig. 1**) are as follows:
- Cystoscope sheath
- Cystoscope obturator
- Bridge
- Light cable
- Telescope

TABLE 1: The old and new schema for Karl Storz cystoscopes sheaths.

Old schema	15.5	17	19	21	23.5
New schema	17	19	20	22	25
Color code	Yellow	Green	Red	Blue	White
Catheter capacities	1 × 5 Fr	2 × 5 Fr or 1 × 6 Fr	2 × 6 Fr 1 × 7 Fr	2 × 7 Fr 1 × 10 Fr	2 × 8 Fr 1 × 12 Fr

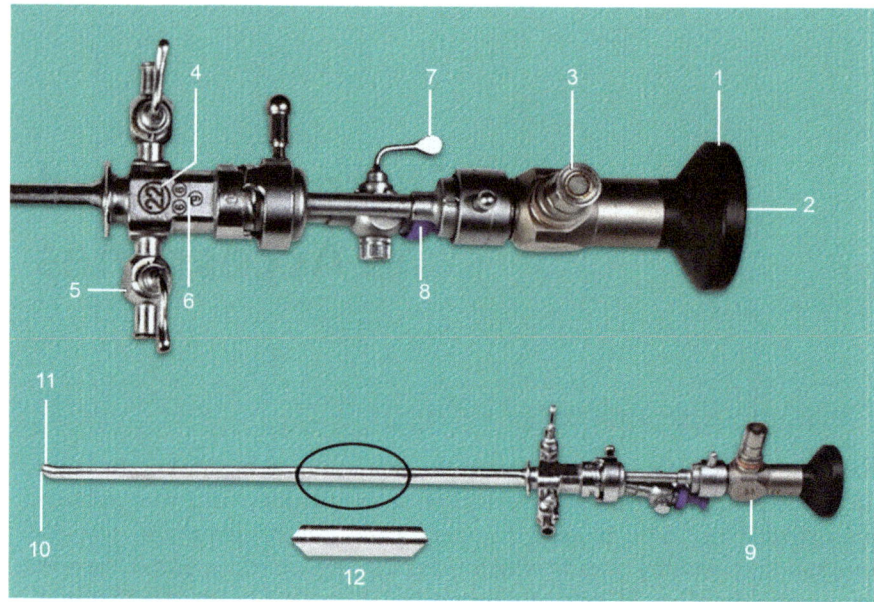

1. Ocular funnel
2. Ocular window
3. Light pillar
4. Number denoting the sheath size
5. Irrigation inlet and outlet
6. Number denoting the size of ureteric catheter that can be passed through the sheet
7. Stop cock of working channel
8. Working channel
9. Color code disk
10. Objective window
11. Beak
12. Marking on the sheath (1 cm apart)

Figure 1: Parts of a cystoscope.

All cystoscopes are made of stainless steel alloy. The cystoscope sheath is calibrated in French (Fr), this is considered to be the outer circumference of the instrument in millimeters (mm). Fr is same as Charrière (Ch). This method of calibration was described by Joseph-Frèdèric-Benoît Charrière. Fr takes into consideration the diameter of the instrument.

1 mm is equal to 3 French. It is also written as F, Fr, or Ch.

THE CYSTOSCOPE SHEATH

The cystoscope sheath (**Fig. 2**) will be discussed under the following headings:
- Cystoscope sheath
- Beak
- Inlet and outlet vent
- Color code disk
- Numbering on the sheath and Albarrans sheath lever

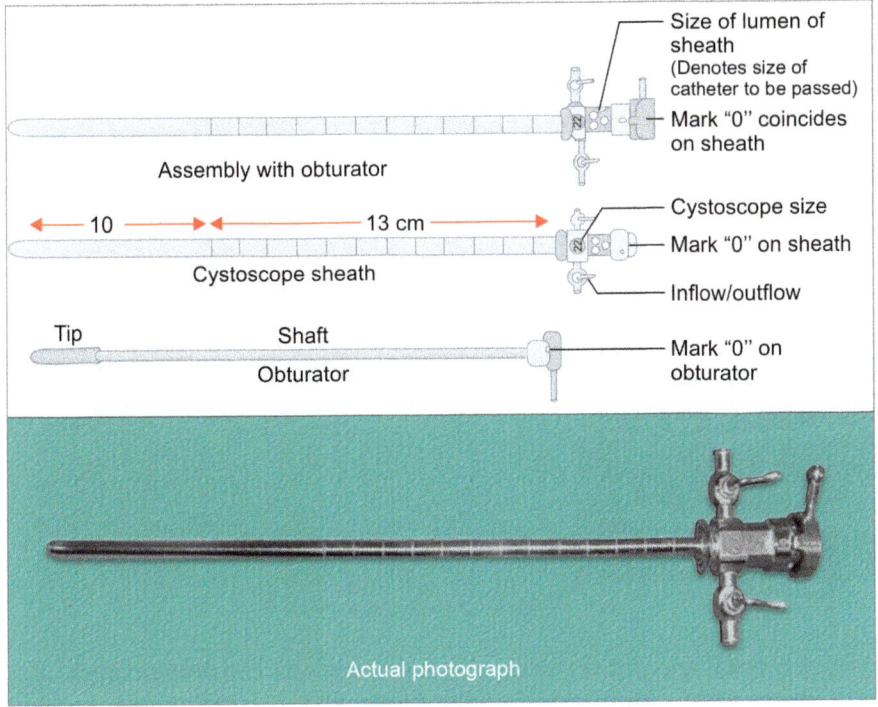

Figure 2: Details of a cystoscope sheath.

- *Cystoscope sheath*: The details of cystoscope sheath (Karl Storz, GmbH) are as follows:
  - Length of an adult cystoscope sheath regardless of size is 22 cm. The cross-section of the sheath is not round but oval. However, the size of the sheath is referred to in Fr, this can be considered as a "misnomer" as mentioned, because if it is to be referred in Fr, it should be circular contrary to its oval shape.
  - *Markings on the shaft* (**Fig. 2**): The proximal 10 cm from the vesical end are devoid of any markings. Markings are engraved on the sheath at every 1 cm thereafter for the next 13 cm. The markings help in estimation of prostatic urethral length [in comparison, 21 Fr optical urethrotome (VIU) sheath has similar markings all along the length of the sheath].
  - *Method to measure prostatic urethral length*: The cystoscope is introduced along the entire length. The cystoscope is withdrawn under endoscopic vision till the bladder neck. The marking on the external meatus is noted (point A). Thereafter, the cystoscope sheath is withdrawn till the verumontanum and a note of the marking is done (point B). The number of markings on the sheath between point A and point B is noted, this is the length of the prostatic urethra.

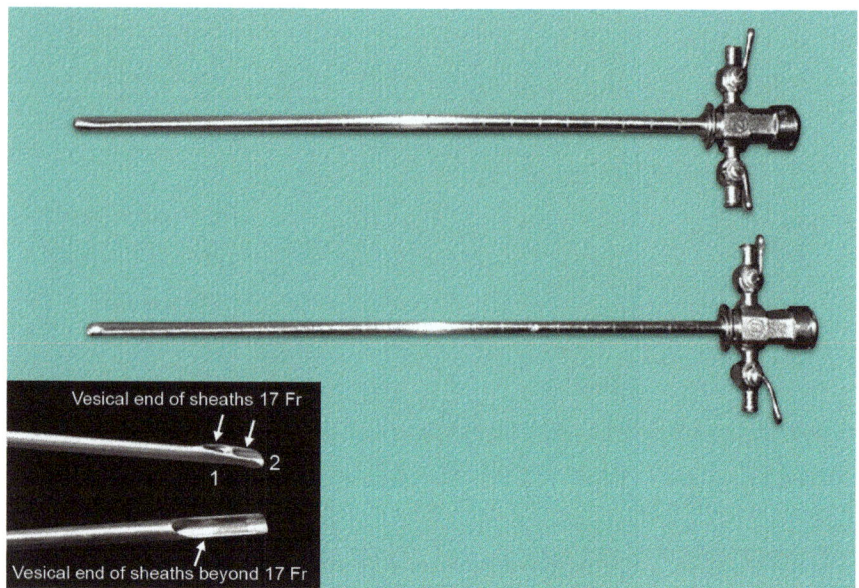

Figure 3: Types of cystoscope beak.

- The distal end of the sheath is bulbous dorsally and smooth without sharp edge. This helps in atraumatic introduction of the scope (**Fig. 3**). Such a design of the tip is essential if an instrument is to be passed under vision (without an obturator), e.g., cystoscope sheath and ureterorenoscope.

  If the beak is not of such design, then that instrument should be passed through the meatus with obturator, e.g., VIU sheath and resectoscope sheath.

  Salient features to remember regarding cystoscope sheath: (1) old and new nomenclature is changed without change in size, (2) all adult sheaths have same length, (3) only 17 Fr sheath has different beak configuration, rest have same configuration, and (4) bridges and telescopes remain same irrespective/regardless of size of sheath.

- *Cystoscope beak*: Sheaths with size 19 Fr onward are long oblique beaks, 17 Fr sheath is short beak sheath, this is used for female cystourethroscopy. The short beak is 2 cm in length (diamond-shaped opening for irrigation at the beak with) while the long beak has a length of 2.5 cm. The gradual withdrawal of the cystoscope sheath helps in visualization of the urethra in females.

  Longer beaks would result in leakage of irrigation fluid after introduction into a short female urethra leading to nondistension of the urethra and poor vision, this problem can be circumvented with shorter 17 Fr sheath (known as female cystoscope sheaths); this problem can also be circumvented by use of (**Fig. 4**) the Nickel adapter used for female urethroscopy.

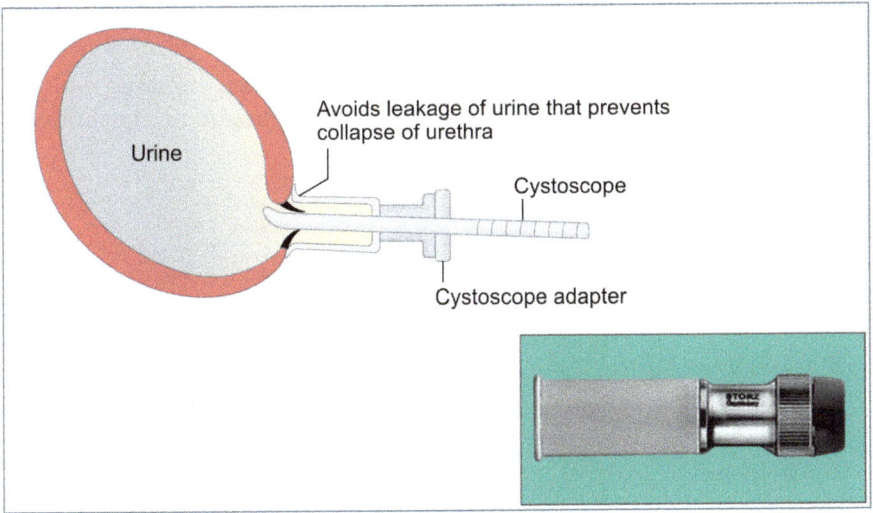

Figure 4: Nickel's adapter.

The adapter should be pressed against the urethral orifice after insertion of the cystoscope to avoid leakage of irrigation fluid and the resultant collapse of the urethra.

- *Inlet and outlet vent*: One for the inlet and one for the outlet allows ingress and egress of the irrigation flow which the surgeon can control (**Fig. 1**).
- *Color code disk*: This is a metal disk on which there is plastic color code cover. With prolonged use or repeated autoclaving, it tends to get damaged.
- Numbering on the sheath and Albarran sheath lever:
  - Size of the sheath is indicated by a number written on the sheath at the level of inlet/outlet channel.
  - The numbers written in two circles behind the above indicate the largest size of the catheter, two of which can be passed simultaneously through the sheath.
  - Behind the above is a single circle with a numerical value, denoting the single largest catheter, which can be passed through the sheath.
  - The above catheter size is the maximum size with scope and Albarrans lever in situ, so if simple bridge is used, maximal permissible catheter size will increase by 1 Fr. So the maximum size of catheter that can be passed through 19 Fr sheath with simple bridge is 7 Fr (for 20 Fr is 8 Fr, for 22 Fr is 11 Fr, and for 25 Fr is 13 Fr).
  - *Albarran lever* (**Fig. 5**): It is bridge with a deflecting lever, which can be used to deflect the ureteric catheter to align the catheter with the ureteric orifice. It has two channels through which two catheters can be passed simultaneously. A circular knob near the eyepiece end of the device is used to deflect the lever and thus, the ureteric catheter to

SECTION 1: Instruments

up to 90°. Pointer on the knob tells the degree of deflection. Albarran lever can be attached to sheath size 19 Fr or more.
- *Locking knob on the sheath*: It has a zero (0) mark engraved which corresponds with same (0) mark on the obturator or the bridge (**Fig. 2**).

BRIDGES (FIG. 6)

Adult cystoscope bridges are universal and can fit into all sizes of sheaths. Length of bridge is 6 cm. Specially designed cystoscopes are available

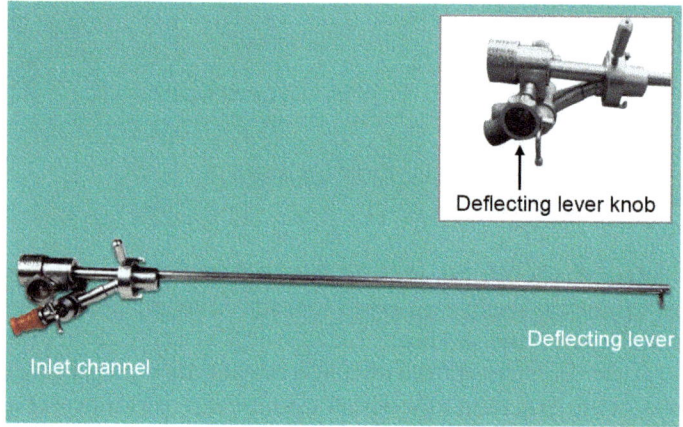

Figure 5: The Albarran lever.

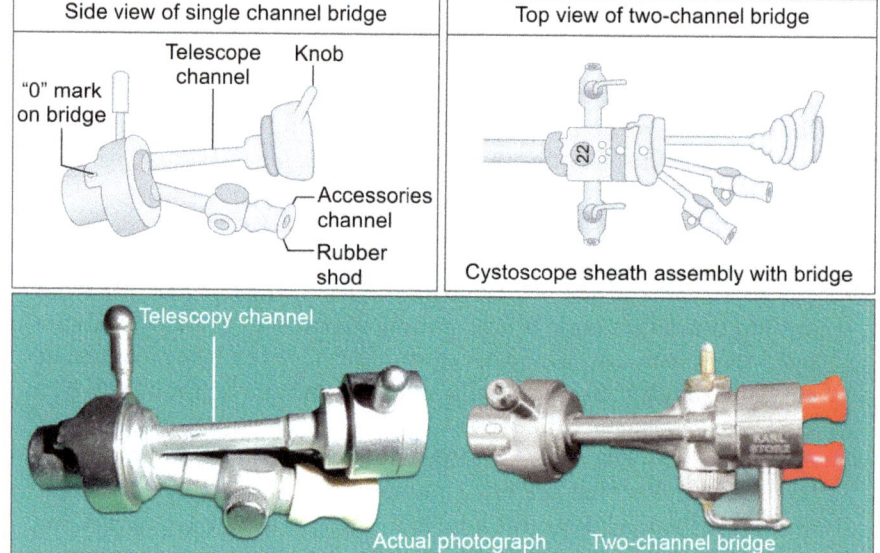

Figure 6: Parts of the bridge.

wherein the bridge and the telescope cannot be detached, they are called as "integrated cystoscopes." These cystoscopes have advantages of having a smaller shaft size with a comparatively larger working channel.

The advantages of detachable bridge are as follows:
- It helps in empting the bladder efficaciously.
- It helps in passing larger size catheter after detaching the bridge.
- It helps in attaching the Ellik evacuator for evacuation of stone fragments/clots/chips, etc.

Types of Bridges (Classification)
- Without side channel
- With one side channel
- With two side channel

Parts of Bridge
- *Telescope channel*: It accommodates the telescope.
- *Accessories channel*: It is meant to pass the accessories such as ureteric catheter and wires forceps. It has a rubber shod which helps in easy passage of the instrument.

OBTURATORS (FIG. 7)

They are specific for a given sheath. Once attached to the sheath, it makes the tip of the sheath smooth thereby snuggly fitting to it. The length of the obturator is 26 cm.

Parts of obturator are as follows:
- *Vesical end knob*: This helps in smooth atraumatic insertion of the cystoscope.
- *Shaft*: It connects the vesical end knob and the locking mechanism.
- *Locking mechanism*: Zero (0) should correspond to zero (0) of the sheath when locked.

Specifications of Obturators (Fig. 7)

The obturator of 17 Fr sheath (new) has a smaller distal end without any groove. In addition, the sheath of 17 Fr sheath has a diamond-shaped opening at the distal end which helps in irrigation egress. The obturator of 19 Fr sheath (new) onward has a groove which helps in egress of irrigation. The sheath size is engraved on the obturator. The 17 Fr obturator has a smaller knob but is same in length. Rest of the obturators have same shape and length but vary in the size according to the size of the sheath. Points which differentiate a cystoscope, Sachse's, and resectoscope obturator are detailed in **Figure 7**. The differentiation is based on size of the knob and the presence and the absence of groove (**Table 2**).

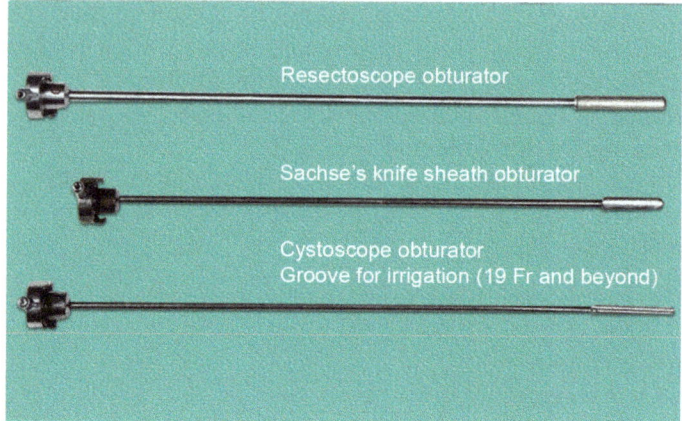

Figure 7: Types of obturator.

TABLE 2: Difference in the types of obturator.

	Cystoscopic sheath obturator	VIU sheath obturator	TURP sheath obturator
Knob	Conforming to the beak of sheath	Rounded	Rounded
Groove	Groove for irrigation is present (19 Fr and beyond). 17 Fr sheath has no groove	Absent	Absent
Length	Equal to the sheath	Projects just beyond the sheath	Projects just beyond the sheath

(TURP: transurethral resection of the prostate)

SPECIAL TYPES OF CYSTOURETHROSCOPES AND THEIR USES

- *Extended length cystoscope-urethroscope*: The working length is 29 cm. It is 22 Fr, the color code is blue. The compatible telescope bridge has one instrument channel; it is for use of 10 Fr instruments. A catheter deflecting mechanism is also compatible with the extended length cystoscope-urethroscope, it is for use of 9 Fr instruments.
- *Continuous flow laser cystoscope-21 Fr (URO-LAS)*: The round tip configuration of the sheath and an 8 Fr working channel helps for easy urethral manipulation and insertion of laser with its accessories. The laser telescope bridge after Fraundorfer is compatible with the cystoscope.

Telescopes

The telescopes are classified depending on the viewing angle. They are available as 0°, 30°, 70°, 120°, and 12° (**Fig. 8**). Adult telescopes can be used with any adult sheaths. They need to be used with a bridge. The color coding for the telescopes are as follows, green code for 0°, red code for 30°, yellow code for 70°, and white code for 120° for Storz (**Fig. 8**). Even though the color codes seem confusing, it is paramount for universal recognition. Straight "forward" telescopes (0°) is focused to view straight ahead. It is usually used for urethroscopy. Forward oblique telescopes (30°) best afford visualization of the base and anterolateral aspect of the bladder, this is the most commonly used telescope. Lateral telescope (70°) is used to view the bladder dome.

It views structures around bladder neck such as postprostatic pouch. Retrospective telescopes (120°) help to visualize the anterior bladder neck from inside. With conventional system, the viewing angle was relevant but with Hopkins 2, the use of 70° and 120° has ebbed. In addition, with the use of flexible cystoscopes on the rise, the 70° and 120° telescopes have become obsolete. These color codes differ with the make (**Fig. 8**). The eyepiece can be fitted with a camera. The eyepiece is black in color and has the catalog number engraved on it. The light cable can be attached to the telescope directly. Size of telescopes available—4 mm and 30 cm (fits in all cystoscope sheaths and VIU sheaths and resectoscope sheaths).

The Rod-lens System (Fig. 9)

In 1966, the collaboration between Karl Storz and professor, HH Hopkins, led to the new design of rod-lens system. This was a major development for the progress of endourology since the description of cystoscope by Maximilian Nitze.

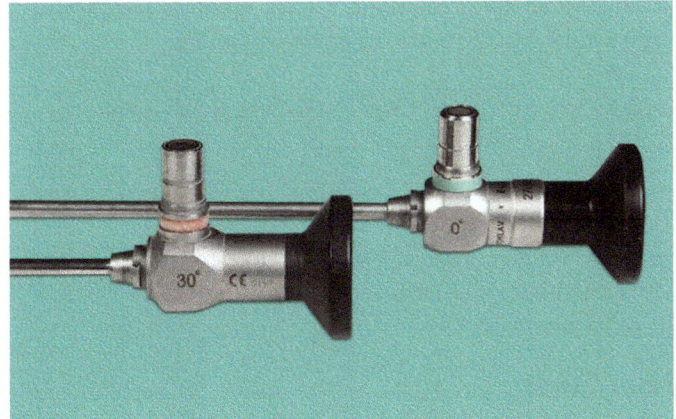

Figure 8: Color coding for cystoscope.

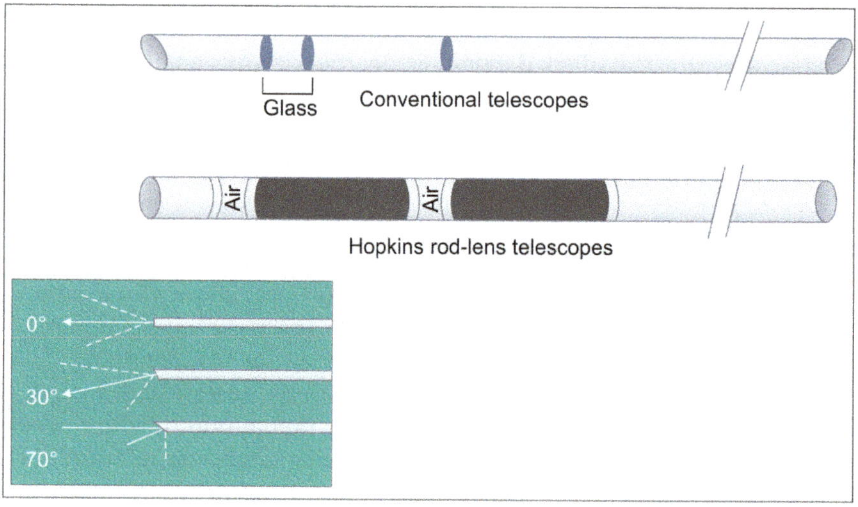

Figure 9: Rod-lens system.

The key difference in the conventional optical system and the rod-lens system is that the Hopkins rod-lens system employs special glass rods with customized finished ends. The rod-lens system reduced the air spaces between lens with long rods of glass which were ground, contoured, and polished at both ends, there are short gaps of air in between. Once this endoscopic image is transported back through the telescope, it is magnified at the ocular lens. The degree of magnification is to some extent dependent on the diameter of the viewing lens.

The image and optical image transmission differs in rigid and flexible endoscopes.[1,2] In the flexible endoscopes, typically there are two sets of fiberoptic glass bundles which are either coherent or noncoherent. The coherent bundles help in transmission of images, as a result the image of a fiberoptic scope has a "honeycomb" appearance. This is called as the "Moiré effect." The noncoherent bundles help in the transmission of light.

Difference Between Conventional and Hopkins Rod-lens System[1] (Table 3)

The Hopkins rod-lens system offers the following advantages over the conventional system:
- Better light transmission offers images of improved quality and contrast.
- Wide viewing angle offers better visualization of the structures.
- Decrease in profile of telescope shaft

Advantages of Hopkins II Lens
- Wider viewing angles
- Lens diameter has been increased and air spaces have been decreased.
- 30° Hopkins II covers areas which could be only seen by a 70° lens earlier.

TABLE 3: Comparison of conventional versus Hopkins rod-lens system.	
Conventional rod-lens	Hopkins rod-lens system
Glass rods act as lens	Air space acts as lens
Thicker shaft profile	Smaller shaft profile
Narrow viewing angle	Wide viewing angle

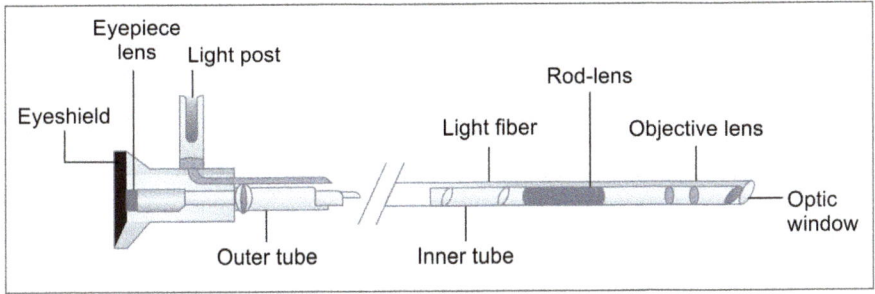

Figure 10: Parts of a cystoscope.

- Autoclavable
- Greater brightness
- Greater brilliance
- Higher resolution

Basic Structure of Telescope (Fig. 10)

Rod-lens are glued with special adhesive cement which is a special alloy, effectively making it waterproof. The special adhesive helps in preventing permeation of water into the rod-lens system.

Light pillar: **Figure 11** shows the adapters and light pillars for various manufacturers. The light cable configuration differs with the make. Hence, the structure of light pillar varies. The use of adapters helps the use interchangeable, e.g., a specific custom made Wolf adapter can be used with the adapter on a Storz instrument.

Parts of Telescope

- *Shaft*: Angulation at the tip varies depending on the viewing angle (diagram).
- *Eyepiece*: It is typically black in color, the size is universal, and adapts to any camera head.

FLEXIBLE CYSTOURETHROSCOPE (FIG. 12)

There are two types of flexible cystourethroscopes:
1. *Fiberoptic cystourethroscopes:* Within the shaft of a flexible cystourethroscope are generally three fiberoptic bundles—two noncoherent bundles

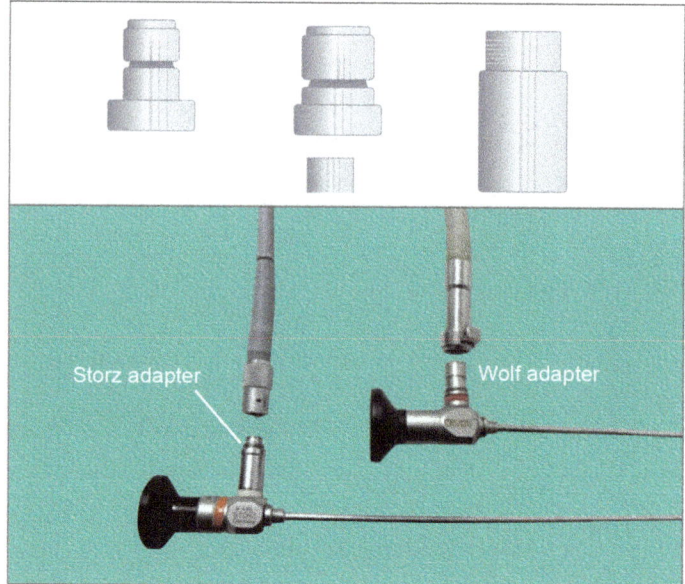

Figure 11: Various adapters.

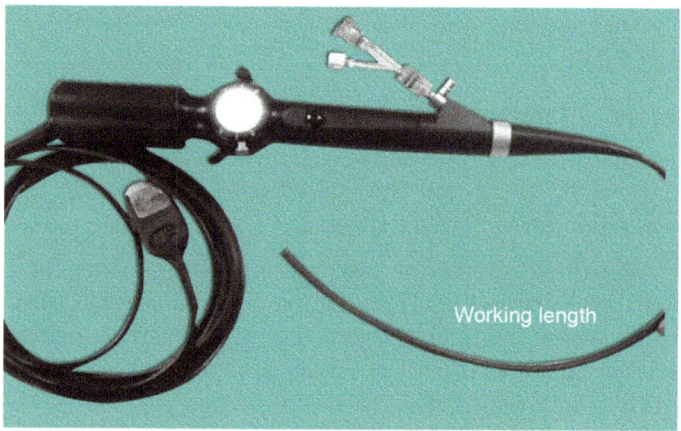

Figure 12: Flexible cystourethroscope.

of fibers that transmit light and a single coherent bundle of glass fibers that constitutes the imaging bundle. Unlike its rigid counterpart, the image obtained by the fiberoptic bundle is not a single image, but rather a composite matrix of each fiber within the bundle. The image obtained is analogous to a newspaper photograph—that is, it is composed of multiple dots merging into a single reconstructed image known as "honeycomb" effect.

2. *Digital cystourethroscopes*: The digital scopes do not need a separate camera or light cable attachment. The digital scopes have chip on the tip of the scope for image capture and led for light source. The two different technologies used for capturing images digitally are:
   i. *Charge coupled device (CCD) sensor*: Every pixel's charge is transferred through an output nodes to be converted to voltage, buffered, and sent off-chip as an analog signal. All the pixels can be devoted to light capture, and the output's uniformity is high.
   ii. *Complementary metal oxide semiconductor (CMOS) image sensors*: Each pixel has its own charge-to-voltage conversion, and the sensor often includes amplifiers, noise-correction, and digitization circuits, so that the chip outputs digital bits. These other functions increase the design complexity and reduce the area available for light capture. With each pixel doing its own conversion, uniformity is lower. They have been developed now even as higher resolution like 4K sensor.

Indications of Flexible Cystourethroscopes

- Ureteral stent removal
- Surveillance for bladder and urethral malignancies
- Evaluation of macroscopic/microscopic hematuria
- Diagnosis of urethral/bladder neck stricture
- Lower urinary tract symptoms evaluation, urethral/bladder fistulae
- Urethral assessment for diverticular disease (women)

Advantages of Flexible Cystourethroscopes

- Ease in patient positioning resulting in better patient comfort under local anaesthesia
- Thus, it can be done as day-care procedure often known as "office cystoscopy."
- Ease of manipulation across difficult curves and high bladder necks and median lobes.
- The ability to flex the endoscope helps in complete visualization of the bladder easily.

The various flexible cystourethroscopes available are given in **Table 4**.

Advancements in flexible cystourethroscopes:
- Single-use flexible scopes
- Like single-use digital flexible ureteroscopes, cystoscopes are also available as single-use flexible digital scope. This has the benefit of decreased initial and maintenance cost as well as decreased chance of transmission of infection.
    - Isiris® from Coloplast (**Fig. 13**) (Coloplast Corp, Minneapolis, USA) is a single-use flexible digital integrated ureteric stent grasper to perform office-based ureteral stent removal under local anesthesia.

TABLE 4: Various flexible cystourethroscopes.

Manu-facturer	Model	Deflection up	Deflection down	Working channel (Fr)	Sheath size (outer diameter—Fr)
Karl Storz	Fiberoptic	210	140	7	15.5
	Digital (CCD technology)	210	140	6.5	16
	Digital with NBI/PDD (CCD technology)	210	140	6.5	16
	Digital (CMOS technology)	210	140	6.5	16
Richard Wolf	Fiberoptic	210	150	7.5	15
	Digital	210	210	7.5	11.5/16.2
	Digital (4k sensor)	210	210	7.5	11.5/16.2
Olympus	Fiberoptic	210	120	7.2	11.7/16.5
	Digital	220	130	6.6	8.1/16.6

Note: The working length of the flexible cystoscopes range from 37 to 40 cm and the field of vision is 110–120°.

(CCD: charge coupled device; CMOS: complementary metal oxide semiconductor; NBI: narrow band imaging; PPD: photodynamic diagnosis)

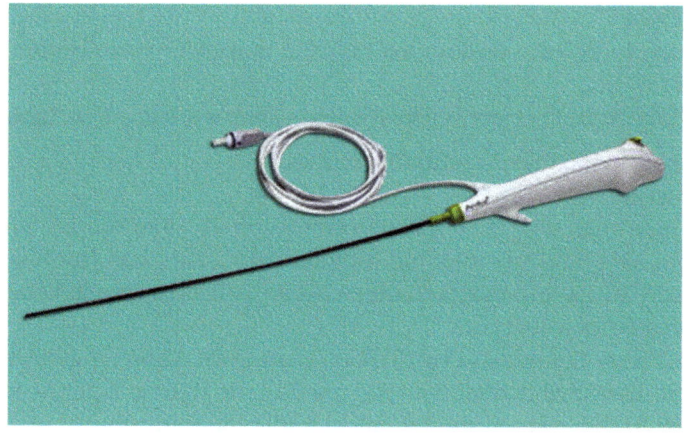

Figure 13: Ambu® aScope™.

- UroViu cystoscope platform (UroViu Corporation, Bellevue, WA) is a single-use flexible female diagnostic cystoscope.
- WISCOPE cystoscope (innoMedicus, Switzerland): It is 9/13.8 Fr scope with 6.6 Fr working channel. It has bidirectional deflection of 180°.

Ambu® aScope™: It is a single-use flexible digital cystourethroscope. It has an outer diameter of 16.2 Fr, with a working channel of 6.6 Fr. It has a bending angle of 210° up and 120° down. It has 120° field of view. It has to be attached to a light-weight, portable, propriety monitor.

- *Blue-light flexible cystoscopy*: Conventional blue-light cystoscopy is photodynamic diagnostic test for bladder cancer surveillance. The procedure involves intravesical instillation of a photoactive porphyrin, such as hexaminolevulinate (HAL), which preferentially accumulates in neoplastic tissue, where it induces an accumulation of protoporphyrin, with fluorescence red when exposed to blue light. This enhancement improves the demarcation between normal and neoplastic tissue, which allows for improved detection of exophytic tumors and flat tumors.

All are digital, they do not need a separate camera or light cable attachment.

The accessories which are compatible with flexible cystoscope are all flexible in nature:
- *Grasping forceps*: 5 Fr, 73 cm
- *Biopsy forceps*: 5 Fr, 73 cm
- *Stone basket*: 5 Fr, 60 cm
- *Ball electrode*: 4 Fr, 73 cm

The flexible cystourethroscope can be sterilized with gas sterilization.[1,3]

Types

Logic (up is up). This means when the lever is turned down, the deflection occurs downward and antilogic (down is up). This means when the lever is turned down, the deflection goes up.

MEATOTOMY SCISSOR

Meatotomy Scissor (Fig. 14)

It is a scissors which can be passed through a cystoscope sheath. It can be used for ureteric meatotomy, for cutting sutures and meshes migrated in the bladder.

Flexible Biopsy Forceps (Fig. 15)

- It is a flexible and reusable forceps made up of stainless steel.
- It has cup-shaped jaws for superior cutting of bladder biopsy.
- It is autoclavable.
- It goes through the working channel of cystoscope sheath.

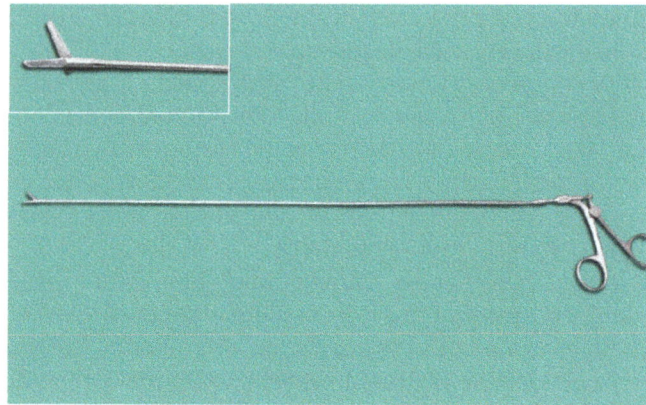

Figure 14: Meatotomy scissor.

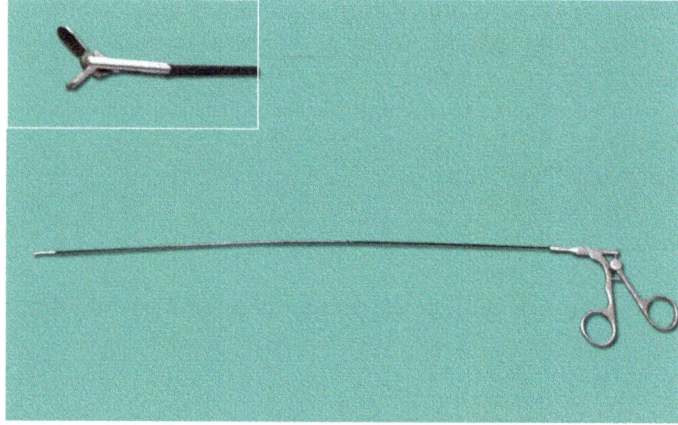

Figure 15: Flexible biopsy forceps.

Rigid Biopsy Forceps (Fig. 16)

- It is a rigid forceps which has a small diameter sheath for passing cystoscope and an integrated bridge.
- It can be used with 20, 22 and 25 sheaths.
- It should preferably used with 0 degree telescope but can also be used with Hopkins II – 30 degree telescope, which has wide angle.
- It has cup-shaped for cutting of bladder biopsy.
- A note to be made is that the tip of forceps projects well-beyond the cystosheath. Hence cystoscope cannot be introduced with forceps in position. Scope should be introduced with bridge and then bridge is replaced with rigid biopsy forceps.
- The procedure:
  - Initially, a diagnostic cystoscopy must be performed with a 25 Fr cystosheath

- The bladder should be distended
- Then keeping the bladder distended, the telescope and bridge to be removed and replaced with the forceps with telescope.
- This prevents inadvertent perforation of empty bladder while insertion of forceps as it projects beyond the cystosheath.

Stent Removal Forceps (Fig. 17)

- It is a reusable and flexible forceps for removal of stents.
- It is strong grasping and has alligator jaw for strong grip.
- It is autoclavable.
- It can also be used for cold cup bladder biopsy, if bladder biopsy forceps is not available.

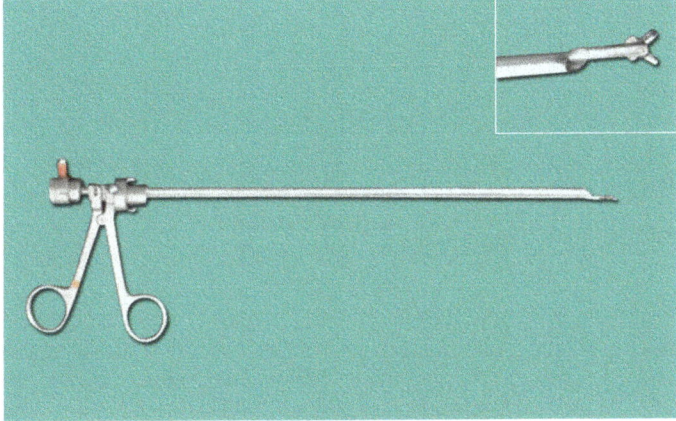

Figure 16: Rigid biopsy forceps.

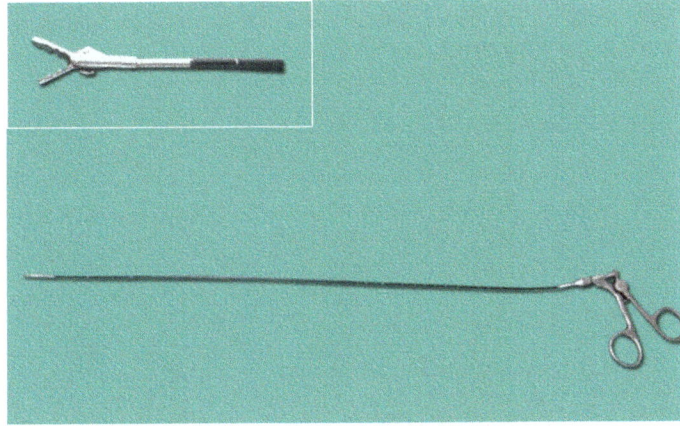

Figure 17: Stent removal forceps.

Bugbee Electrode (Fig. 18)

The electrode has to be connected to a conventional underwater cautery. It is used for fulguration of small bleeders with the ball electrode.

The hook electrode can be used for ureterocele incision or for meatotomy of the ureteric orifice when a stone is impacted at the VUJ.

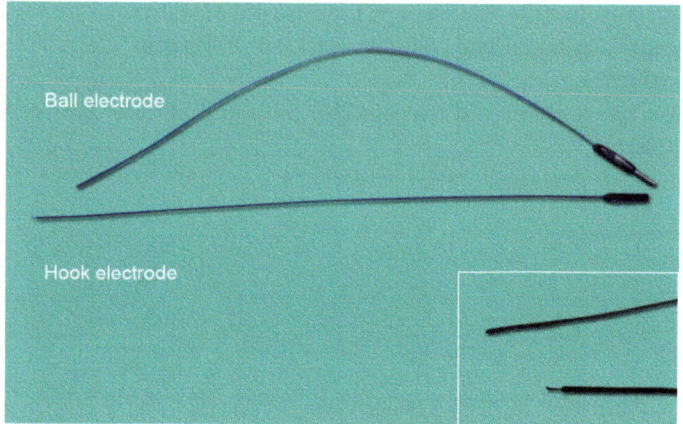

Figure 18: Bugbee electrode.

REFERENCES

1. Karl Storz. Catalogue (Endourology), 5th edition. [online] Available from: https://www.karlstorz.com/in/en/human-medicine.htm. [Last Accessed march, 2021].
2. Babyan RK, Wang DS. Basic principles optics of flexible and rigid endoscopes. Smith endourology, 2nd edition. New York: Wiley-Blackwell; 2019. pp. 3.
3. Karl Storz. Catalogue (Cyst 1B), 5th edition. [online] Available from: https://www.karlstorz.com/in/en/laparoscopy.htm. [Last Accessed march, 2021].

CHAPTER 2

Visual Internal Urethrotomy, Otis Urethrotome

SACHSE'S OPTICAL URETHROTOMY (FIG. 1)

The Sachse's optical urethrotome assembly includes the outer sheath, obturator, zero degree telescope, and a working element.

The details are as follows:
- *Sheath*: The size of the Sachse's optical urethrotome sheath is 21 Fr (1 Fr or Ch is equal to 0.33 mm). This refers to the outer circumference of the metal sheath. The cross sectional shape of the sheath is oval and not circular. The length of the sheath is 20 cm. In contrast to the cystoscope sheath, the Sachse's sheath has markings throughout the length (20 markings) each at a distance of 1 cm. The sheath has a side working

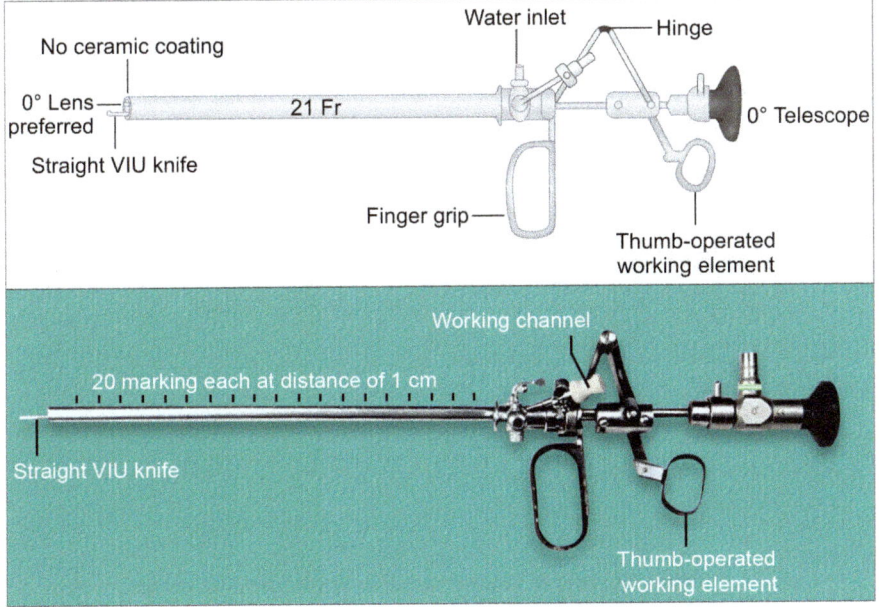

Figure 1: Sachse's optical urethrotome.

channel (top left side for right-handed). The channel admits instruments up to 5 Fr. Cross-section of the tip of the sheath is straight (not oblique or bulbous). A left-handed surgeon can order a customized sheath (top right side instrument channel).
- *Obturator*: The obturator of a Sachse's urethrotome is required while negotiating the meatus as the tip of the sheath is straight, thus a sheath introduced without obturator would be traumatic. The obturator in place smoothens the tip and helps in easy introduction of the urethrotome through the external urethral meatus. Once this is done, obturator can be replaced by working element with lens *in situ*.
- *Working element*: The thumb-operated working element is used as this helps in maintaining the knife inside the sheath at rest and avoids injury to the urethra. The working element is same as used for transurethral resection of the prostate (TURP).

BLADES (FIG. 2)

The blades are usually double stem. They cannot be used with high frequency current.

The types of blades are as follows:
- *Sachse's cold knife straight*: This is the most commonly used knife used for short segment bulbar stricture.
- Cold knife hook-shaped
- *Cold knife round-shaped (half-moon)*: It is useful for cases with bladder neck stenosis. Half-moon knife because of its design cannot be passed under vision. It needs to be deployed when the Sachse's urethrotome is in place in the urethra. It cuts to and fro (while going in and coming out).
- *Ludwik's straight knife waveform (Serrated)*: It is useful for dense strictures or core through urethrotomy.

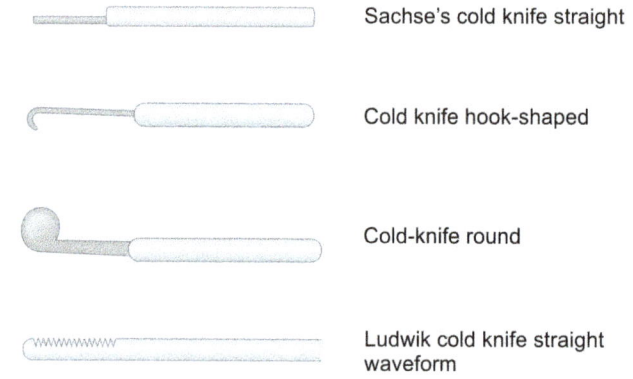

Sachse's cold knife straight

Cold knife hook-shaped

Cold-knife round

Ludwik cold knife straight waveform

Figure 2: Different types of visual internal urethrotomy (VIU) blades.

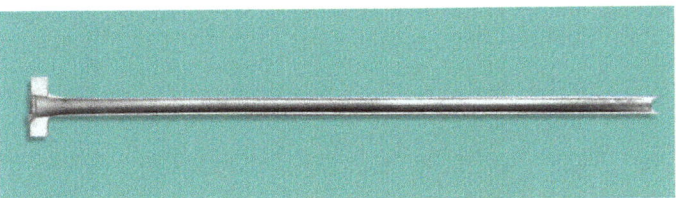

Figure 3: Half sheath: Can be used during optical urethrotomy.

Inlet Channel

The Sachse's optical urethrotome sheath does not have an outlet channel, it only has an inlet channel.

Accessories for a Sachse's Urethrotomy Sheath

- *Half sheath (Fig. 3)*: It is to be attached over the sheath. It increases the circumference and should be deployed in position prior to insertion. The size of this assembly becomes 23 Fr. After removal of the sheath, it accommodates 16 Fr or less Foley catheter. It is used when one anticipates a difficult introduction of Foley's catheter.
- *Continuous irrigation sheath*: It is an outer sheath to visual internal urethrotomy (VIU) sheath, similar to TURP outer sheath. It has multiple holes akin to a resectoscope sheath and an outlet channel for egress of irrigating fluid. It is useful in difficult urethrotomies when bleeding occurs and vision gets hampered, because in VIU sheath, there is no outlet to irrigation fluid and also fluid is not able to enter the bladder due to tight stricture.

OTIS MAURMYERS URETHROTOME[1] (FIG. 4)

The instrument is commonly used to incise a narrow urethra. It is also used for managing urethral stenosis in females. The knife is inserted through the hub of the urethrotome and incises only tough tissues. The knife does not protrude beyond the surface of the instrument in a fully deployed position. The prerequisite for use of this instrument is the presence of a full bladder to avoid inadvertent incision of the bladder. The knife should be inserted with thumb pressing on the shaft of the knife as the knife enters the groove as shown in **Figure 4**.

The parts of an otis urethrotome are as follows:
- *Shaft*: The shaft is 16 cm in length and houses a hub/groove for passage of knife. The tip of the shaft is smooth, this avoids injury to the bladder. The shaft on the dorsal aspect houses a hinged calibrating device which maximally can dilate the urethra to 15–45 Fr. This is connected

SECTION 1: Instruments

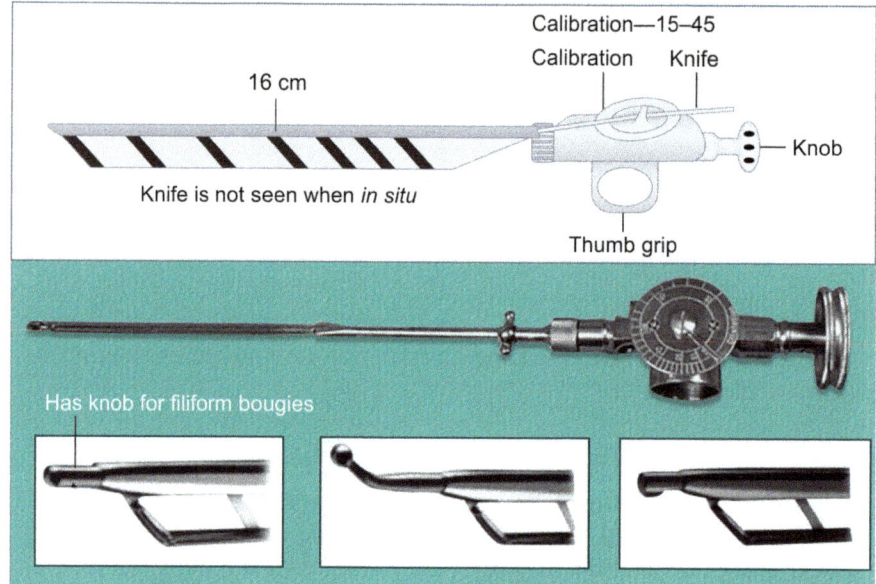

Figure 4: Otis urethrotome.

to the calibrating gauge on the external end. The knob at the tip of the instrument helps in passage of a filiform bougie. Size of the shaft is 14 Fr on rotating end, the knob at external end helps the shaft to open up. Once open, maximum size achieved is 45 Fr. The minimal diameter of the urethra should be at least 16 Fr to admit this instrument. The bulbous tip gets detached and there is a threaded area which can be connected to filiform dilators and followers (**Fig. 4**).

- *The external end*: The external end has a calibration gauge, a rotating knob, thumb grip, and a knife hub. The maximum dilatation and incision that can be achieved is 45 Fr.

  Knife has to be slided through the V-shaped guider located over disk. Knife has to go into the groove.

REFERENCE

1. ELMED Medical. (2013). [online]. Available from: http://www.elmed.ro/upload/products/product_1319.pdf. [Last accessed February 2020].

CHAPTER 3

Transurethral Resection of the Prostate Instruments

INTRODUCTION AND HISTORY OF TRANSURETHRAL RESECTION OF THE PROSTATE INSTRUMENTS

In 1909, Hugh Hampton Young developed a cold-cut punch for prostate resection, which was used blindly. Electrical cautery that could work underwater was first demonstrated by Edwin Beer in 1909. The second invention was amalgamated with the first in 1911, but the diathermy and resulting hemostasis was of poor quality, which limited its usefulness. It was Maximilian Stern who designed and named the first instrument as resectoscope. It had a tungsten wire. The idea of foot switch was first put forth by Davis. In 1932, Joseph F. McCarthy introduced the first modern resectoscope. His landmark contribution to innovation of the resectoscope was development of Bakelite sheath. Iglesias, who happened to be McCarthy student, developed continuous irrigating resectoscope. Further, Captain George Baumrucker designed a spring mechanism for the working element with an action that was the reverse of the Iglesias mechanism (resectoscope).[1]

RESECTOSCOPE SHEATH (MONOPOLAR)

The resectoscopes are available from a variety of manufacturers. The available sheath sizes are 22, 24, 26, 27, and 28 Fr.

Parts of Resectoscope

Different Ways of Classifying Resectoscopes
- Depending on size 24 Fr, 26 (yellow) Fr, 27 Fr, and 28 Fr (black)
- Depending on beak (short or long or oblique)
- Depending on sheath material [Teflon or MTC (metal, ceramic, and Teflon)]
- Depending on type of irrigation (conventional or continuous)

Depending on size: Standard resectoscope sizes available are 24, 26, 27, and 28 Fr. The 24 and 26 Fr are color coded yellow and used same loops which are

Figure 1: Various shapes of vesical end of resectoscopes.

also color coded yellow. The 27 and 28 Fr are color coded black and use the same loop which is colored brown. Now, a 22 Fr integrated resectoscope is also available for small size urethra and its color coded white.

Depending on types of beaks:
- *Long beak*: These are similar to cystoscope beak but have no bulbous end. The long beak supposedly occludes the bleeders during resection. However, this design of the beak led to poor vision and is not commonly used.
- *Short beak*: Optimization of the length was done to prevent the mentioned drawback of the long beak. This design has gone out of fashion.
- *Oblique beak*: It has a short oblique end. Most modern resectoscopes have this design.

Vesical end of the resectoscope is shown in **Figure 1**.

Depending on materials of sheath: During transurethral resection if the loop is still active (foot pedal pressed) and if it comes in contact with the sheath, it can damage and erode the sheath because of very high temperature. In addition, it can transmit the current through the sheath if the insulation is breached or the sheath is conductive. Previously sheaths were made up of Bakelite, this material was fragile and hence susceptible to easy breakage. Then came Teflon which had better durability and was nonconductive of electricity. Later, metal sheath was tried, it gave good strength to the sheath but since metal sheath would conduct electricity, it resulted in current leakage. In addition, metal made the sheath heavy.

Modern resectoscope sheaths are made of MTC. The distal portion is made of Teflon which is nonconductor, rest of the sheath is metal, which gives strength, and the inner portion of beak is coated with ceramic which is heat resistant and nonconductor.

Depending on type of irrigation: Depending on irrigation system mechanism, they are classified as:
- *Conventional irrigation*: They do not have an outer sheath resulting in requirement for frequent emptying of the bladder.
- *Continuous irrigation (**Figs. 2A and B**)*: Outer sheath is added for drainage of irrigation fluid. It was first described by Iglesias in 1975. It enables resection to be undertaken as a continuous, uninterrupted process. It can

CHAPTER 3: Transurethral Resection of the Prostate Instruments | 27

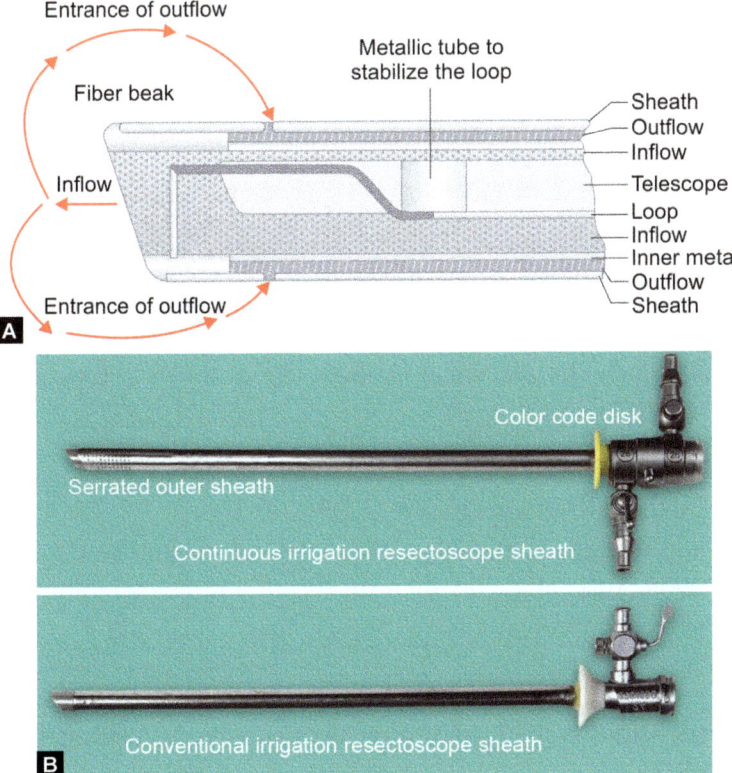

Figures 2A and B: (A) Continuous flow resectoscope top figure working mechanism; (B) Actual photograph of the resectoscope.
Source: Adapted from Thompson P. Blandy's Textbook of Operative Urology. New York: Wiley–Blackwell; 2006.

be used as a conventional resectoscope after removing the outer sheath. It works on the principle of two concentric sheaths so that the irrigation channel passes down the central sheath over the telescope and active electrode.

The return flow enters the outer sheath just proximal to the beak of the instrument; the flow then passes between the two concentrically arranged sheaths to the exit tap. The advantages include the following: It avoids any buildup of pressure inside the bladder, keeps field clear, quickens the procedure of transurethral resection, and it will maintain the volume of bladder at a constant capacity for resecting bladder tumors (**Fig. 2**).

WHAT IS A ROTATING RESECTOSCOPE?

Rotating resectoscope is a resectoscope that enables the urologist to rotate the working element and telescope to the desired position independently of the sheath. The result is no rotating components in the urethra and no entangled tubings due to rotation. This makes the procedure simpler.

Parts of Resectoscope Sheath

The resectoscope sheath generally consists of a cylindrical metal tube, the internal (vesical) end, which is protected from the current by a ring of insulating material. The vesical end is available in varying contours ranging from long beak to minimal obliquity. The insulating coating helps in preventing burns. At times, a metal sheath may be responsible for burns to the urethral mucosa.

The types of insulated coatings are as follows:
- *Bakelite*: The sheath for the original Stern McCarthy instrument was made of insulated material.
- *Teflon*: In Teflon sheaths, small leakages can give rise to large leak of current.
- *Ceramic*: This material is currently used as an insulation coating.

External End of the Resectoscope (Fig. 3)

It closes and smoothens the vesical end of the sheath and helps in instrumentation. This snugly fits into the sheath and helps in atraumatic insertion of the instrument.

They are of three types:
1. *Viewing obturator (SCHMIEDT)*: It helps in introduction of sheath under direct vision, thus avoiding trauma to the urethra due to instrumentation and irrigation.
2. *Straight distending obturator (Leusch obturator)*: Locking the obturator causes the rubber cuff to distend distal to edge of the sheath thus, covering its sharp edges, this reliably protects the urethra from trauma, by eliminating the "little step" seen because of the gap between the sheath and the obturator, which avoids trauma due to the alignment because of the rubber.
3. *Hinged obturator (Timberlake)*: Helpful for blind insertion of instruments, particularly in obstructing median lobe. When pressed, obturator

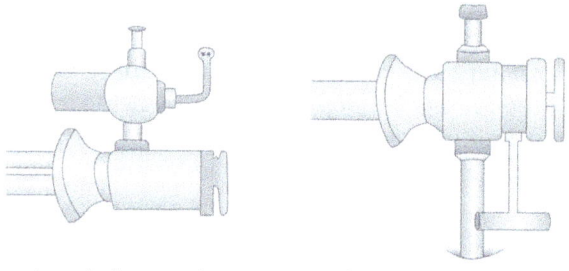

Luer-lock connector   Central three-way cock

Figure 3: External end of the resectoscope (without central valve or with central valve) obturator (**Fig. 4**).

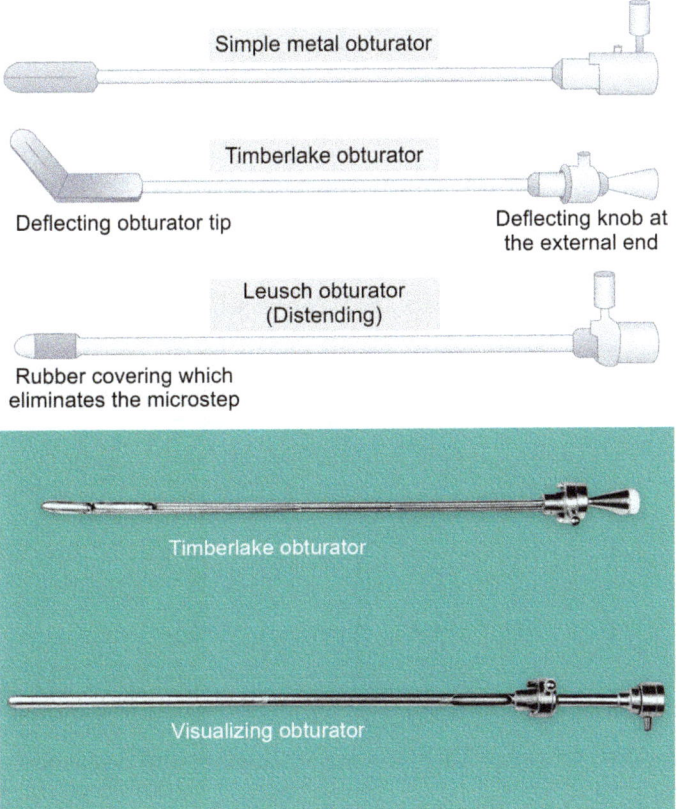

Figure 4: Resectoscope obturator.

becomes angulated, thus allowing negotiation at bulbar urethra and bladder neck.

WORKING ELEMENT

Loop Control Mechanism

Three different types of loop control mechanisms are described. They are classified as passive or active or either as thumb-operated or finger-operated.

The individual description is as follows:
- *Rack and pinion system (**Fig. 5**)*: This was the original loop described by McCarthy. It works by to and fro movement of the lever. The loop requires a longer practice to master the art of resection. Not commonly in use.
- *Thumb-operated (Nesbit system) (passive) (**Fig. 6**)*: In this loop control mechanism, the spring retracts the loop into the sheath, thus for cutting a tissue, it requires the loop to be extended out of the sheath by pressure against the spring, the loop thereafter retracts on its own. This implies that

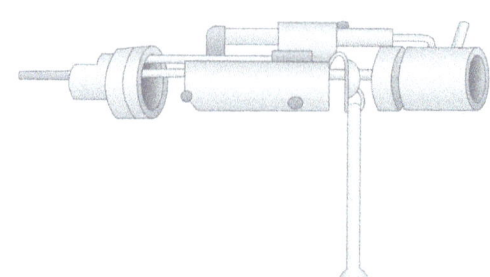

Figure 5: The rack and pinion working element.

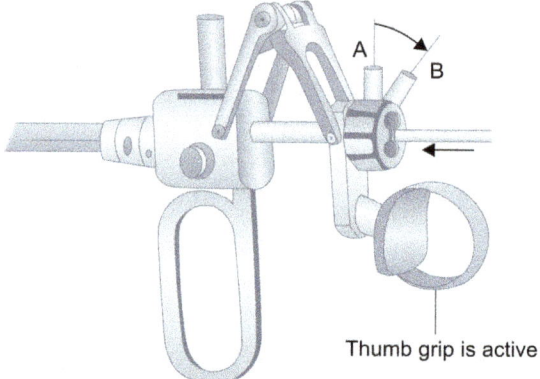

Thumb grip is active

Figure 6: Schematic diagram of thumb-operated working element.

cutting of the tissue is by passive retraction of the spring and hence the term "passive." In a resting state, the loop is inside the sheath.
- *Finger-operated (Baumrucker system) (active)* (**Figs. 7A and B**): In this loop control mechanism, the spring extends the loop out of sheath, the cutting is achieved by the manual retraction of the loop into the sheath. The cutting of tissue is by active retraction of the working element by the surgeon and hence the term "active." In a resting state, the loop remains outside the sheath. The preference of the loop to be used is a matter of surgeon preference.

What are the Advantages and Disadvantages of Active and Passive Working Element?

Advantage of Active Element
As the movement is active, the resection is supposedly fast.

Disadvantage of Active Element
As the loop remains outside the sheath in resting state, the surgeon should be careful while operating. Since the cutting is active if surgeon exerts more pressure, resection can become deep.

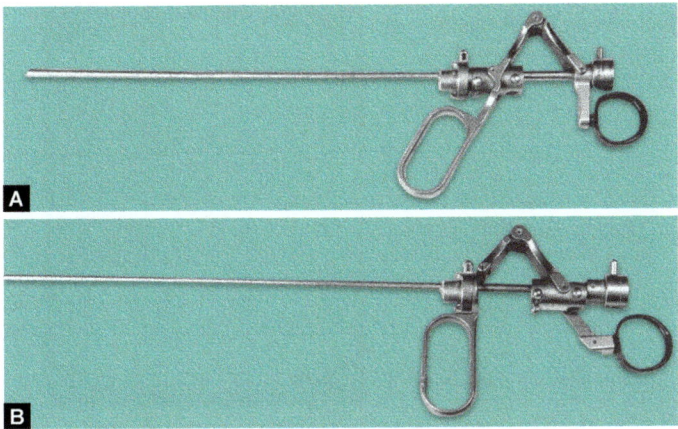

Figures 7A and B: (A) Finger-operated working element; (B) Thumb-operated working element.

Advantages of Passive Element

In resting position, the loop remains inside, hence inadvertent damage to bladder is avoided if foot pedal is inadvertently pressed by the surgeon or the assistant.

Since the cutting is passive, the chips are cut in a controlled fashion. The same working element can be used for optical urethrotomy.

Disadvantage of Passive Element

Since cutting is passive, speed of resection is slightly slower.

Cutting Loops

The loops are made of fine tungsten wire. The size is measured in millimeters (mm). The size ranges from 0.35 mm (standard) to 0.30 mm (thin) and 0.40 mm (thick).

Classification of Loops
- Depending on size of sheath—24 and 27 Fr
- Depending on color coding, yellow is 24 and brown is 27.
- Depending on size of wire—standard, thick, and thin. The sizes of the loops are as follows: 0.35 mm (standard) and 0.25 mm (thin), 0.40 mm (thick).
- Depending on the telescope used (0° or 30°)

Most resections of prostate are done with 30° telescope, some bladder tumors at the dome are resected with 0° telescope. The loop for 0° is straight and 30° is curved. All loops are color coded. 24 and 26 Fr resectoscopes used yellow-colored loops. 27 and 28 Fr resectoscopes used brown color loop. The path of passage of current is shown in **Figure 8**.

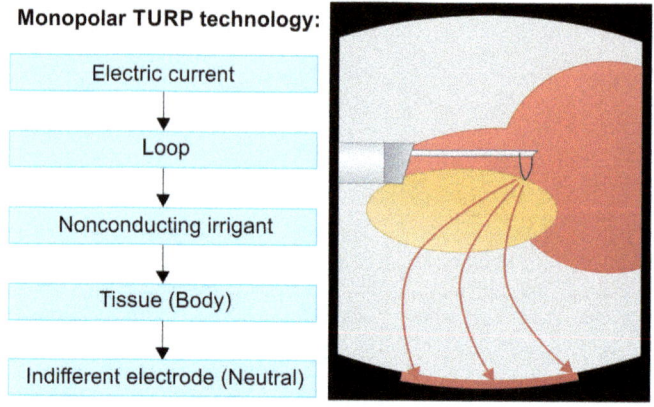

Figure 8: Path of current in monopolar circuit.

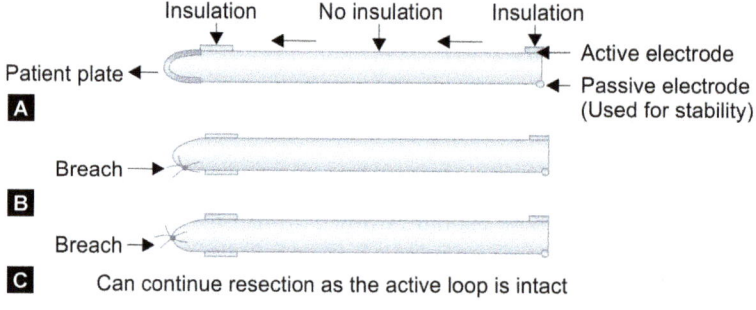

Figures 9A to C: Diagram showing what happens if a broken loop is used.

Broken Loop (Figs. 9A to C)

If the loop breaks on passive arm, what happens?

*If loop is broken at passive arm (**Fig. 9B**)*: Current will continue to flow, resection can be done; however, loop will not be stable and will get angulated. Coagulation can be done without any problem.

*If the loop is broken at middle of the curve (**Fig. 9C**)*: The current will continue to flow; however, resection cannot be done as only half part of loop is active.

What are the uses of broken loop?
- It can be used if active arm is connected, for ureteric meatotomy.
- It can be used for bladder neck incision (BNI).
- It can be used for posterior valve fulguration.

Salient features for use include the following:
- The thinner the loop, the less the current required to cut, hence they are used when less charring is required. They are useful in resection of bladder tumor.

- *Single stem or double stem*: Single or double stems do not make any difference in resection. In double stem, the current only flows through active arms and passive arms give stability.
- Depending on sides of wire that standard, thick, and thin

Uses of Thin Loop
- When precise and sharp cut is required
- Used for bladder tumor resection
- Resection during transurethral resection of the prostate (TURP) at the verumontanum (apical lobe resection)

Uses of Thick Loop
- Used for resection of bulk of adenoma
- Eventually, the thick loop becomes a thin loop after repeated use.

Types of Loops (Figs. 10A and B)
- *Standard cutting loop*: The standard loops are useful for TURP, whereas surgery to a prostatic adenoma demands the almost exclusive use of thicker loops so as to avoid change of loop during operation. Wear and tear occur at the convex part of the loop and usually breaks in the center.
- *Collins knife*: It is used to incise bladder necks or transurethral incision of the prostate (TUIP). The incision is made in cutting mode, thus achieving sharp linear cuts at the bladder neck.
- *Ball electrode (rolly ball/roller ball)*: This is used for achieving hemostasis after completion of the resection.
- *Conical electrode for point coagulation*: Helps in hemostasis
- *Blunt curette*: This is for scraping off necrotic tissue.
- *Sharp curette*: This is for removing more firmly adherent slough and for drawing calculous debris into the sheath.
- *Mowing loop*: This is for resecting bladder tumors on the posterior wall.

Problems in Loop Angles
The loop electrode used for cutting should never be at more than a right angle to the insulated shoulders carrying the loop. The angle of the loop exactly corresponds to the angle of the beak, and the window of the telescope. The loop should retract <1 mm inside the sheath so that it cannot approximate too closely to the telescope. The loop should retract inside the sheath to ensure that each cut of tissue is complete. If the loop is found to be at an obtuse angle to the insulated shoulder, it will not retract inside the sheath and small tags of uncut tissue will remain.

High Frequency Cable
It gets attached on working element, the active arc of loop is longer and has insulation, right hole on high frequency cable accommodates the active long

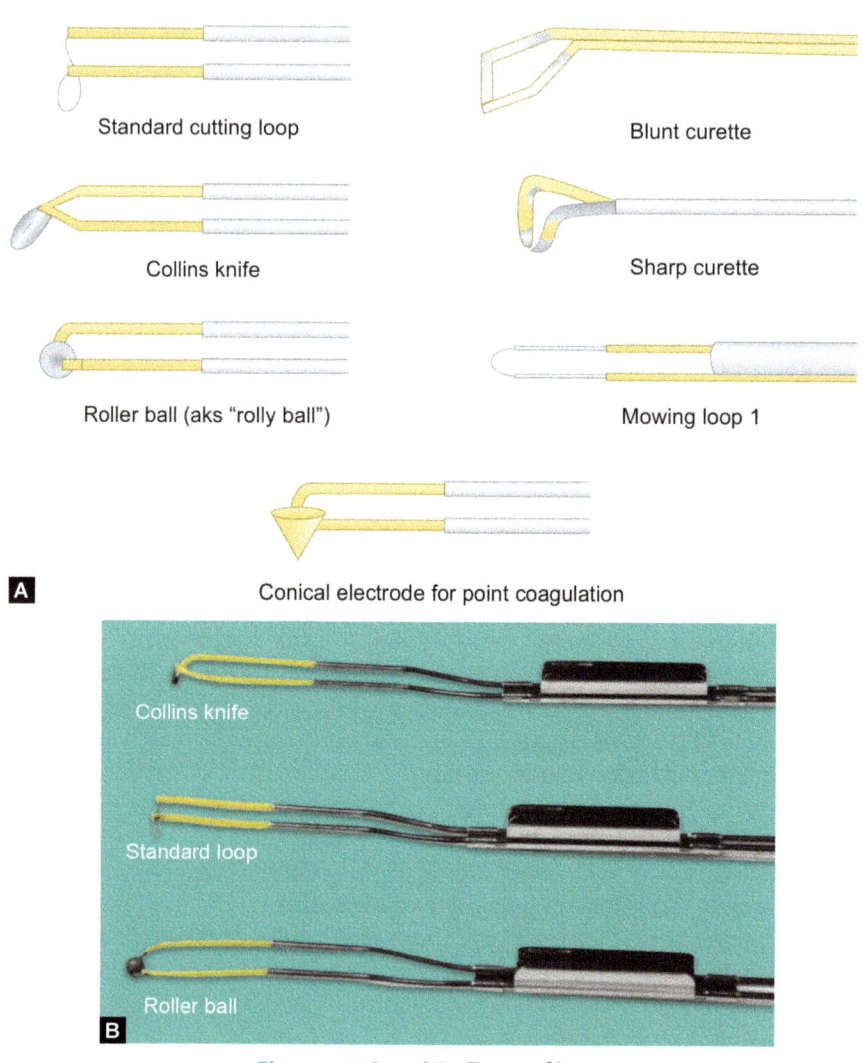

Figures 10A and B: Types of loops.

arm of loop. On the left side, there is no hole and the passive arm does not go inside and remain at the surface (**Fig. 11**).

The active loop in adults is on the right side, 4 mm, 300 cm. In pediatrics, the active loop is on the left side (surgeons' view).

IRRIGATING FLUIDS IN TRANSURETHRAL RESECTION OF THE PROSTATE

Most commonly used fluids are glycine 1.5% in water (230 mOsm/L), sterile water. Other fluid which can be used are: 5% dextrose, mannitol, sorbitol, and combination of mannitol and sorbitol.

CHAPTER 3: Transurethral Resection of the Prostate Instruments | 35

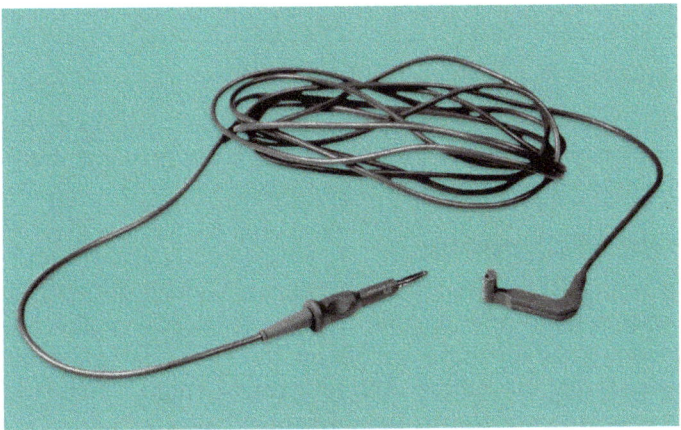

Figure 11: High frequency cable.

Salient Features Related to Absorption

- 20 mL/min absorbed
- If 1 L fluid absorbed, then the drop in sodium level 5-8 mmol/L
- Height of 60-100 cm above the patient is needed for irrigation and pressure of 2 kPa at the operative site is critical for fluid absorption.
- Not >300 mL/min required for good vision—excessive irrigation pushed by the assistant avoided

Fluid absorption is proportional to the number of prostatic sinuses opened. Main driving force is hydrostatic force in operating area.

TRANSURETHRAL RESECTION OF THE PROSTATE SYNDROME

Definition

Sodium level after TURP of <125 mmol/L with two or more symptoms or signs of TURP syndrome (nausea, vomiting, bradycardia, hypotension, hypertension, chest pain, mental confusion, anxiety, paresthesia, and visual disturbance).

Risk reduction strategies to prevent TURP syndrome:
- Proper use of irrigating fluids
- Proper selection of patients
- Increased wariness in the part of anesthetist
- Newer modalities—bipolar TURP, laser TURP.

ACCESSORIES TO EVACUATE PROSTATE CHIPS

Ellik Evacuator

Milo Ellik invented Ellik evacuator, he was resident under Alcock at University of Iowa. It consists of two glass bulbs connected to a rubber bulb and a connector for attachment to resectoscope sheath.

Method to Use Ellik Evacuator

It is to put in basin full of normal saline, rubber bulb is to be disconnected and filled with normal saline after creating negative suction, once this is done, it is reconnected to glass apparatus and placed under normal saline and again filled by compressing the rubber bulb (creating suction). Once ready, it is connected to resectoscope sheath and the rubber bulb is compressed and tip of the sheath is elevated in the bladder by depressing the shaft. The negative suction thus created sucks out all the prostatic chips and clots. It has to be filled completely with normal saline, if air enters, evacuation does not take place properly (**Fig. 12A**).

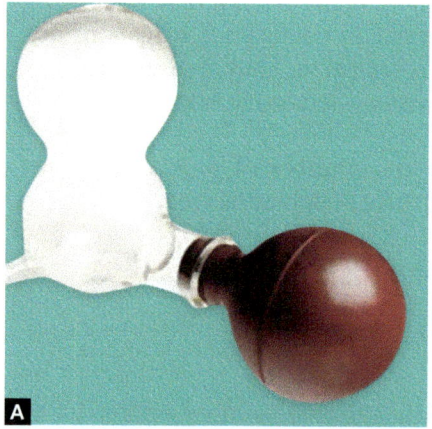
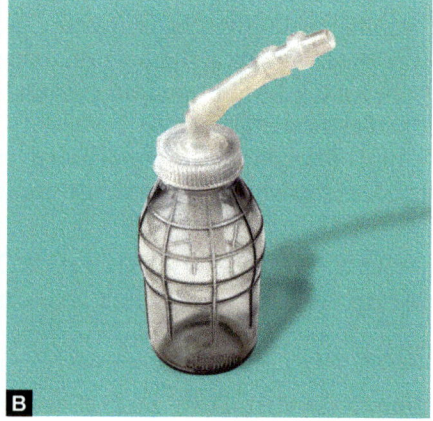
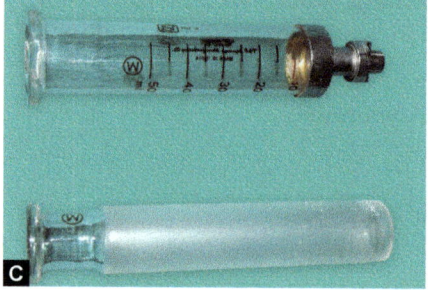

Figures 12A to C: (A) Ellik evacuator; (B) Modification of bladder evacuator; (C) Toomey syringe.

Modification of Bladder Evacuator

It is commonly available. Normal saline is filled by pouring into the bottle after opening the cap, it has to be filled up to the brim of the connector. If air enters, evacuation does not take place properly (**Fig. 12B**).

Toomey Syringe

They are glass syringes and have a metal catheter adapter. They are graduated with a 50 cc capacity. The metal adapter fits onto the resectoscope sheath and it is used for evacuation of prostatic chips and clots by creating suction (**Fig. 12C**).

REFERENCE

1. Blandy JP, Notley RG, Reynard JM. History. In: Blandy Transurethral Resection, 5th edition. Oxford: Taylor and Francis; 2005. pp. 11-27.

CHAPTER 4

Bipolar Transurethral Resection of the Prostate

INTRODUCTION

A bipolar electrode is defined as an electrode that has two active electrodes attached to a single support, and a structure that allows high-frequency electric current to pass through these two electrodes when electrified.

The bipolar technology uses the plasma arc for resection of tissue. The plasma is the fourth state of matter. It is a partially ionized gas containing *free electrons and cations*. The plasma is conductive. These gas molecules in plasma return to their initial state with emission of electromagnetic radiation of specific color which is orange for sodium and blue or purple for potassium. The principles behind the resection in bipolar transurethral resection of the prostate (TURP) are given in **Figure 1**.

As the electrode is activated, the current flows in the irrigation fluid as impedance is low in the saline. As the electrode is heated, the air bubble forms around the electrode and the whole electrode gets covered with air bubbles. Later current is conducted to air surrounding the electrode and then the plasma arc covers the electrode. Resection is done by the heat of plasma around the electrode.

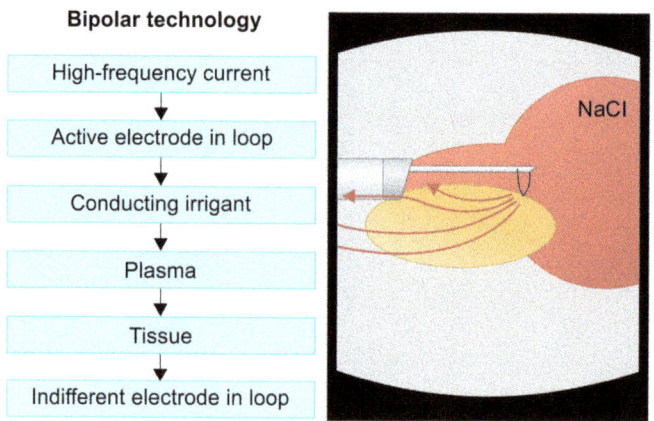

Figure 1: Bipolar technology of transurethral resection of the prostate.

IRRIGATION IN BIPOLAR TRANSURETHRAL RESECTION OF THE PROSTATE

As the irrigating solution used in bipolar TURP is normal saline, there is no risk of transurethral resection (TUR) syndrome. However, it is to be remembered that this does not mean that there is no fluid absorption in bipolar TURP. So resection time has to be limited in patients who have comorbidities which may decompensate in fluid overload stage like congestive cardiac failure or renal failures.

ADVANTAGES OF BIPOLAR TRANSURETHRAL RESECTION OF THE PROSTATE

- Less conductive trauma, so a lower rate of bladder neck stenosis or urethral strictures due to thermal change of urethra
- Less chance of TURP syndrome
- Lower risk of capsular perforation as there is decreased stimulation of pelvic floor
- Better visual orientation by reduced coagulation depth
- Self-cleaning of the loop by high energy level at plasma ignition

LIMITATIONS OF BIPOLAR TECHNOLOGY

- Higher risk of conductive trauma if current is deviated via sheath and insufficient lubrication. Risk of recurrent bleeding due to smaller coagulation zone.
- There are different types of bipolar electrodes: These differences are by the way in which the active and indifferent electrodes are arranged:
  - Two different loops (parallel or opposite)
  - Using the distal end of the resection loop
  - Using the working element of the resection shaft

TYPES

Quasi-bipolar

The current does not flow exclusively between two electrodes (i.e., definition of bipolar electrosurgery). Instead the current runs to a negative pole through sheath of the resectoscope, e.g., Olympus TURis system (**Fig. 2**).

Olympus TURis System (Transurethral Resection in Saline)

Both the active and return electrode are within the resectoscope in the bipolar electrosurgical system. As there is conductive saline, small fraction of the current passes through the tissue, and no neutral electrode is required. In this system, high-frequency current is used to create a plasma corona. After plasma ignition, cutting or vaporization can be performed.

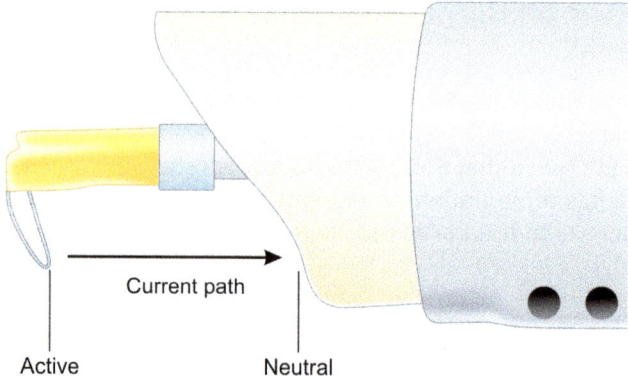

Figure 2: Olympus electrode.

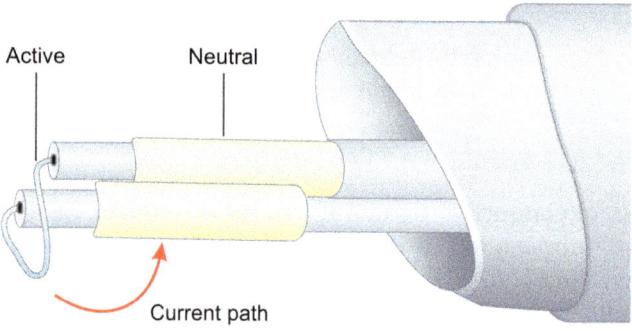

Figure 3: Gyrus loop.

Plasma Kinetic Resection Loop by Gyrus

It uses a single platinum-iridium loop as active electrode, whereas on the same axis (axipolar), the distal end of the loop (stainless steel electrode separated by a ceramic insulator) serves as a neutral electrode. This loop is designed for single use (**Fig. 3**).

Karl Storz Bipolar Resectoscope Loop

It has two oppositely facing loops with passive electrode as counterpart. This loop is designed for multiple uses (**Fig. 4**).

The flat cuneiform probe allows dissection of inner prostate gland from the outer prostatic capsule. This is done by mechanical dissection in correct plane. The hemostasis is achieved by coagulation along with vaporization properties of the electrode. This combines mechanical dissection with bipolar coagulation and vaporization of prostatic tissue in one instrument.

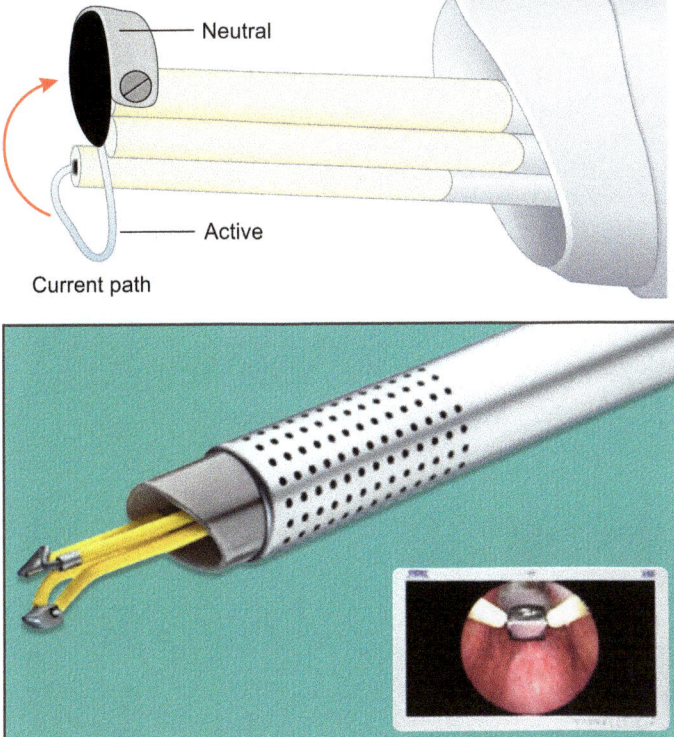

Figure 4: Karl Storz electrode.

Bipolar Button Electrode for Transurethral Vaporization of Prostate (Fig. 5)

This oval electrode causes vaporization of prostatic tissue by plasma technique as described previously in this chapter. Tissue is vaporized by a locally confined denaturation process, while surrounding tissue heating effects are minor.

In this technique, the electrode's wire loop is only used to locate the layers and coagulate any bleeding (**Fig. 6**). The black runner is used to gently peel off the prostate lobes as a whole, to remain in right planes. The next electrode is used to coagulate any bleeding points after peeling of the lobes. The lobes are then pushed into the bladder, where they are cut and eventually removed.

Differences between bipolar and monopolar TURP
- Bipolar TURP has less chances of bleeding and less chances of clot retention
- Catherization time can be less in bipolar.
- Duration of surgery can be extended and hence larger glands can be resected.

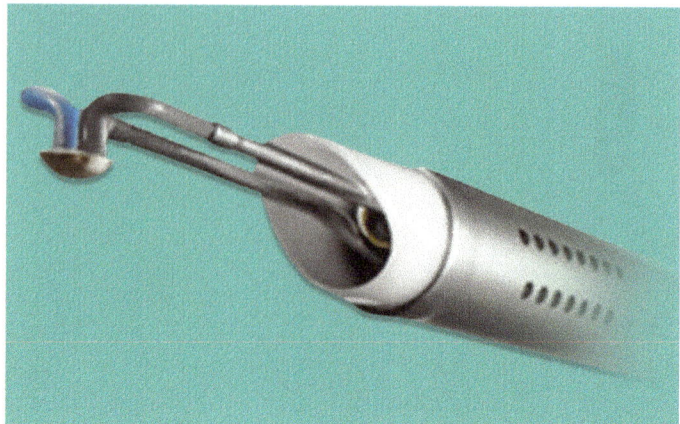

Figure 5: Button electrode.

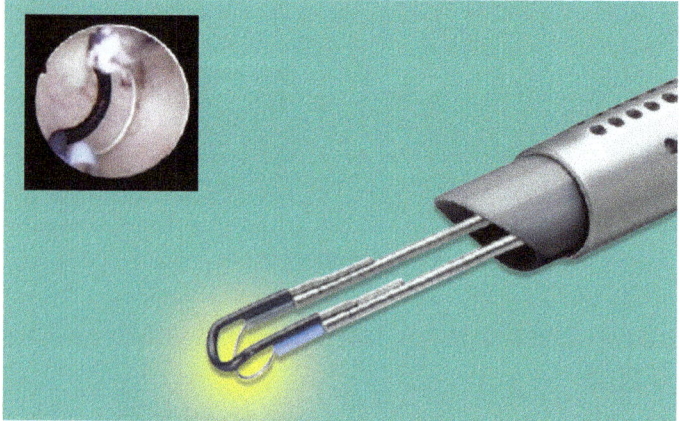

Figure 6: Transurethral enucleation of the prostate—bipolar (TUEB).

- TUR syndrome is not observed in bipolar in Bipolar TURP saline is used which is isotonic fluid. However significant quantity of fluid can still be absorbed which can cause fluid overload and its consequences. However unlike in TUR syndrome Hyponatremia, hemolysis (if water is used) will not occur that is main difference.
- Bipolar TURP can be slightly slow as plasma (corona) has to generate and then cutting starts which takes little time
- Many studies have shown post-incidence of urethral stricture is higher in bipolar than monopolar. It is probably due to prolonged time of instrumentation.

CHAPTER 5

Cystolithotrity Instruments

HISTORY AND BRIEF INTRODUCTION

Jean Civiale was a urologist practicing in France in the 19th century and is credited with the invention of surgical instrument lithotrite and performed transurethral lithotripsy. This is considered to be the first minimally invasive surgery. The instrument which he developed contained three prongs to grasp a stone. The instrument was capable of making a number of holes in the stone. Bladder stones can be managed either by urethral route, suprapubic route, or by open approach. The suprapubic approach is preferred in multiple stones or large stone bulk. The transurethral route offers a plethora of options with regard to the energy source. The stone can either be crushed with stone-crushing forceps or broken by ultrasound, pneumatic, or laser energy lithotrite. In pediatric age group laser and pneumatic are preferred energy sources.

Nomenclature of Various Procedures
- *Cystolitholapaxy*: Intact removal of stone
- *Cystolithotrity*: Mechanical crushing of the stone
- *Cystolithotripsy*: Breakage of stone with energy source
- *Cystolithotomy*: Open removal of stone

Stone-crushing Forceps (Fig. 1)

It is available as a single action jaw. The stone-crushing forceps fits in 25 Fr cystoscope sheath. This forceps can be used for smaller stones and for crushing fragments after use of lithotrite. After removal of forceps, evacuation is possible through the sheath with evacuator. The surgeon should not grasp stones larger than the size of the jaw, as it may damage the instrument. The assembly requires 30° telescope. It is less robust than Mauermayer stone punch. While crushing stones it is important that bladder is not empty, stone is grasped, instrument is rotated to ensure that the mucosa is not caught in the jaws.

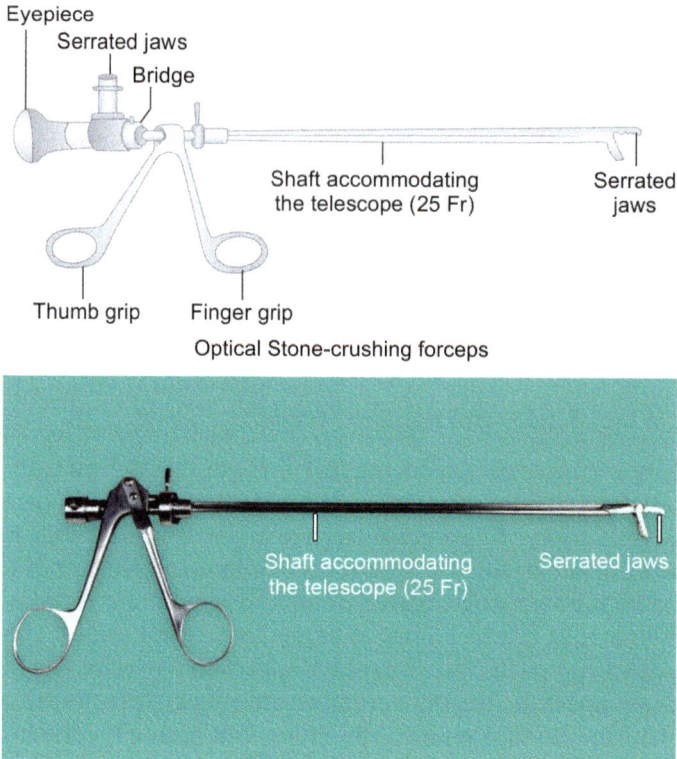

Figure 1: Stone-crushing forceps.

Hendrickson's Classical Lithotrite (Fig. 2)

This instrument has to be passed blindly; it has to be used with 70° scope. It is cumbersome to use. It is passed blindly like a dilator, hence there is a high chance of creating a false passage in urethra. If jaws get stuck, it may even need open surgical removal. This instrument is not used nowadays because of high rate of complications and availability of better instruments.

Mauermayer Stone Punch (Figs. 3A and B)

It is complete with its own sheath, working element, and inserting obturator (with bridge). Hence, becomes costly. It is sturdy therefore bigger stones can be crushed. Movement is forward and backward (vis-à vis-upward and downward movement in stone crushing). The instrument requires a zero-degree telescope.

The parts of the instrument include (**Figs. 3A and B**):
- A punch working element
- Punch sheath with central valve, 25 Fr straight beak with obturator

CHAPTER 5: Cystolithotrity Instruments | 45

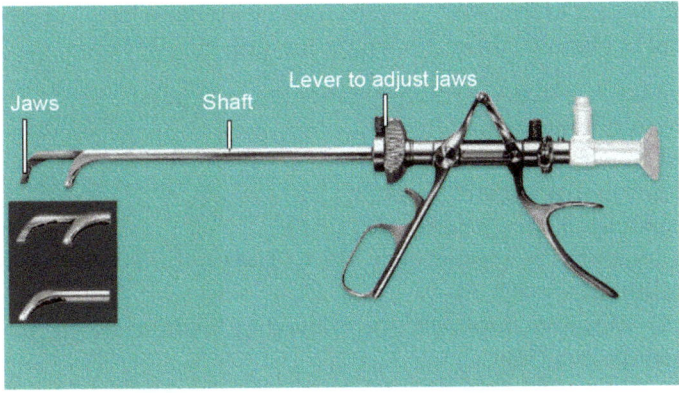

Figure 2: Hendrickson's classical lithotrite.

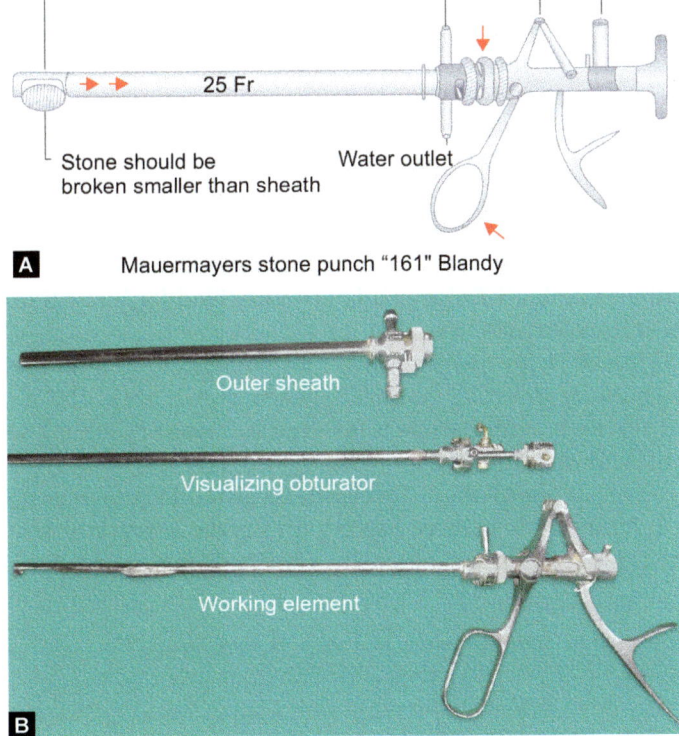

Figures 3A and B: Mauermayers stone punch.

The stone can be broken so that it becomes small enough so that the stone can be pulled out through the punch sheath or can be washed with the evacuator. It requires to be introduced with visualizing obturator.

With the advent of lithoclast, nephroscope with lithoclast is used for the management of bladder stones, making stone-crushing devices less popular.

The different ways of treating bladder stones are as follows:
- Open cystolithotomy
- Laparoscopic cystolithotomy
- Endoscopic management
  - Transurethral cystolithotripsy (TUCL)
  - Percutaneous cystolithotripsy (PCCL). Also called as suprapubic cystolithotripsy (SPCL)

The most common approach for managing bladder stones in adults currently is endoscopically.

The various ways of performing TUCL are as follows:
- Cystolithotrity
- *Laser TUCL*: The bladder stones can be lased with laser fiber inserted through ureteric catheter.
- *TUCL using cystolithotripsy sheath and lithoclast*: The cystolithotripsy is performed using lithoclast probe inserted through a cystolithotripsy adapter (**Fig. 4**) in a 25 Fr sheath.
- *Iglesias outer sheath with nephroscope*: In males, cystolithotripsy with lithoclast or laser can be done especially for large stones by inserting nephroscope in Iglesias outer sheath. The modified Iglesias sheath is first inserted and then inner sheath is removed. Then, nephroscope is inserted. Even newer technology energy sources can be used for larger stones such as ShockPulse or EMS Trilogy. This prevents bladder distention which occurs if only nephroscope is used.
- *Amplatz sheath with nephroscope*: In females, cystolithotripsy can be performed by inserting Amplatz sheath over dilator. The dilator is removed and then nephroscope is inserted and stone is either lased with laser or blasted with lithoclast.
- *PCCL or SPCL*: In this method, the bladder is distended under cystoscopic guidance. Puncture is achieved with pun needle suprapubically and a glidewire is passed in the bladder. The tract is dilated under cystoscopic

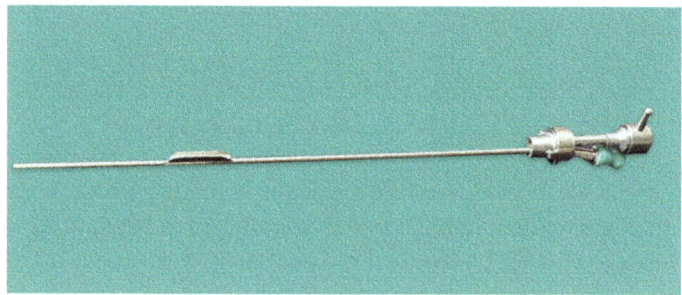

Figure 4: Cystolithotripsy adapter.

vision with Amplatz dilator and sheath over guide rod. Amplatz sheath is placed and dilator is removed leaving back the glidewire. Nephroscope is then inserted via Amplatz sheath and stone is blasted with lithoclast or laser. The stone fragments can be removed through cystoscope by Ellik evacuator.

While doing this procedure, precaution should be taken so that Amplatz sheath does not slip out of the bladder when it collapses.

Pediatric Instruments

Depending upon size of urethra, nephroscope can be used for breaking bladder stones.
- In infants MIPXS can be used with laser disintegration of stones.
- Minimicroperc sheath can be used with microperc instruments by laser disintegration
- In elder children miniperc can be used.

All these are nephroscopes and they do not have outlet channel. Hence while using these instruments, bladder needs to be drained by inserting large bore angiocath which can keep bladder draining continuously.

If stone is bigger, it is better to do Suprapubic cystolithotripsy (SPCL). Miniperc nephroscope with either miniperc sheath or amplatz can be used.

CHAPTER 6

Percutaneous Nephrolithotomy Instruments

INSTRUMENTS

The key instruments required for successful completion of a percutaneous nephrolithotomy (PCNL) are as follows:
- Access needles
- Tract dilators
- Nephroscope (rigid and flexible)
- Accessories, guidewires, forceps, etc.

ACCESS NEEDLES (FIG. 1)

The access needle helps in gaining optimal access and also offers space for passage of guidewire. Typically, the needle has two parts, a shaft and a stylet. Traditionally, they are classified as a two-part and three-part needle (**Fig. 1**). The needles can also be classified depending on the configuration of the

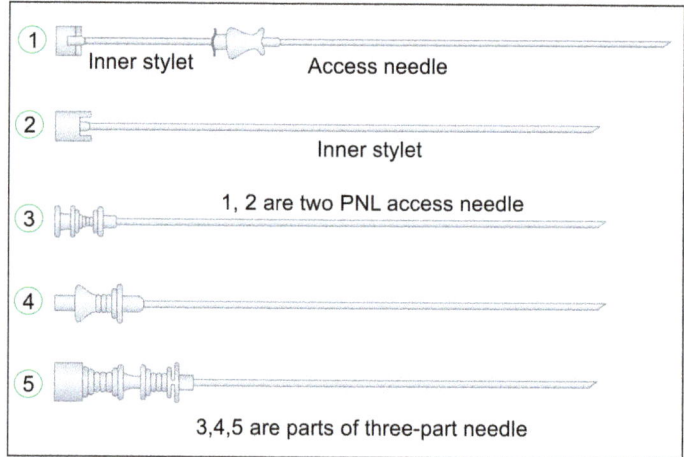

(PNL: percutaneous nephrolithotomy)

Figure 1: Access needles.

tip which can be either beveled or diamond tipped. In general, the shorter needles have better control. Longer needles are necessary for obese patients and in a situation where an ultrasound-guided puncture is contemplated. The triangulation technique requires a longer tract and hence it requires a longer needle. The alternative access needle system uses a 21-gauge primary access needle; these needles are compatible with a 0.018 guidewire.

Types of Needles (Fig. 2)

Initial Puncture Needle—Three-part Bevel Tip

These are the first instruments used for gaining access. A 0.035" guidewire is used with it. Initial puncture needle is 18 gauge, it is 20 cm in length, and has three part with a bevel tip. The bevel helps in ensuring entry of guidewire into the pelvicalyceal system (PCS). The beveled tip should be facing the crystals in the ultrasound for acoustic visualization of the needle. The disadvantage of using a beveled needle is that the needle tends to bend toward the bevel. In contrast, the diamond-tipped needle does not deviate in either direction. This is not used nowadays as there is no specific advantage of three-part needle over two-part needle.

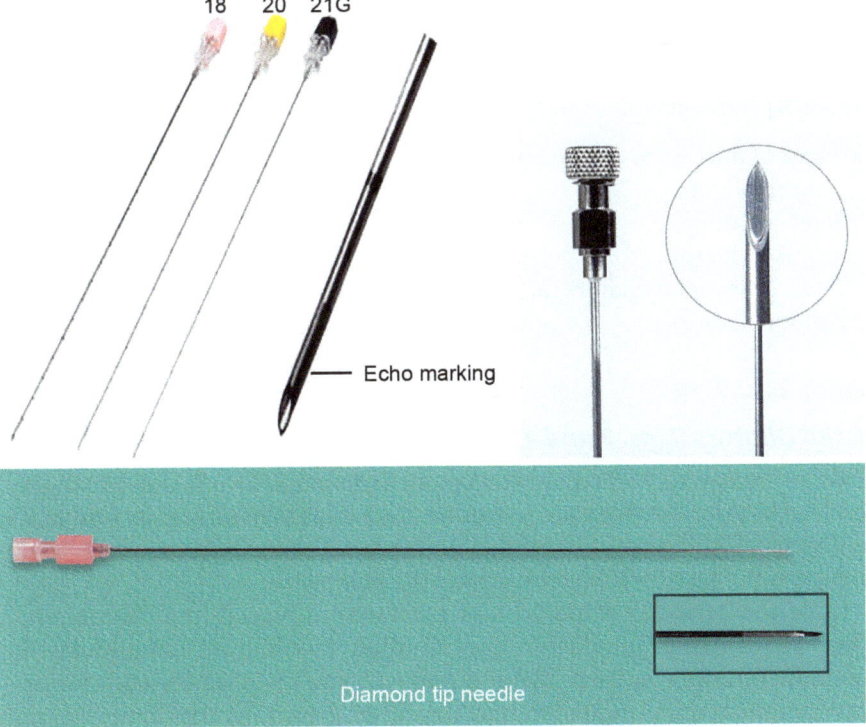

Figure 2: Types of needles.

Initial Puncture Needle—Two-part Trocar Tip (Diamond)

This is the most popular needle. The needle is 20 cm in length; it is 18 gauge, two-part trocar tip. The color code is pink for 18 gauge, yellow for 20, and black for 21 (**Fig. 2**).

Chiba Needle—Three-part Bevel Tip[1]

It has stylet, inner sheath, and outer sheath. Outer sheath is of shorter length. It is used for fluoroscopy-guided puncture. Puncture is made with 21-gauge needle since it is longer in length. When perfect puncture is made as confirmed by efflux of urine on withdrawal of stylet, outer sheath is advanced over the inner sheath. Once it reaches PCS, the stylet and inner sheath is taken out and the operator proceeds for dilatation. Advantage of 21-gauge needle is that even when multiple attempts are made to obtain PCS access, it would theoretically cause less damage to kidney, less bleeding and less chance of arteriovenous (AV) fistula as compared to 18-gauge needle, though this has not been proven in any study. The needle was developed at the University of Chiba, Japan. This needle is also called as a skinny needle and is used for opacification of the PCS.

PERCUTANEOUS NEPHROLITHOTOMY TRACT DILATORS

The dilators are used for creation of PCNL tract. The types of dilators to be used are dictated by the size of stone and the degree of hydronephrosis and size of tract you want to make. The type of dilator to be used is a matter of surgeon's preference.

The types of dilators to be used are as follows:
- Fascial dilators
- Screw dilators
- Amplatz dilators
- Telescopic metal dilators (also known as Alken dilators)
- Balloon dilators.

Tract Dilators

Fascial Dilators (Figs. 3 and 4)[2]

Available from 6 to 16 Fr polytetrafluoroethylene (PTFE), (Cook Medicals Inc., IN, USA) in size, they are useful for tract dilatation after puncture and placement of guidewire. Fascial dilators have an elongated conical tip and opening at the tip which accommodates the guidewire.

Once the access is achieved and guidewire is placed, the dilators are passed sequentially. The dilators are cheap but theoretically are associated with more bleeding, as each dilator is removed and replaced with one larger dilator until complete dilatation is achieved. As every time the dilator has to

CHAPTER 6: Percutaneous Nephrolithotomy Instruments | 51

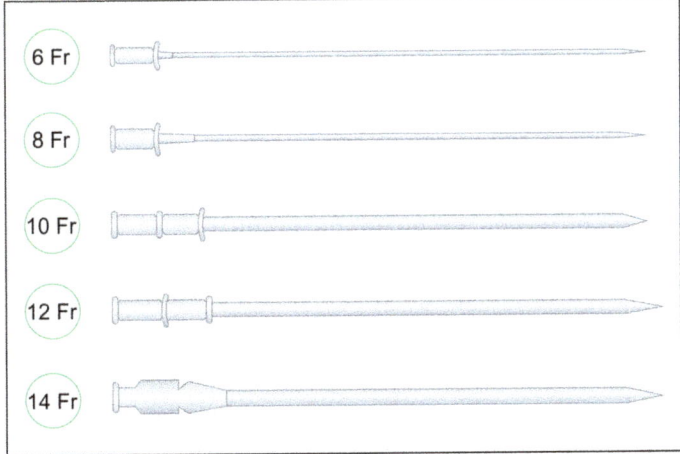

Figure 3: Fascial dilators: Dimension of the tip varies at shaft and tip.

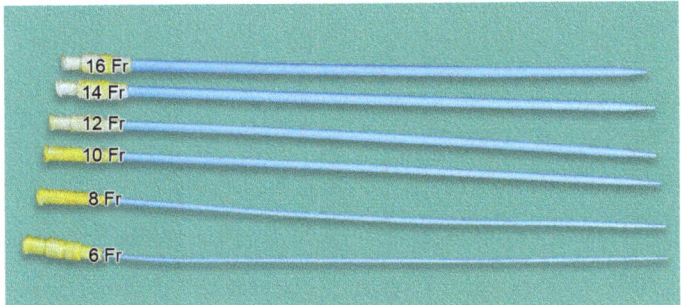

Figure 4: Fascial dilator.

be removed and replaced, the chance of bleeding due to loss of tamponade of the tract being dilated increases.

Screw Dilators (Figs. 5A and B)[3]

They have a screw-shaped tip. They are available in 3 sizes—size 6–12 Fr, 6–14 Fr, and 6–16 Fr (6 implies the size of tip and 12 implies the size of the shaft). Even bigger dilators are available.

Amplatz Renal Dilator Set (Fig. 6)

They are used for progressive dilatation of nephrostomy tract prior to percutaneous kidney stone removal. They are radiopaque dilators and sheaths. They have a short-tapered tip with smooth surface to reduce tissue trauma. A typical dilator set consists of an 8 Fr radiopaque tetrafluoroethylene (TFE) catheter (also known as Cobra catheter), the dilators range from 12 to 30 Fr, the Amplatz sheaths range for 24, 26, 28, and 30 Fr dilators. The sheaths

52 | SECTION 1: Instruments

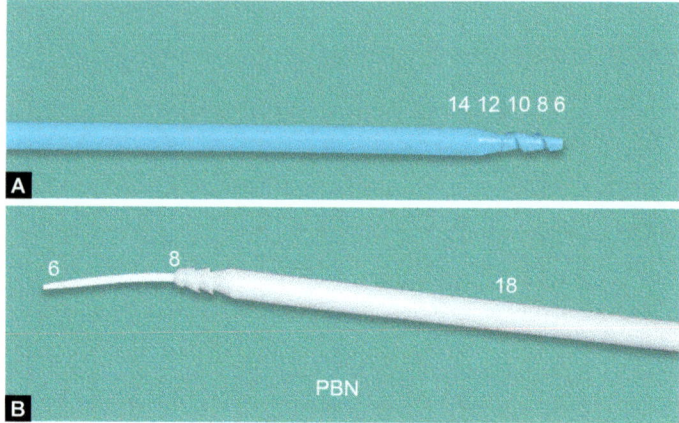

Figures 5A and B: Screw dilators.

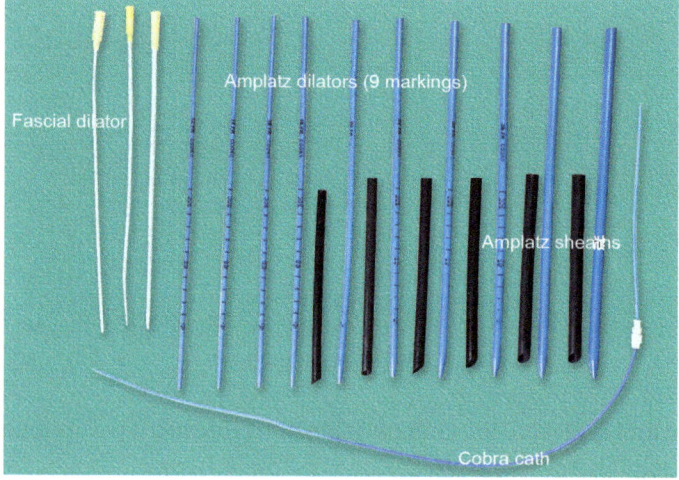

Figure 6: Amplatz dilator.

are not numbered; however, conventionally same size Amplatz sheath snugly fits over same size Amplatz dilator, e.g., 24 Fr Amplatz sheath will fit over 24 Fr Amplatz dilator. Radiopaque TFE catheter (Cobra catheter) acts as a guide for dilators 12–30 Fr, radiopaque TFE catheter (8 Fr) allows safety wire placement. They are 30 cm in length, however, long Amplatz dilators with length of 32 and 40 cm are available (for obese patients). Smaller sheaths 14–20 Fr are now available. The length of sheath is 16 cm. The length of longer sheath is 20 and 30 cm (use for obese patients). Thus, once the puncture is made, guidewire is passed, tract dilated up to 10 Fr by using serial fascial dilators 6 Fr-8 Fr-10 Fr. Then, Cobra catheter (8 Fr) is passed in PCS. Over this catheter, Amplatz dilators are passed sequentially one by one. Once the desired size dilatation is achieved by a dilator, over it corresponding Amplatz sheath is passed and dilator removed.

Metallic Serial Telescopic Dilators (Figs. 7A and B)

The set consists of a central rod and serial metal dilators. The rod is 58 cm and can be either rigid or flexible. The most commonly used are the rigid rod which gives sturdiness required during dilatation. The entire unit resembles an assembled collapsed radio antenna after all the dilators are assembled. The dilators are advanced over a central rod which is 7 Fr in diameter and with a rounded knob which is 9 Fr in diameter. The central rod is placed over a stiff guidewire; the dilators are available in an increment of 3 Fr depending on the make (starting from 9 Fr up to 24 Fr). Additionally, 27 and 30 Fr size dilators can be ordered (Karl Storz, GmBh). After placement of guidewire, rod

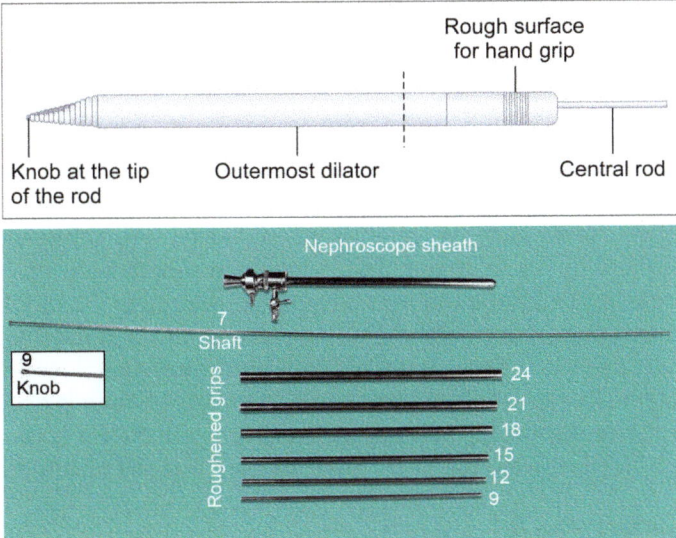

Figure 7A: Upper: Schematic of Alken dilators over Alken rod; Lower: Alken telescopic metal dilator.

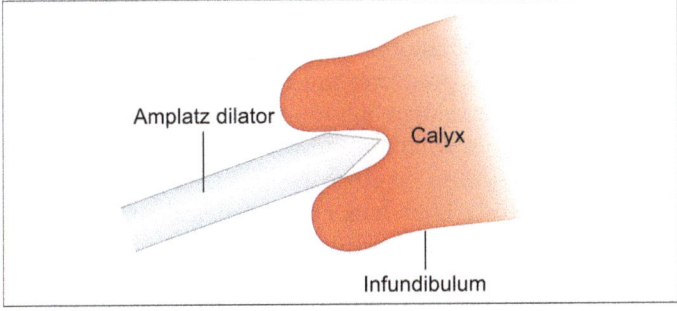

Figure 7B: Amplatz dilator entering calyx.

is passed with the advancing bulbar end. The first dilator being 9 Fr, it does not overshoot the knob of the central rod. The inner end of each dilator is designed in such a way that it does not go beyond the previous dilator and hence beyond the knob of the rod. Outer end of each dilator has serrations (holding grip) (approximately 1 inch) which allows optimal grip while dilating the tract. Each dilator is designed in such a way that they snugly fit over one another and do not traumatize the tissue during dilatation. Since the dilators snugly fit over each other and do not overshoot the knob of the rod, on withdrawing the rod all the dilators come out with the rod.

These dilators are cheap and allow complete dilatation up to calyx. The rigidity of this system offers it to be an effective dilator even in tough tissues such as in previously operated cases. The dilatation can be done up to the desired size and a sheath placed thereafter. Over the last dilator either a snugly fitting nephroscope sheath or an appropriately sized Amplatz sheath can be passed. Alternatively, after removing all the dilators, Amplatz dilator and its sheath can be introduced over a rod.

The operator should be aware of the shortcomings of this system which include possibility of kinking the glidewire. In Amplatz system, initial Cobra catheter is passed. Over this catheter sequential, Amplatz dilatation is done up to desired size and then Amplatz sheath placed. While in Alken system, a rod is passed over the guidewire and then serial dilatation done over which a nephroscope sheath is passed and PCNL is carried out. However, often dilatation is done by Alken system and over which Amplatz sheath is kept. If more force is applied, then rod may advance further up to the medial wall of pelvis causing perforation. In the Amplatz system, the tip of the dilator is 1 inch conical and hence the tract is underdilated as the full shaft does not enter the PCS system. This assumes importance particularly if stone is occupying the whole calyx or narrow infundibulum. Every time the dilator is taken out, there may be bleeding from the tract. This dilatation is time consuming.

Balloon Dilators (Fig. 8)[4]

These are radial dilators unlike other dilators which are axial dilators. The balloon dilators work by lateral compressive force rather than a lateral shearing force. After the initial puncture and placement of wire, the tract has to be dilated up to 8 Fr with facial dilators and then balloon dilation catheter is introduced. High-pressure balloons are capable of developing pressures up to 15–30 atmospheres of pressure; the length varies up to 15 cm and diameters of 10–12 mm. With single balloon inflation, the entire access tract is dilated. They are placed over stiff guidewire. The distal end of balloon is placed close to collecting system (as close to stone bearing calyx as possible) and balloon is inflated by a Luer lock-controlled inflation device. Before introduction of catheter, the Amplatz sheath should be back loaded from the renal end (it is not possible to pass the Amplatz sheath later). Finally, Amplatz sheath is placed over the balloon and balloon is removed. The advantage of these dilators is that dilatation is rapidly achieved and they are easy to use.

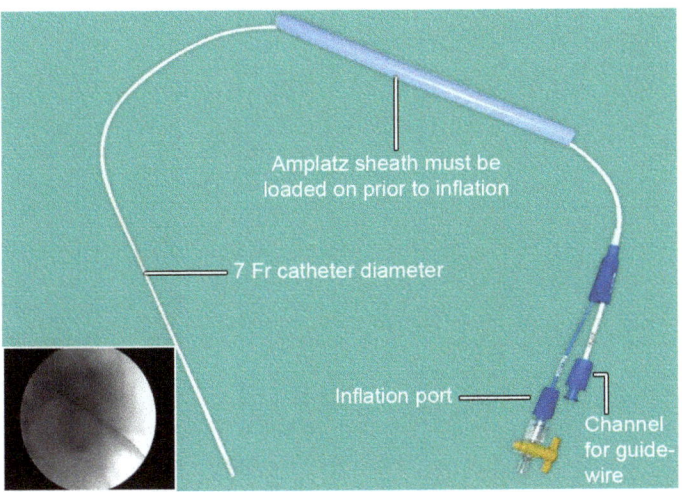

Figure 8: Parts of a balloon dilator inset shows the fluoroscopic view.

The disadvantage is that balloon has a tapered end, so dilatation up to entry calyx may not be complete, especially when enough length of glidewire is not parked in kidney. Balloon dilators tend to be less effective in dense retroperitoneal scarred tissue, in addition, they are expensive.

Guidewires or glidewires: The guidewires are key accessories in preparation of any endourological procedure. The type of guidewire to be used depends on the access to be gained. The details have been mentioned in chapter on accessories.

Accessories for PCNL: These would be discussed in chapter on accessories.

NEPHROSCOPES

Varieties of rigid and flexible nephroscopes from different manufacturers are available. It is necessary to know the advantages and disadvantages of each to select a best instrument in a given case.

The rigid nephroscopes have a rod-lens system for imaging. The eyepiece can be parallel to the nephroscope working channel or it can be oblique. The eyepiece of oblique variety is suitable for direct viewing as accessories can be inserted easily. The eyepiece of parallel variety is useful when endovision is used (this fact holds true when one is using a camera without a beam splitter). Oblique eyepiece suits a beam splitter camera.

Types of Nephroscopes (Fig. 9)

Classification

The nephroscopes can be classified as:
- *Depending on the make*: Karl Storz, Richard Wolf, ACMI (Olympus)
- Size of the nephroscope

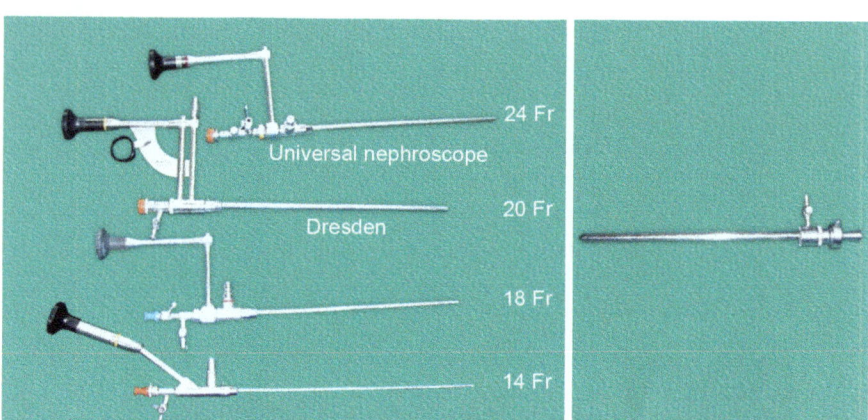

Figure 9: Nephroscopes: Wolf.

Major differences in Wolf and Storz nephroscopes are:
- All Wolf telescopes (of a nephroscope) are integrated with a sheath and hence can be used as an independent unit without the sheath over it.
- Storz nephroscopes have a sheath and the telescope and hence are not integrated, Storz recently has introduced a similar design of a slender nephroscope.

The parts of nephroscope are:
- Sheath
- Telescope

Traditionally, the sizes of nephroscope mean the size of the sheath. Richard Wolf nephroscope models are called as universal nephroscope and are available in various sizes.

Adult Nephroscopes by Richard Wolf, GmBh, Tuttlingen, Germany.
- *Percutaneous low pressure universal nephroscope (Model Marberger)*[4]: It is 27 Fr in size and has a 25° down viewing telescope. It has an oval working channel through which 4 mm instrument can be used.
- *Percutaneous universal nephroscope*[5]: The available size is 24 Fr sheath with channel accommodating 3.5 mm instrument. The viewing angle is 20°.
- *Percutaneous universal nephroscope (Model Dresden)*[6]: It has a 20.8 Fr sheath with larger working channel for instruments up to 3.5 mm. The working channel is oval in cross section. Angle of vision is 12° down (diagram of the grip). Although slender it has the same sturdiness as bigger nephroscope. The channel size is 3.5 mm and the design is ergonomically better because of the valve retainer.
- Invisio® Smith Digital Percutaneous Nephroscope[7]

This is an advanced scope, much lighter than traditional scope (470 g vs. 935 g) effectively decreasing the fatigue during long procedure This also helps the surgeon to use nondominant hand-to-hold scope and use dominant hand-to-manipulate instruments.

Difference in 24 Fr, 27 Fr, and 20.8 Fr is 20.8 is to be Held in a Vertical Manner (Figs. 10A to C)

The terminology "continuous irrigation" irrigation nephroscopes.

All nephroscopes if used with sheath become continuous. The sheaths have side holes at the distal tip which allows egress of irrigation through the

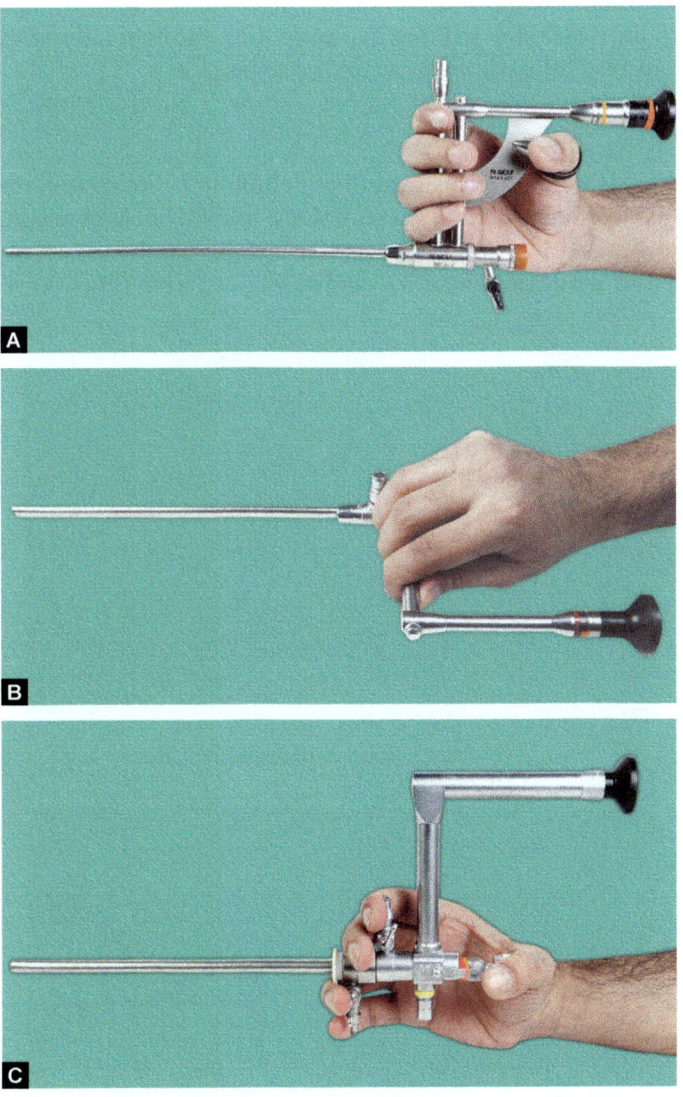

Figures 10A to C: Different grips of nephroscopes: (A) Wolf Dresden; (B) Wolf 24 Fr nephroscope; (C) Storz 24 Fr nephroscope.

outlet channel. The nephroscope with sheath can be used with Amplatz of size >24 Fr.

Nephroscopes by Storz[8] (Fig. 10C)

The angle of vision in all Storz nephroscope is 6°, regardless of size. The available sizes are 22, 24, and 26 Fr. The eyepiece can be either parallel or oblique to the axis of the nephroscope (length available: 19 cm or 24 cm or 25 cm). Unlike Wolf, these nephroscopes cannot be used without sheath, as they are not integrated, hence the water from the irrigating channel comes out at the proximal end and also accessories from the straight channel are not aligned with the distal end. In Storz nephroscopes, the light pillar is directed to the floor and the inlet channel toward the ceiling.

Miniperc

Although there is no consensus regarding definition for Miniperc, tract size <20 Fr is considered miniperc. Storz miniperc nephroscope is conceptualized by Naegle, whereas the Wolf is conceptualized by Lamhe. Storz miniperc is also called as modular miniature nephroscope system (**Figs. 11 and 12**)

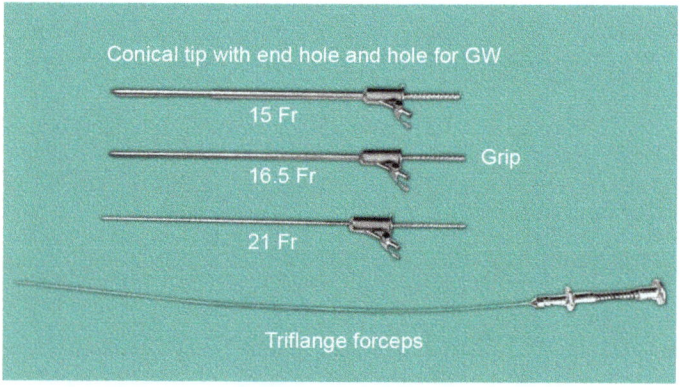

Figure 11: Storz miniperc sheath with dilator.

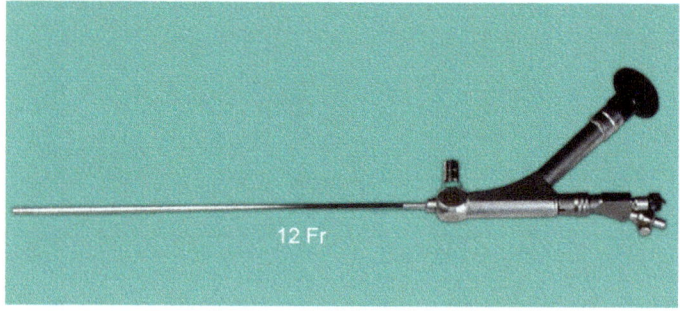

Figure 12: Storz miniperc dilator with Amplatz sheath.

CHAPTER 6: Percutaneous Nephrolithotomy Instruments | 59

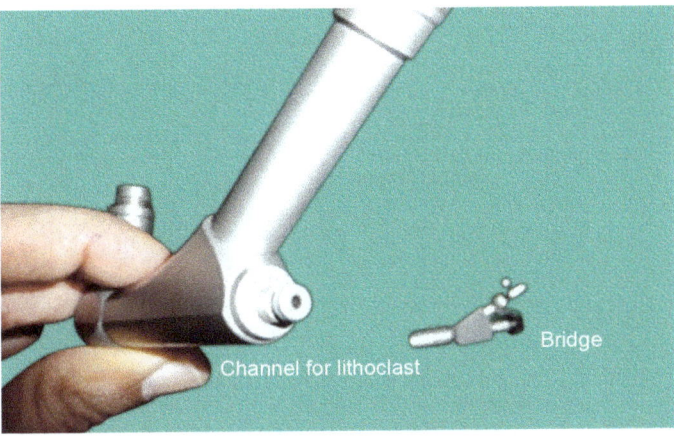

Figure 13: Storz nephroscope.

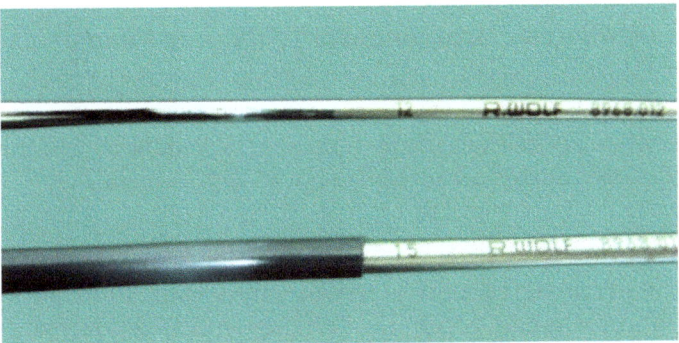

Figure 14: Wolf miniperc dilators and sheath.

with automatic pressure control. It is available in three sizes; 15/18 Fr and 16.5/19.5 Fr and 21/24 Fr sheaths are available (**Fig. 13**). This describes inner and outer circumference of the sheath. It comes with its own dilators with end hole accommodating the guidewire. Each sheath has its own dilator which has got end hole accommodating guidewire. The other component of the assembly includes telescope with 6.7 Fr working channel for instrument up to 5 Fr with 22 cm length. There is an irrigation channel on sheath as well as on the working channel. However, the telescope can be used with any appropriate size Amplatz sheath. Eyepiece is oblique.

Wolf miniperc nephroscopes are available in two sizes. Outer sheath size of 15 and 18 Fr (**Figs. 14 and 15**). It comes with its own dilators with end hole accommodating the glidewire. Nephroscope is common with 12-degree angle and 6 Fr working channel and 14 Fr in size. However, the telescope can be used with any appropriate size Amplatz sheath. Very useful for stones in renal pelvis and staghorn calculi, can be used in children and adults, made up of titanium and stainless steel to decrease the weight of instrument. It has offset eyepiece.[9]

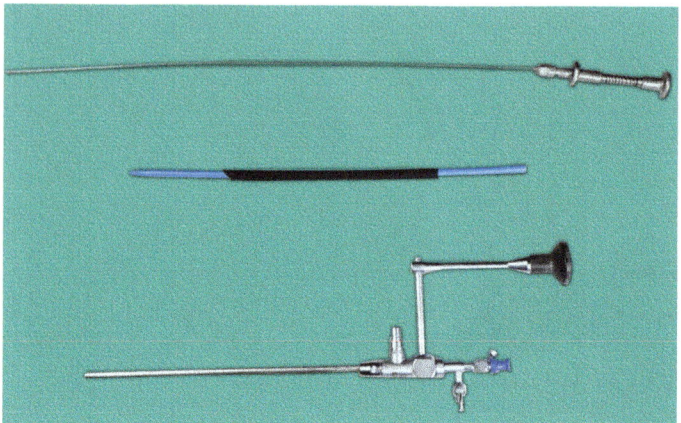

Figure 15: Wolf miniperc nephroscope.

Accessories of Miniperc (Storz and Wolf)[10] (Figs. 16A and B)

Two and five mm diameter forceps are available (alligator type or triflange type or mouse tooth type).

Because of small size of forceps these are very delicate and liable to damage very easily. Stones can also be removed with baskets.

Microperc[11]

The parts of microperc assembly include: Three-part all-seeing needle, consisting of micro-optics 0.9 mm in diameter with a 120-degree angle of view and resolution up to 10,000 pixels (**Fig. 17**). Needle, including the shaft, with outer diameter of 1.6 mm (4.85 Fr), slightly larger than the diameter of a standard 1.3-mm needle. The highly flexible fiberoptic telescope contains 10,000 fiberoptic bundles and can be bent over itself without causing damage (**Fig. 18**).

There is an outlet from the connector to an irrigation pump (**Fig. 19**).

ULTRAMINI PERCUTANEOUS NEPHROLITHOTOMY

It consists 3.5 Fr telescope which is mounted inside a 6 Fr sheath (LUT-GmbH, Germany). The inner telescope sheath has two side ports. One is used for irrigation and the other one for passing laser fiber. Telescope is connected to standard camera system. The outer sheath is 11–13 Fr sheath (**Figs. 20A to C**).

Minimally Invasive Percutaneous Nephrolithotomy XS/S

Karl Storz™ 7.5 Fr nephroscope, 2 Fr working channel, and 3 Fr irrigation channel. Uses fiberoptic system and is 24 cm in length. It has prefabricated dilator and sheath 8.5 Fr/9.5 Fr and 11/12 Fr (**Figs. 21A and B**).

CHAPTER 6: Percutaneous Nephrolithotomy Instruments | 61

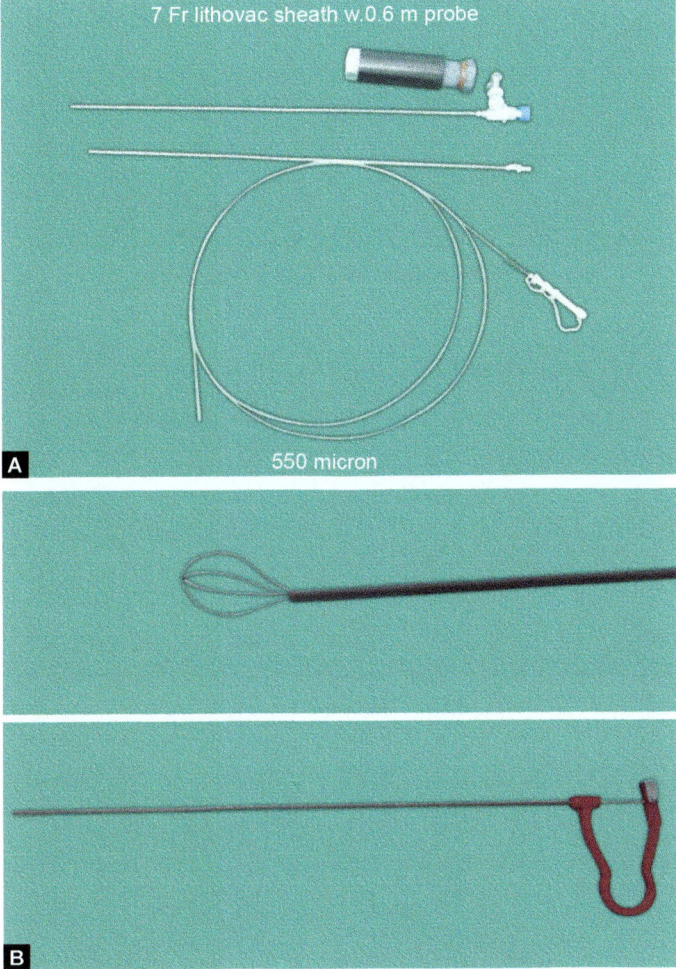

Figures 16A and B: Miniperc accessories.

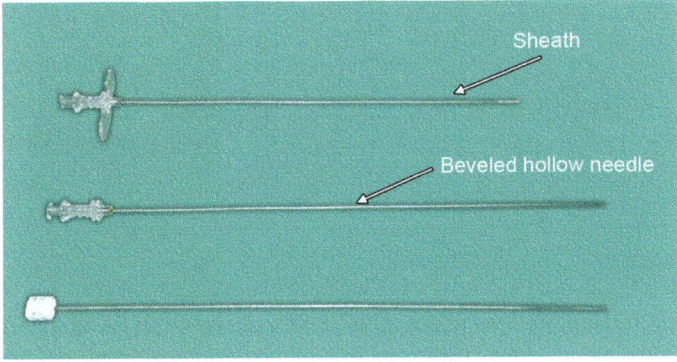

Figure 17: Three-part needle.

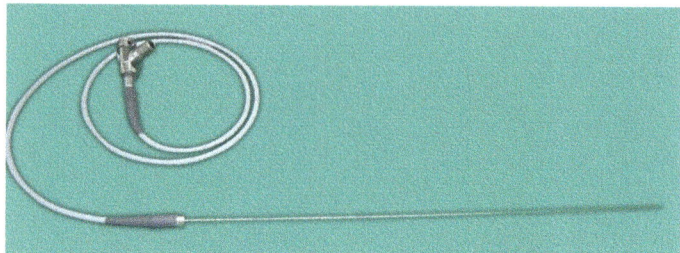

Figure 18: Fiberoptic telescope for microperc.

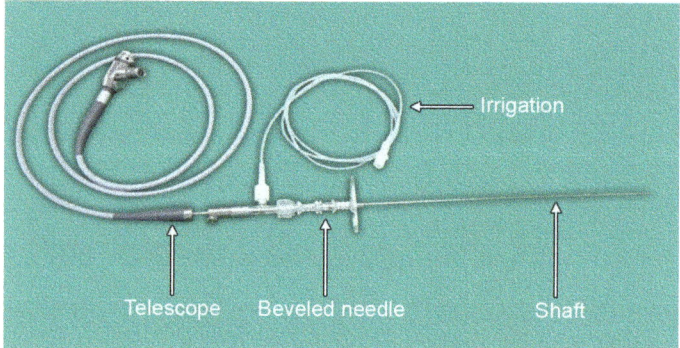

Figure 19: Microperc assembly.

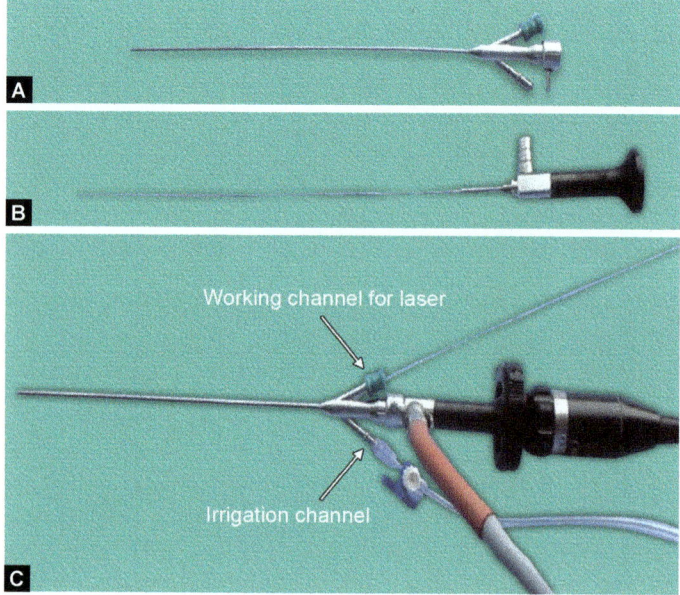

Figures 20A to C: Ultramini percutaneous nephrolithotomy (PCNL) assembly: (A) Inner sheath; (B) Telescope; (C) Inner sheath with telescope attached to camera light and irrigation.

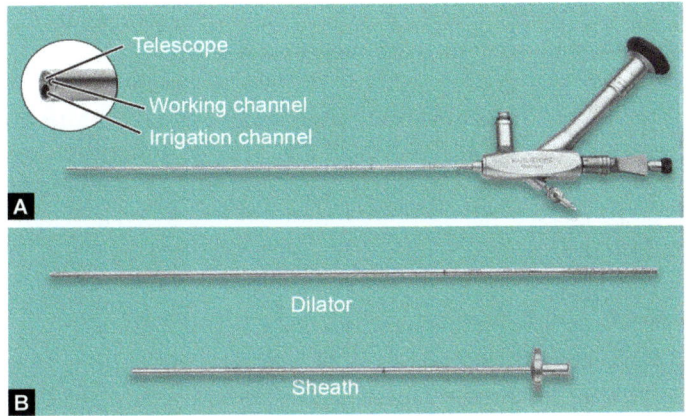

Figures 21A and B: Minimally invasive percutaneous nephrolithotomy (MIP) XS/S: (A) Telescope; (B) Sheath.

Miniaturized Percutaneous Nephrolithotomies

Since the introduction of miniperc, in year 2000, several newer instruments are designed and are being used. They have different sizes of sheaths and telescopes. Several names such as superminiperc, ultraminiperc, microperc, and microminiperc are confusing and do not give idea of what sheath size is being talked about. Uniformity of nomenclature is attempted by Shilling et al. by describing all scopes in uniform format.

XXL—size >30 F
XL—size 25–30 F
L—size 20–25 F
M—size 15–20 F—miniperc
S—size 10–15 F—ultraminiperc, superminiperc, minimally invasive percutaneous nephrolithotomy (MIP) S
XS—size 5–10 F—minimicroperc, MIP S
XXS - size <5 F—microperc

Storz adopted this system and all Storz nephroscopes now are described in above nomenclature.

Storz New Minimally Invasive Percutaneous Nephrolithotomy System

Storz new minimally invasive percutaneous nephrolithotomy system has different design than old. Irrigation channel on sheath is removed, outer end design is changed, and two lengths are available—longer sheath for supine PCNL and shorter length for prone. In supine PCNL, teract tend to be longer, hence longer sheath.

Sheath sizes are 15/16, 16.5/17.5, and 21/22 which represent inner and outer diameter. All sheaths come with their own dilators.

Storz has three nephroscopes: MIP L—19.5 F, which can be used in conventional PCNL, and has a working channel size of 12.5 F, MIP M—12 F, which has working channel of 6.7 F, MIP XS—it is 7.5 F nephroscope with two working separate channels in single space. 3 F and 2 F—benefit of two is that even if you pass laser—space of irrigation is not reduced and hence flow remains unaffected.

Superminiperc

This system is developed by Zeng et al. Sheath size varies from 10 to 14 F. Sheath has oblique channel—which is for suction attachment. Straight channel is used to pass instrument, laser, etc. This is a closed system—unlike miniperc where irrigation fluid comes by the side of nephroscope. In closed system, fluid comes out through oblique channel, and when suction is applied. Along with suction, fragments are supposed to get sucked out.

Ultraminiperc

Ultramini percutaneous (UMP)—this developed by Janak Desai et al. for LUT, Germany. The sheath size is 11 and 13 F. It has its own 3.5 F telescope. Stones come out with whirlpool effect. It is an open system.

Superperc (Figs. 22 to 24)

These sheaths are developed by Kaushik Shah et al. from India. Multiple sheaths are available with this technology i.e 10Fr, 12 Fr and 15 Fr. The sheath has been innovated by Shah et al. and the length of the sheath may vary from 8-20 cm. The key feature of this technology is that the master suction is attached to the sheath rather than the scope and this channels is at right angles to the sheath. The authors described used of a multi-hole ureteric catheter for retrograde irrigation while using this sheath. The ureteric catheter has holes at every 10 cm allowing a free retrograde flow of saline. Enabling a better irritant flow even with suction. The suction tubing is attached to the outlet of the superperc sheath. The suction is controlled using a suction port which is finger controlled, on occlusion of port with finger suction gets activated. It allows larger fragment size retrieval. A short ureteroscope can be used as nephroscope with this sheath for mini PCNL's as described by the author and other nephroscopes compatible with the size of the sheaths can also be used. Microperc telescope, micro nephroscope from Apple life sciences, UMP (ultra mini perc) telescope with inner sheath or Karl StorzTM nephroscope can be all used with 10 and 12 F sheath. Miniperc nephroscope from Karl StorzTM, Olympus TM or Richard Wolf TM can be used with 15 F sheath size.

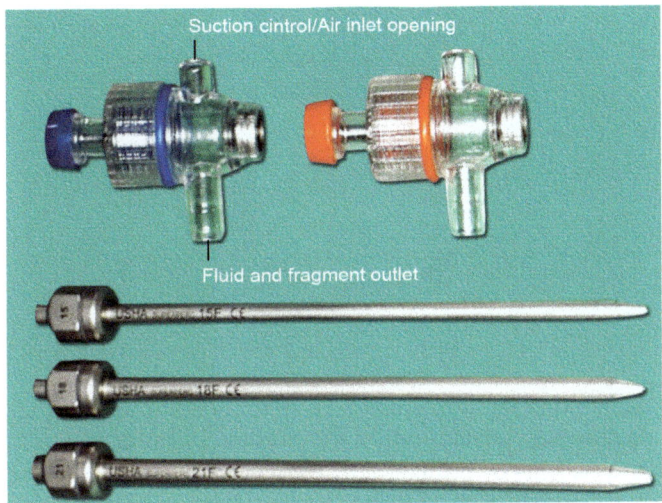

Figure 22: Shah Superperc sheaths (Autoclavable)

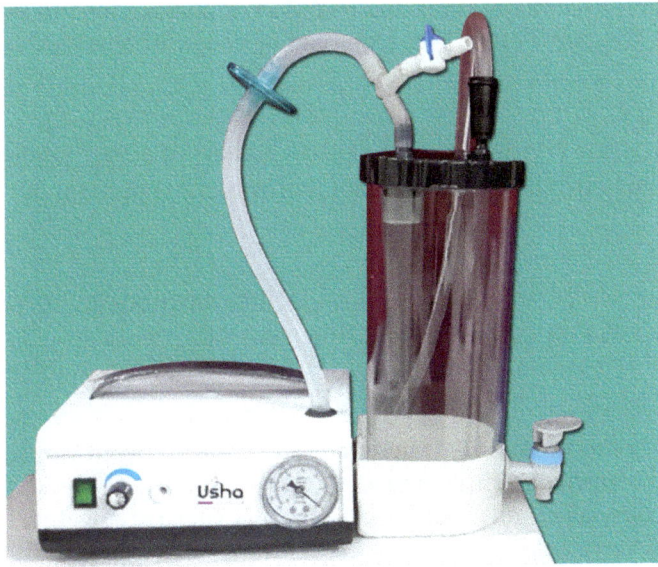

Figure 23: Low Power Suction with Drainage.

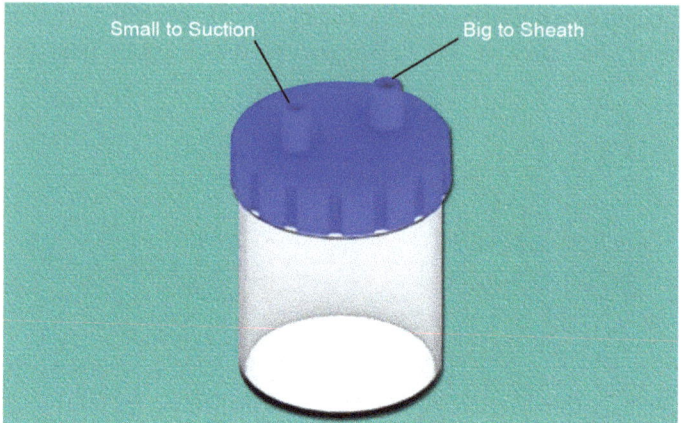

Figure 24: Stone Catcher.

Clear Petra Sheath

Clear Petra sheath was developed by the Welllead group. It is a 12, 14,16 and 18 fr sheath with its own dilator . The sheath has a large offset channel for suction to be attached. It can suction out fragments upto 3 mm. The transparent suction channel and the terminal sheath allows visualization of the fragments being sucked out as the scope is withdrawn. The suction channel is an offset channel making a smoother passage for the stone out once it is sucked. Any 12 fr or 14 fr scope can be used with this sheath.

MIP S/XS

MIP S sheath size is 11/12 and MIPXS sheath size is 8.5/9.5 and 5 nephroscope can be used in both. Since there is no suction, this is an open system.

Microperc

As described earlier, it is the smallest possible instrument. 16 G which accounts for 4.85 F. Telescope is 9 mm which is 2.7 F.

Mini-microperc

This system is modification of Microperc—where 8 F sheath is developed, which has its own dilator. Three-part adapter is attached to 8 F sheath through which telescope, laser, and irrigation can go. Since space of irrigation is less, it requires pressure irrigation.

ENERGY SOURCES

Under this section we will describe various energy sources used for stone disintegration apart from Lasers.

1. Swiss Lithoclast (Lithotripter)

This intracorporeal lithotripter was first introduced in 1990. The principle of lithoclast is based on the law of Newton's cradle, which demonstrates the transfer of energy between the projectile, probe and the stone. Compressed air is used to generate ballistic energy in the handpiece (**Fig. 25**). A projectile is accelerated to a high speed which is precision guided to less than one micrometer with the help of accurately controlled burst of compressed air. When the projectile hits the probe in the handpiece, a shock wave is transmitted through the probe to the calculus. The different acoustic characteristics of the metal probe and the stone leads to fragmentation of stones. The lithotripter can operate from frequency of 1 Hz to 12 Hz and release energy output of 85 mJ.

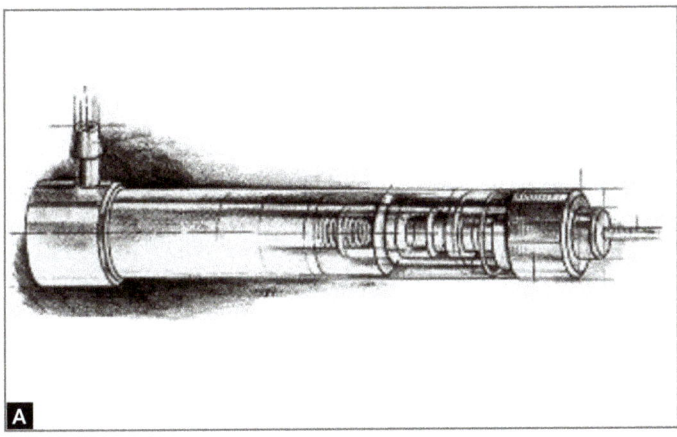

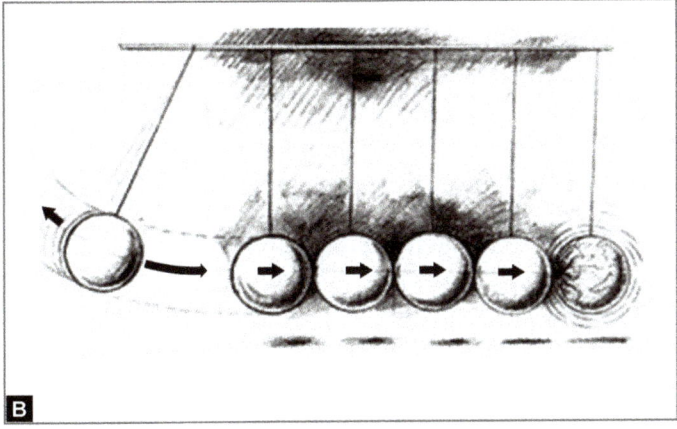

Figures 25A and B: Mechanism of action of lithoclast.

Advantages
- No heat generation
- Low risk of damage to mucosal surface
- Low cost
- Low maintenance

Disadvantages
- Large fragments
- Fly back effect of stones
- Bending of probe can lead to loss of effective fragmentation of stones.

Lithoclast with Suction (Lithovac) (Fig. 26)

After the development of pneumatic ballistic lithoclast, improvements in design led to lithoclast added with suction. Small (<2 mm) fragments can be removed easily during lithotripsy. Fragments upto 3.5 mm can be evacuated with the Lithovac after removing the Lithoclast probe. Using the suction, clear vision can be achieved and push back of stones can be avoided.

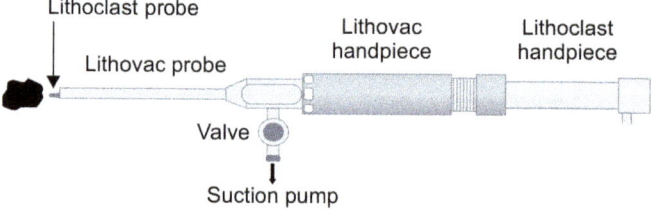

Figure 26: Lithoclast with suction.

2. Swiss Lithoclast Master (Fig. 27)

The Swiss Lithoclast Master integrates three basic intracorporeal lithotripsy tools and methods into one single device.
- Pneumatic effect for fast coarse fragmentation
- Ultrasonic lithotripsy for fine fragmentation and pulverization
- Controlled suction for complete evacuation of stone fragments

Concurrent use of both technologies has superior efficacy

The energy output of the Ballistic component is approximately 85 mJ while that of ultrasonic component is 78 W. The Ballistic component operates from 1 to 12 Hz and ultrasonic component operates on a continuous mode (**Fig. 28**).

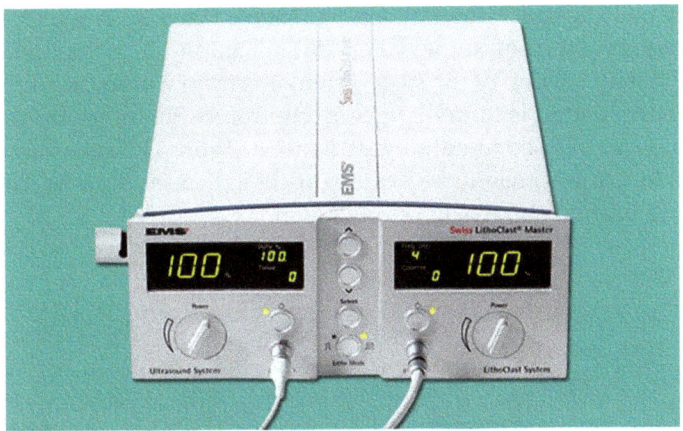

Figure 27: Lithoclast Master.

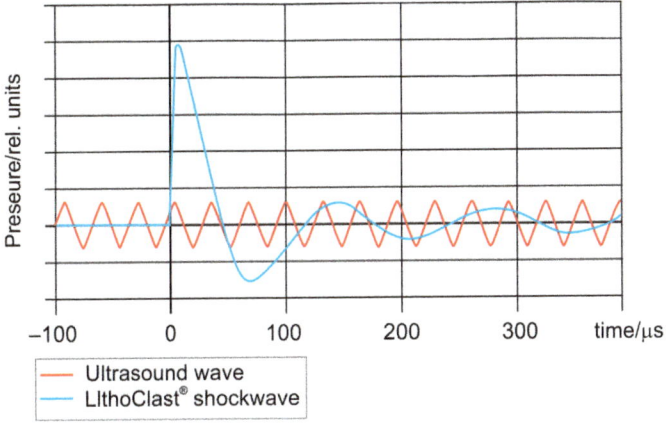

Figure 28: Shockwaves of Swiss Lithoclast Master.

It has clinically proven four times faster than standard lithoclast and more than twice as fast compared to standard ultrasound lithotripters
The suction component also prevents stone fragment blockage in the ultrasound handpiece and probes

3. ShockPulse-SE™ Lithotripter (Fig. 29)

It is a dual action lithotripsy system developed by Olympus™. In this system, there is a constant emission ultrasonic wave energy and intermittently there are bursts of ballistic shockwaves at 300 Hz (**Tables 1 and 2**). This high energy leads to fragmentation of stones (**Fig. 30**). In addition to fragmentation there is a constant suction of the stone fragliments from within the probe. The pressure of the suction is under surgeons control. Different probe sizes are available and can be used in different situations (**Table 1**). Probes are of two types it can be either single use or can be used in 5 cases. Can be sterilized with heat sterilization and plasma sterilization.

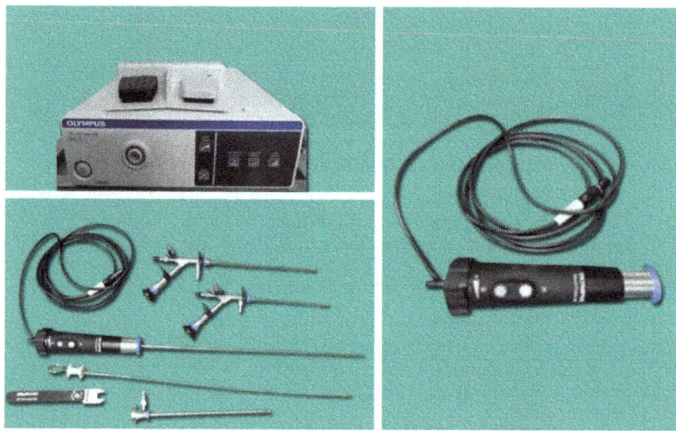

Figure 29: ShockPulse Lithotripter.

TABLE 1: Showing all the probe sizes.

Color	Size	Use
Silver	3.76 mm	PCNL, Bladder Stone
Blue	3.40 mm	PCNL, Bladder Stone
Red	1.83 mm	Mini PCNL
Green	1.50 mm	Semi-rigid URS
Gold	0.97 mm	Semi-rigid URS

TABLE 2: Difference between ShockPulse and Lithoclast Master

ShockPulse	Lithoclast Master
Ballistic Mechanical: 300 Hz	Pnuematic ballistic 12 Hz
Single probe: larger suction channel	Dual probe design
Single generator: fast setup	Dual generato
• USG- 21,000 Hz • Ballistic -300 Hz	• Outter : 21,000 Hz • Inner- 11 Hz

CHAPTER 6: Percutaneous Nephrolithotomy Instruments | 71

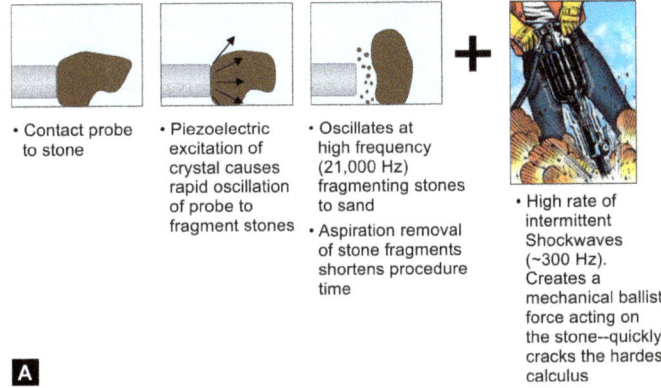

Figure 30A: Mechanism of action of ShockPulse Lithotripter.

ShockPulse-SE Technology

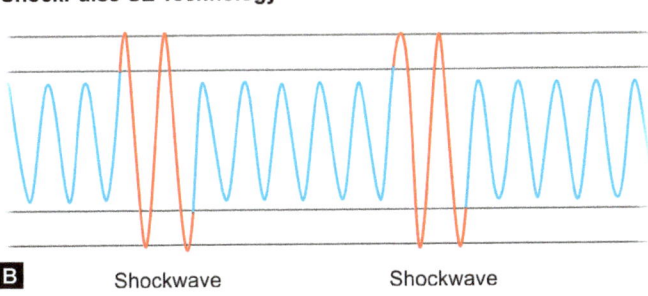

Figure 30B: Shockwaves of ShockPulse.

4. Trilogy by EMS™ (Fig. 31)

It is similar device developed by EMS™. This device consists of a hollow single probe which delivers a constant ultrasonic energy for fine fragmentation of stones. This is boosted by strong ballistic impacts delivered by an

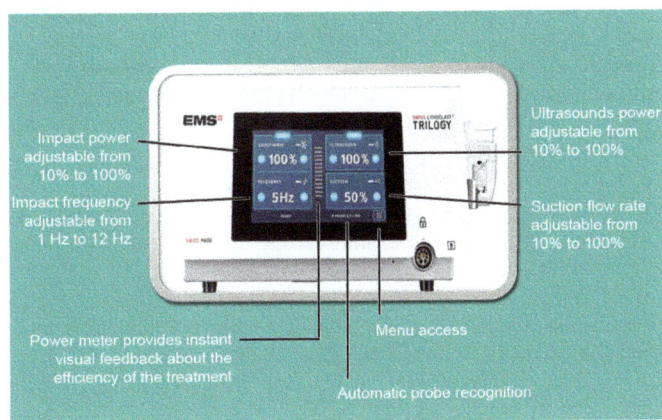

Figure 31: Trilogy by EMS.

electromagnetic generator. There is a constant suction of all the fragments through the hollow probe. Probes are available for standard and mini PCNL functionality. Impact, ultrasound power and suction flow is adjustable from 10% to 100%. Frequency is adjustable from 1 to 12 Hz. The handle is gun shaped may be more ergonomic.

REFERENCES

1. Cookmedical.com. Cook Urology, 2010—Domestic Product Catalogue (pp. 124). Available from: https://www.cookmedical.com/urology/. [Last Accessed February, 2021].
2. Cookmedical.com. Cook Urology, 2010—Domestic Product Catalogue (pp. 50). Available from: https://www.cookmedical.com/urology/. [Last Accessed February, 2021].
3. Devon Innovations. Dilators Sets. [online] Available from: http://www.devoncath.com/Urology_dilatorssets.html. [Last Accessed February, 2021].
4. Boston Scientific. Urology. Available from: https://www.bostonscientific.com/en-EU/medical-specialties/urology.html. [Last Accessed February, 2021].
5. Richard-Wolf.com. Richard Wolf Catalogue (pp. D740.305). [online] Available from: https://www.richard-wolf.com/en/disciplines/urology/. [Last Accessed February, 2021].
6. Richard-Wolf.com. Richard Wolf Catalogue (pp. D740.303). [online] Available from: https://www.richard-wolf.com/en/disciplines/urology/. [Last Accessed February, 2021].
7. GYRUS ACMI Medical Systems. Percutaneous Nephroscopes. [online] Available from: http://www.gyrusacmi.com/user/display.cfm?display=product&pid=9849&catid=76&maincat = Video&catname = Percutaneous% 20Nephroscopes. [Last Accessed February, 2021].
8. karlstorz.com. Karl-Storz Urology product catalogue (pp. 150/151). [online] Available from: https://www.karlstorz.com/in/en/online-catalog.htm. [Last Accessed February, 2021].
9. Richard-Wolf.com. Richard Wolf Catalogue (pp. D740.501). [online] Available from: https://www.richard-wolf.com/en/disciplines/urology/. [Last Accessed February, 2021].
10. Richard-Wolf.com. Richard Wolf Catalogue (pp. D780.901). https://www.richard-wolf.com/en/disciplines/urology/. [Last Accessed February, 2021]. [Last Accessed February, 2021].
11. Desai MR, Sharma R, Mishra S, Sabnis RB, Stief C, Bader M. Single-step percutaneous nephrolithotomy Microperc: the initial clinical report. J Urol. 2011;186(1):140-5.

FURTHER READING

1. Agarwal M, Agrawal MS, Jaiiswal A, Kumar D, Yadav H, Lavania P. Safety and efficacy of ultrasonography as an adjunct to fluoroscopy for renal access in percutaneous nephrolithotomy (PCNL). BJU Int. 2011;108(8):1346-9.
2. Aminsharifi A, Alavi, M, Sadeghi G, Shakeri S, Afsar F. Renal parenchymal damage after percutaneous nephrolithotomy with one-stage tract dilation technique: a randomized clinical trial. J Endourol 25(6);2011:927-31.

3. Castaneda WR, Espenan GD. Chapter 3: How to protect yourself and others from radiation In: Smith AD, Badlani G, Bagley D (Eds). Smiths Textbook of Endourology, 1st edition, Section 1. St Louis: Quality Medical. 1996. pp. 21-8.
4. Cook medical systems. [online] Available from: http://www.cookmedical.com/uro/familyListingAction.do?family=Wire+Guides). [Last accessed February 2021].
5. Cook medical. [online] Available from: http://www.cookmedical.com/uro/dataSheet.do?id=1940. [Last accessed February 2021].
6. Cook medical/ catalog page: [online] Available from: http://www.cookmedical.com/uro/dataSheet.do?id=1941. [Last accessed February 2021].
7. Desai M. Ultrasonography guided punctures with and without puncture guide. J Endourol. 2009;23(10):1641-3.
8. Desai MR, Jasani A. Percutaneous nephrolithotripsy in ectopic kidneys. J Endourol. 2000;14(3):289-92.
9. Desai MR, Sharma R, Mishra S, Sabnis RB, Stief C, Bader M. Single step percutaneous nephrolithotomy (Microperc): the initial clinical report. J Urol. 2011;186(1):140-5.
10. Desai MR, Sharma R, Mishra S, Sabnis RB, Stief C, Bader M. Single-step percutaneous nephrolithotomy (Microperc): the initial clinical report. J Urol. 2011;186(1):140-5.
11. Falahatkar S, Neiroomand H, Akbarpour M, Emadi SA, Khaki N. One-shot versus metal telescopic dilation technique for tract creation in percutaneous nephrolithotomy: comparison of safety and efficacy. J Endourol. 2009;23(4):615-8.
12. Grasso M, Lang G, Taylor FC. Flexible ureteroscopically assisted percutaneous renal access. Tech Urol. 1995;1(1):39-43.
13. GYRUS ACMI Medical Systems. Nephroscopes [online] Available from: http://www.gyrusacmi.com/acmi/user/display.cfm?display=product&pid=9849&catid=76&maincat=Urology&catname=Percuta neous%20Nephroscopes. [Last accessed February 2021].
14. Kahn F, Borin JF, Pearle MS, McDougall EM, Clayman RV. Endoscopically guided percutaneous renal access: "Seeing is believing". J Endourol. 2006;20(7):451-5.
15. Karami H, Rezaei A, Mohamaddahosseni M, Javanmard B, Mazloomfard M, Lotfi B. Ultrasonography guided percutaneous nephrolithotomy in the flank position versus fluoroscopy guided percutaneous nephrolithotomy in the prone position: A comparative study. J Endourol. 2010;24(8):1357-61.
16. Mishra S, Sabnis RB, Desai M. Staghorn morphometry: a new tool for clinical classification and prediction model for percutaneous nephrolithotomy monotherapy. J Endourol. 2012;26(1):6-14.
17. Olcott EW, Sommer FG, Nape S. Accuracy of detection and measurement of renal calculi: In vitro comparison of three dimensional spiral CT, radiography and nephrotomography. Radiology. 1997;204(1):19-25.
18. Rassweiler J. I-pad assisted percutaneous access to the kidney using marker based navigation: Initial clinical experience. Eur Urol. 2012;61(3):627-31.
19. Richard wolf medical systems. Urology [online] Available from: www.richard-wolf.com/en/human-medicine/urology.html. [Last accessed February 2021].
20. Sountoulides PG, Kaufmann OG, Louie MK, Beck S, Jain N, Kaplan A, et al. Endoscopy guided percutaneous nephrostolithotomy: Benefits of ureteroscopic access and therapy. J Endourol. 2009;23(10):1649-54.
21. Surgimedik medical systems [online] Available from: http://www.surgimedik.com/ProductDetails.aspx?PID=86&CID=yYut//BrHa8=). [Last accessed February 2021].
22. Xu Y, Wu Z, Yu J, Wang S, Li F, Chen J, et al. Doppler ultrasound guided percutaneous nephrolithotomy with two step tract dilatation for management of complex renal stones. Urology. 2012;79(6):1247-51.

CHAPTER 7

Semirigid Ureteroscopy

INTRODUCTION

Hugh Hampton Young visualized upper urinary tract using a 9.5 Fr cystoscope in a male child with megaureter in 1912.[1] In 1979, Lyon et al. used the first dedicated ureteroscope that was made by Richard Wolf Medical Instruments.[2] The original ureteroscopes used rod-lens system for image transmission. These instruments were larger in size and caused "half-moon" effect while reaching the upper ureter. The later generations of ureteroscopes used flexible fiberoptic bundles for both image (coherent) and light transmission (noncoherent). These ureteroscopes were smaller in caliber and did not distort the image even while bending. These ureteroscopes were called semirigid or mini-ureteroscopes. Dretler and Cho described the first semirigid ureteroscope or "mini-scope" in 1989.[3]

EVOLUTION OF URETEROSCOPES

Goodman first reported rigid ureteroscopy in 1977 using a pediatric cystoscope.[4] The first endoscope specifically for ureteroscopy was designed by Richard Wolf Medical Instruments in 1979.[2] This instrument was 23 cm long and had 13 Fr sheath for inspection and 14.5/16 Fr sheath to allow insertion of instruments for stone removal. In 1980, Enrique Pérez Castro in collaboration with Karl Storz Endoscopy, developed a 39 cm ureteroscope which could reach renal pelvis.[5] Most of the initial ureteroscopes had interchangeable 0° and 70° telescopes. With the development of 8 Fr ultrasonic probes, these probes were used blindly to fragment stones after an initial inspection using ureteroscope. In order to allow small rigid probes through a straight channel in ureteroscope, telescopes with offset eyepiece were developed. The first ureteroscope with fiberoptic imaging system was introduced by ACMI in 1985.[5] Once the rod-lens imaging system was replaced with fiberoptic, the half-moon effect was eliminated. Later on, compact ureteroscopes, which integrated rod-lens telescope into the ureteroscope to reduce the outer diameter without compromising the size of working channel, were developed. Initially pneumatic and subsequently laser came into the picture. Once laser was developed, the need for a large working channel decreased and dual channel ureteroscopes with separate channels for flow and accessories were developed. Recent ureteroscopes have a high density of coherent fiberoptic bundles to improve vision and smaller outer diameter. All modern ureteroscopes are semirigid and have optical fibers. Old rigid ureteroscopes had rod lens system which is now obsolete. This is the reason why ureteroscopes are called semirigid.

CLASSIFICATION (TABLE 1)

All semirigid ureteroscopes have size described as two digits, e.g., 7/8.5 which means the tip is 7 Fr and shaft is 8.5 Fr. Every scope is small in size at tip and increases in size proximally. Each make has a different way of transition of this size from tip to base. Common size of a ureteroscopes are 6/7.5, 7/8.5, 8/9, 8, etc. Length of URS can be short or long. Short are generally 35 cm and used for females, whereas long are generally 45 cm and are used for males.

Semirigid ureteroscopes can be classified based on size, make, and channel.
- According to make (Storz, Wolf, Olympus, Scholly)
- According to size—4.5/6 Fr, 6/7.5 Fr, etc.

TABLE 1: Semi-rigid ureteroscopes.

Manufacturer	Eyepiece	Shaft diameter (Fr)	Working channel (Fr)
Features of different semirigid ureteroscope			
Karl Storz (All stepwise sheath)	Angled	6.5–9.9	4.8
		7.0–12.0	5.0
		8.0–12.0	5.0
		9.0–12.0	3.0 and 3.0
	Straight	7.0–9.9	3.4
		7.0–13.5	5.0
		8.0–13.5	6.0
Richard Wolf (All stepless sheath)	Straight	6.0–7.5	4.0
		8.0–9.8	5.0
		6.5–8.5	4.2 and 2.55
	Oblique	6.0–7.5	4.0
		8.0–9.8	5.0
		8.5–11.5	6.0
	Lateral	4.5–6.5	3.0
		6.0–7.5	4.0
		8.0–9.8	5.0
		6.5–8.5	4.2 and 2.55

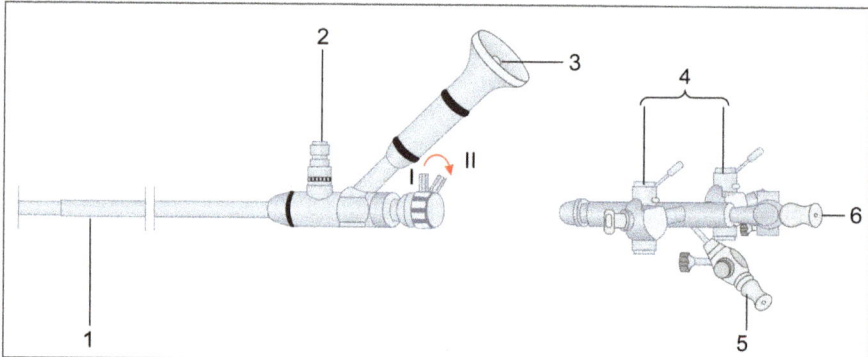

Figure 1: Parts of semirigid ureteroscope. (1) Shaft; (2) Light pillar; (3) Eyepiece; (4) Inlet + outlet top; (5 and 6) Working channel.

- According to eye piece—straight eyepiece (almost obsolete) and angulated eyepiece-—has a straight channel as well as an oblique channel.
  Straight channel: Allows use of rigid pneumatic lithotripsy probes.

Parts (Fig. 1)

- *Eyepiece*: Straight, oblique or lateral offset
- *Body*: It has a light post and working channels
- *Working channels*: Ureteroscopes have either a single larger channel or two separate channels. Dual channel also allows the simultaneous use of laser fiber and a basket.
- *Sheath*: 7/8.5 There are different measurement schema used by different companies. For instance 7/8.5 Fr ureteroscope by wolf means, the shaft is 8.5 Fr and the tip is 7 Fr. While in a Storz ureteroscope it means that the diameter of the shaft is 8.5 Fr and diameter of the ureterscope at the point where working channel ends is 7 Fr (**Figures 2A and B**).
- Currently, Wolf has three varieties of ureteroscope—needle (4.5/6 Fr), ultrathin (6/7.5 Fr), and dual-channel (6.5/8.5 Fr).
- *Tip design*: General principles of tip of the instruments:
  - *Angulated tip*: This helps to negotiate stricture and any meatus in atraumatic manner, e.g., cystoscopes and ureteroscopes. The angulated end is engaged initially and then the instrument is lifted up.

Majority of the semirigid ureteroscopes are available in 34 and 43 cm length, while some scopes of Wolf Company are available in 31.5 cm length.

KARL STORZ 7/9.9 FR SEMIRIGID URETEROSCOPE

It is available in two lengths—34 and 43 cm. The distal end is angulated, rounded tip for smooth insertion into ureteric orifice. The telescope is of fiberoptic system with a 6° angle of view at the tip. The tip measures 6.5 Fr without the working channel. The instrument sheath is 7 Fr in size for the distal 6 cm length, with an unobtrusive step to 9.9 Fr toward the proximal

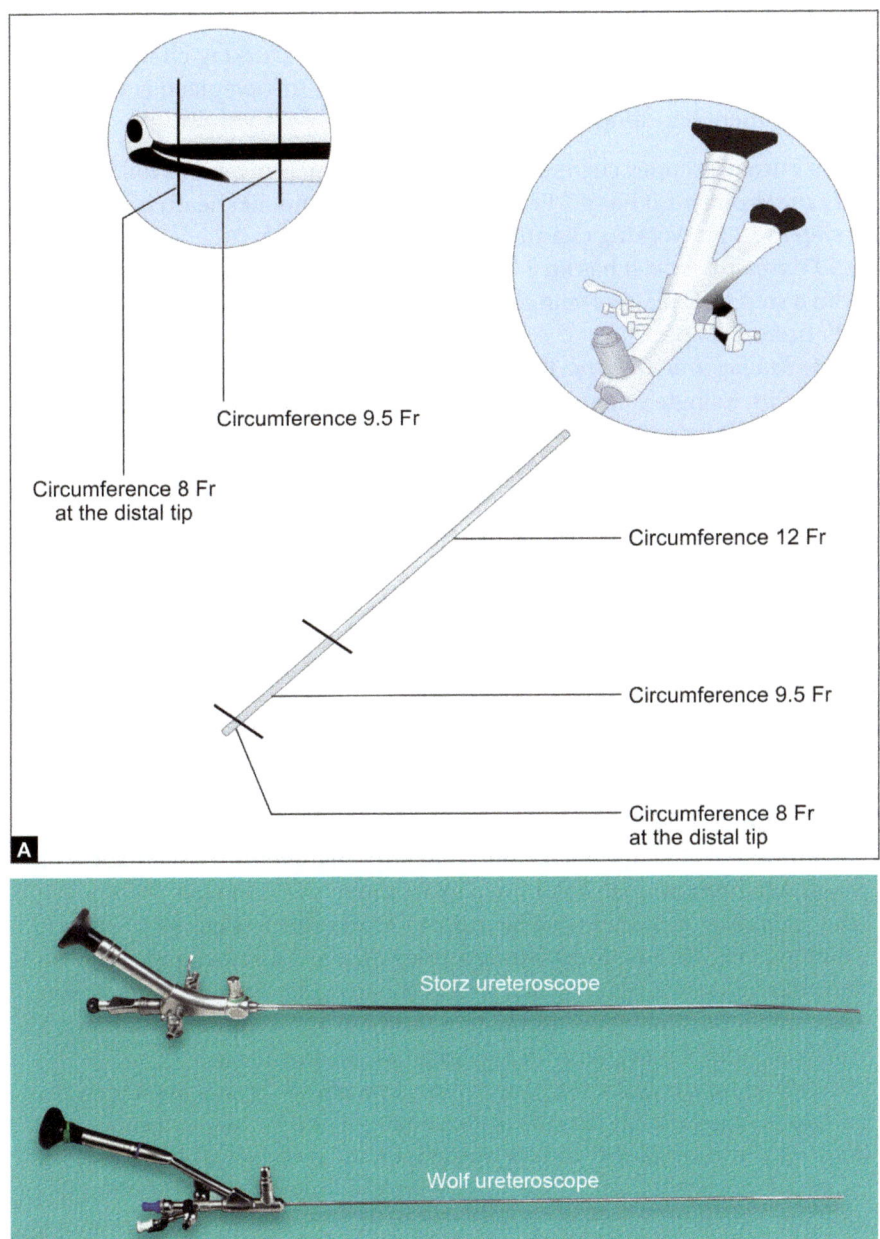

Figures 2A and B: Specifications of Karl Storz endoscopes.

part. The sheath is conical in shape for strength and durability. The light post is just proximal to the proximal end of the sheath. There are two irrigation ports which open into the large working channel for maximum flow.

They are at right angles to the instrument to avoid cluttering of tubings and instruments. The irrigation port has an optional flow control stop cock for precise control of irrigation. The instrument ports are variable with quick release coupling and self-closing sealing system. The working channel is 4.8 Fr in size and allows rigid instruments up to 4 Fr. The eyepiece is offset to make instrument handling easier (**Fig. 2**).

The other ureteroscopes currently available with Karl Storz are as follows:
- *8 Fr ureteroscope*: It has a 7 Fr distal tip. The instrument sheath is 8 Fr with a step to 12 Fr. Working channel is 5 Fr.
- *9.5 Fr ureteroscope*: It has an 8 Fr distal tip. The instrument sheath is 9.5 Fr with a step to 12 Fr. Working channel is 6 Fr. Otherwise, it is similar to the 7 Fr ureteroscope.
- *9.5 Fr Michel ureteroscope*: It has a 9 Fr distal tip. The instrument sheath is 9.5 Fr with a single step to 12 Fr. It has a large central working channel with right-angled irrigation port and an additional separate 2.3 Fr irrigation port on the underside. The working channel allows simultaneous use of 2 and 3 Fr instruments or a single 6 Fr instrument.
- *7 Fr "Laserscope"*: 8.4–9.9 Fr conical sheath with a 7 Fr tip diameter. It has a 2.4 Fr irrigation channel on the left side. The 3.4 Fr working channel allows instruments up to 3 Fr. The eyepiece is straight. It is especially suitable for laser ureterolithotripsy (**Fig. 3A**). This is slowly becoming obsolete.

RICHARD WOLF URETEROSCOPES

- *6/7.5 Fr compact operating fiberureterorenoscope*: This ureteroscope has a distal sheath tip of 6 Fr with atraumatic head shape and 5° angle of view and size increases to 7.5 Fr proximally. The sheath is stepless. There is a common oval-shaped irrigation and working channel which allows a single instrument up to 4 Fr or two instruments of 2.4 Fr size.
  The eyepiece is either angled offset (Marberger) (**Fig. 3B**), oblique (Bichler) (**Fig. 3C**), or direct (straight) view. There is an automatic valve for introducing instruments which avoids the need for opening and closing instrument port and leak of irrigation fluid during instrument exchanges. This instrument is available in two lengths—34 and 43 cm.
- *8/9.8 Fr compact operating fiber ureterorenoscope*: This is similar to the previous scope except that the distal sheath tip is 8 Fr; angle of view is 12° and with oval irrigation and instrument channel allows one 5 Fr or 2 × 3 Fr auxiliary instruments. The eyepiece is either angled offset (Marberger), oblique (Bichler), or direct straight view. It is available with a working length of 43 cm.
- *8.5/11.5 Fr Marberger compact operating fiber ureterorenoscope*: In this instrument, the distal sheath tip is 8.5 Fr, angle of view is 12°, and with oval irrigation and instrument channel allows one 6 Fr or 2 × 4 Fr auxiliary instruments. This ureteroscope is available only with angled offset eye piece.
- *6.5/8.5 Fr dual-operating channel (DOC) ureteroscope*: This instrument is available with a straight or oblique (Bichler) eyepiece and with 34 or 43 cm length. Its channel allows one 4 Fr or 2 × 2.4 Fr instruments.

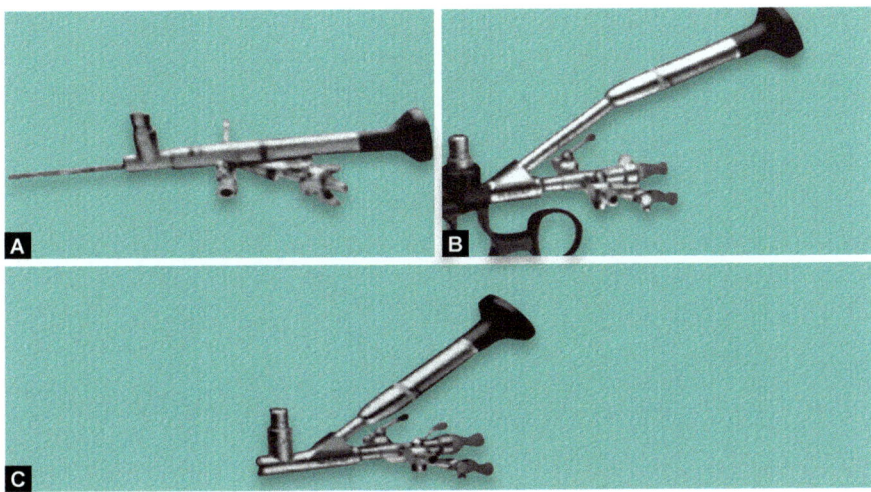

Figures 3A to C: Types of eyepieces. (A) Direct view eyepiece (Straight); (B) Marberger type eyepiece (Angled offset); (C) Bichler type eyepiece (Oblique).

- *4.5/6.5 ultrathin ureteroscope:* This ureteroscope has a tip design which is similar to other Wolf ureteroscopes. The tip is 4.5 Fr and shaft is 6 Fr. The viewing angle is 5° and insert capacity is 3 Fr. It is available with oblique or angled offset eyepiece and 34/43 cm length.

OLYMPUS URETEROSCOPES

The tip is atraumatic and sheath is stepless. The direction of view is 7°. The available sizes are 6.4/7.8 Fr shaft with 4.2 Fr channel and 8.6/9.8 Fr shaft with 6.4 Fr channel. These ureteroscopes are available with angles or straight eyepieces. The available lengths are 33 and 43 cm.

ACCESSORIES

These will be described in accessories chapter (cup biopsy forceps, spring forceps, alligator forceps, brush biopsy basket, bugbee, etc.).

INSTRUMENTS USED IN RETROGRADE ENDOPYELOTOMY

Retrograde endopyelotomy can be performed using ureteral resectoscope, acucise device with holmium laser. Among these, holmium laser endopyelotomy is the most commonly used nowadays.

Ureteroresectoscope

The overall arrangement is similar to a routine resectoscope. This instrument can be used to incise strictures, resect ureteral tumors, or perform

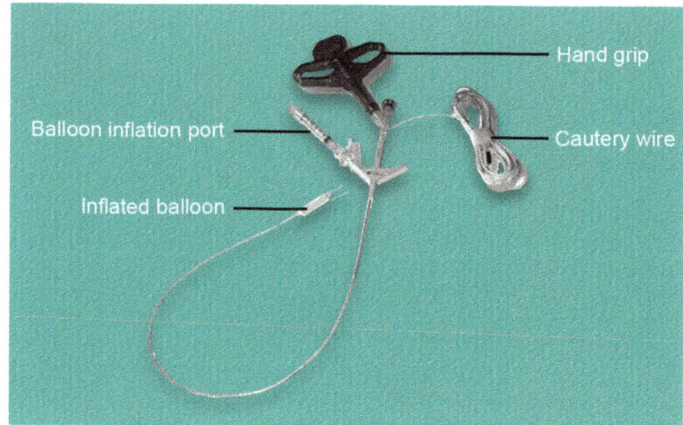

Figure 4: Acucise endopyelotomy.

endopyelotomies or ureteral meatotomies. It has an 11.5 Fr sheath with irrigation channels, working element with attachments for cold knife or insulated electrocautery knife and a telescope. It was available in 27 and 43 cm working lengths. These instruments are not in use now and are no longer available.

Acucise Endopyelotomy (Fig. 4)

Acucise device has a diameter of 6 Fr and length of 78 cm. The balloon is 10/24 Fr and cutting wire is 150 µm diameter and 3 cm in length. There is a side port for instillation of contrast. A radiofrequency cable is attached to the underside of the catheter. The balloon has radiopaque markers to properly align the balloon across pelviureteric junction after contrast study. The wire is placed posterolaterally and pure cutting current activated at 75 watts for incision and balloon left inflated for 2 minutes. Then, an endopyelotomy stent is placed over guidewire. A tamponade catheter of 7 Fr in size and 78 cm long with a balloon of 13/30 Fr size and 4 cm length is supplied along with the device for tamponading bleeding.

REFERENCES

1. Young HH, McKay RW. Congenital valvular obstruction of the prostatic urethra. Surg Gynecol Obstet. 1929;48:509-35.
2. Lyon ES, Banno JJ, Schoenberg HW. Transurethral ureteroscopy in men using juvenile cystoscopy equipment. J Urol. 1979;122(2):152-3.
3. Dretler SP, Cho G. Semirigid ureteroscopy: a new genre. J Urol. 1989;141(6):1314-6.
4. Goodman TM. Ureteroscopy with paediatric cystoscope in adults. Urology. 1977;9(4):394.
5. Pérez-Castro Ellendt E, Martinez-Piñeiro JA. Transurethral ureteroscopy. A current urological procedure. Arch Esp Urol. 1980;33(5):445-60.

CHAPTER 8

Flexible Ureteroscope

EVOLUTION OF FLEXIBLE URETEROSCOPES

The use of a fURS (9 Fr) was first reported by Marshall in 1964.[1] In 1970s, a cystoscopically placed guide tube into the ureter (access sheath) was developed to allow flow of irrigation fluid around the instrument to improve visibility. In the 1980s, irrigation channel and a working channel were combined and incorporated into the next generation of ureteroscopes along with an active deflection mechanism. ACMI DUR-8 ureteroscope had an upward deflection angle of 175° and downward deflection angle of 185°. With this angle of deflection, it was difficult to enter lower pole calyces that were highly angulated. Then, ACMI DUR-8 elite was introduced with a secondary active deflection of 130° controlled by a second lever. Then, newer ureteroscopes with better primary angle of defection (e.g., Flex-X2) were developed. The most recent development is the availability of digital ureteroscopes with clear, magnified image and better depth perception (e.g., Flex-Xc).

TYPES OF FLEXIBLE URETEROSCOPES

- *Conventional*: It is a fiberoptic flexible ureteroscope (fURS). The light is carried to the tip by a set of noncoherent fiberoptic bundles and image is carried back by a set of coherent fiberoptic bundles.
- *Digital*: The newer generation of fURSs has replaced the image-carrying fiberoptic bundles with a camera sensor at the tip of the instrument. The image is thus carried as electronic signals. In these ureteroscopes, the camera is placed at the tip of the ureteroscope and the image is carried as electrical (digital) signal to the processing unit. Thus, the coherent fiberoptic bundle is replaced by electric fibers. It is also called chip-at-the-tip technology (**Figs. 1A to C**).

On basis of use:
1. Reusable eg P6, V[2]
2. Single use : Pusen, Lithovue
3. Limited Use: Indovasive

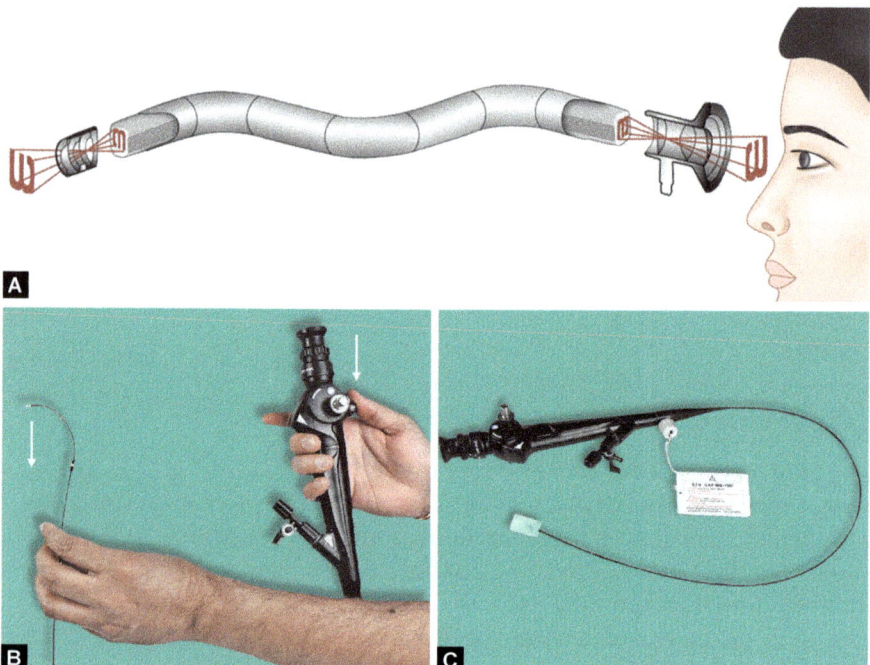

Figures 1A to C: (A) Schematic representation of flexible ureteroscopes; (B) Logic type flexible ureteroscope; and (C) Flexible ureteroscope.

BASIC DESIGN OF A FLEXIBLE FIBEROPTIC URETEROSCOPE

Flexible ureteroscope consists of an elongated plastic-coated endoscope sheath containing optical components such as the objective lens and the image guide as well as the light-transmitting glass fibers. It also has one or two channels for insertion of instruments and irrigation of fluid.

OPTICAL SYSTEM

It is comprised of three different parts:
1. Objective lens
2. Image guide, a precisely arranged glass fiber bundle for transmitting the image
3. Ocular lens

PARTS OF A CONVENTIONAL FIBEROPTIC FLEXIBLE URETEROSCOPE

- *Eye piece (ocular lens) and focusing component*: The eyepiece magnifies the virtual image and makes the image visible for the viewer. It allows for image focus adjustment.

- *Hand piece*: Hand piece has the following components:
  - *Deflecting lever*: Based on the direction of deflection of the tip of ureteroscope with respect to the direction of movement of deflecting lever, the deflection mechanism has been classified into two types.

    In logic (intuitive, positive, or American) type, direction of deflection of tip corresponds to that of the lever, i.e., down is down and up is up. In antilogic (counterintuitive, contrapositive, or European) type, direction of deflection of tip is opposite to that of the lever. In India, logic type is more popular.
  - *Working channel*: Working channel is used to insert graspers, baskets, wires, and laser fibers. The inner diameter of working channel is 3.6 Fr. This allows the use of instruments of size up to 3 Fr with concurrent irrigation. Irrigation port is connected to the working channel port at a right angle.
  - *Seal*: The seal is fitted on the inlet channel. The device consists of an O-ring that fits the size of the instruments inserted into the working channel. It prevents loss of irrigation fluid around the instrument and can be used to fix the laser fiber at a particular distance from the tip of the instrument.
  - *Light post*: The fiberoptic light cable is attached to the light post.
- *Shaft*: The shaft encases fiberoptic bundles for image and light transmission, working channel, and wires for deflection mechanism. The size of fURS is quoted by its tip diameter, which is 7.5 Fr in the case of Storz Flex-X2. The working length of the instrument is 67 cm and working channel is 3.6 Fr. The shock absorbing system is a form of secondary deflection, which is present in modern fURSs. It is located proximal to the active deflecting system and allows for gentle rolling of the distal end for approximately 10 cm enabling access more deeply into the calyces **(Fig. 2)**.
- *Tip*: The objective lens is made of 2-9 lenses as well as a prism if different viewing directions are required. No prism is required if the viewing angle is 0°. It changes the incident light into an image, projecting it onto the

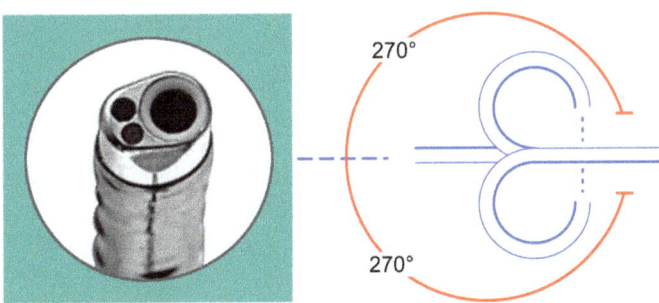

Figure 2: Tip of flexible ureteroscope.

image guide. The tip has the distal ends of fiberoptic bundles carrying image to camera and light from the light source. The distal end of working channel opens below the fiberoptic bundles. The 1.5 cm Laserite™ ceramic-coated tip at the distal end of the working channel prevents thermal damage to the flexible ureterorenoscope during laser usage.[2] The direction of view is 0° and angle of view is 88°. The tip can be deflected 270° in either direction.

WHY DUAL DEFLECTION HAS DISAPPEARED?

The primary purpose of dual deflection was to improve access to lower pole calyces. The older fURSs had a primary deflection angle <200°. Dual-deflection mechanism achieves a deflection angle around 300° by deflecting the scope at two places. Newer ureteroscopes have a larger deflection angle with a single deflection mechanism, which allows easy entry into lower calyces. Moreover, dual-deflection levers are more cumbersome to use.

WHAT DO YOU MEAN BY ACTIVE AND PASSIVE DEFLECTION?

When the tip of the fURS is deflected using the deflecting lever, which controls the tip through wires, it is called active deflection. When the tip of the fURS bends against the wall of the pelvis to enter the calyx, especially the lower calyx, it is called passive deflection.

WHAT IS LEAKAGE TESTER?

Leakage tester is used to verify the integrity of the fURS's working channel. The leakage tester is connected to the special port located at the body of the ureteroscope and scope is pressurized to approximately 140–200 mm Hg by pumping the bulb. Monitor the indicator to detect any fall in pressure, which indicates a leak (**Fig. 3**).

Flexible Ureteroscopes

There are two types of flexible ureteroscopes:
1. Reusable flexible ureteroscopes (**Table 1**)
2. Single-use flexible ureteroscopes (**Table 2**)

Parts of Digital Flexible Ureteroscopes
- *Body*: The body is attached to an integrated cable containing wires to carry electronic signals of image and fiberoptic bundles to carry light. It has a working channel port and deflection lever. In contrast to fiberoptic scopes, there is no focusing component.

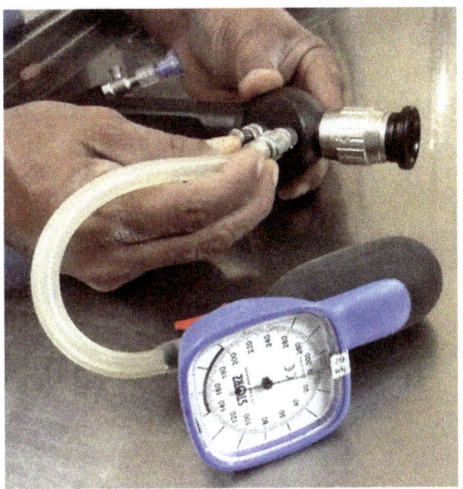

Figure 3: Leakage tester for flexible ureteroscopy.

TABLE 1: Reusable flexible ureteroscopes.						
Manufacturer	Optics	Model	Proximal Tip (Fr)	Distal Tip (Fr)	Deflection up (degree)	Deflection down (degree)
Storz	Fiberoptic	Flex X	8.4	7.5	120	170
		Flex-X2	8.5	7.5	270	270
	Digital	Flex-Xc	8.4	8.4	270	270
Wolf	Fiberoptic	Viper	8.8	6.0	270	270
		Cobra*	9.9	6.0	270	270
	Digital	Boa	9.5	8.5	270	270
Olympus	Fiberoptic	URF-P5	8.4	8.4	180	275
		URF-P6	7.95	7.0	275	275
	Digital	URF-V1	9.9	8.5	180	270
		URF-V2	8.4	8.5	275	275

Note: All the above scopes have working length of 64–70 majority being 67 cm long. All above scopes have working channel of 3.6 Fr except *Cobra—which has two working channels 3.6/2.4 Fr.

- *Shaft*: The shaft has a slightly larger diameter than those of fiberoptic ureteroscopes.
- *Tip*: The tip design of Flex-Xc has a working channel below the objective lens in the middle. The light bundles are divided into two and end on either side of the objective lens. This provides more uniform lighting in the operative field.

TABLE 2: Single-use flexible ureteroscopes.

	LithoVue	Uscope	Indoscope	Wiscope	Neoflex
Imaging	Digital	Digital	Digital	Digital	Digital
Field of view		120°	110°	100°	
Proximal shaft size (Fr)	9.5	9.5	9.9	8.6	9
Distal shaft size (Fr)	7.7	9	9.9	7.4	9
Working channel (Fr)	3.6	3.6	3.3	3.6	3.6
Working length (cm)	68	65	67	67	
Deflection	270° (Both directions)	270° (Both directions)	270° (Both directions)	275° (Both directions)	270° (Both directions)
Handling type	Regular	Regular	Regular	Regular	Regular
Usage hours locked	4 hours	4 hours	21 hours		

How Does A Digital Flexible Ureteroscope Differ from A Fiberoptic Ureteroscope?

In a digital fURS, the image is captured by the camera sensor at the tip of the ureteroscope just behind the objective lens. This image is carried as electronic signals through wires. In a fiberoptic system, the image from objective lens is carried by fiberoptic bundles to the eyepiece.

What is "Chip-on-the-Tip" Principle?

In chip-on-tip, the ureteroscope tip itself contains a camera sensor. The image generated in the objective lens is projected onto to the video chip, which converts the optical signals into electrical signals and transmits them to the camera controller. With the chip-on-tip, there is superior appreciation of depth of field and no need for focusing.

The two different technologies used for capturing images digitally are: (1) charge-coupled device (CCD) and (2) complementary metal oxide semiconductor (CMOS) image sensors. In a CCD sensor, every pixel's charge is transferred through an output nodes to be converted to voltage, buffered, and sent off-chip as an analog signal. All of the pixel can be devoted to light capture, and the output's uniformity is high. In a CMOS sensor, each pixel has its own charge-to-voltage conversion, and the sensor often includes amplifiers, noise correction, and digitization circuits, so that the chip outputs digital bits. These other functions increase the design complexity and reduce the area available for light capture. With each pixel doing its own conversion, uniformity is lower.

Advantages of Digital Flexible Ureteroscope

The image transfer is better since the chip at the tip directly receives it. Image quality is equivalent to 10 times the pixel resolution of standard fiberoptic endoscopes. Since there is no need for attaching a camera, the instrument becomes light and easy to manipulate. The wear and tear is lower as there is no fiberoptic bundle in this ureteroscope.

Disadvantages of Digital Flexible Ureteroscope

Since tip size increases because of chip at the tip, patients require more ureteric dilatation with larger access sheaths and there is an increased chance of staging the procedure if ureter could not be adequately dilated. Even the smallest digital fURS is 8.5 Fr in size. Further, these ureteroscopes are more expensive.

ACCESSORIES (SEE CHAPTER ON ACCESSORIES)

Various accessories required are:
- Access sheath
- Wires-Bi wire and glide wires
- Baskets-engage, entrap, etc.
- Laser fiber

Single-use Flexible Digital Ureteroscope

Advantages of single use flexible scopes:
- Less initial purchase cost
- No repair cost
- No worry of damaging of deflection of scope
- No lengthy sterilization process needed
- Decrease in case turnover time as new scope is available every time
- No risk of transmission of infection to next patient

The basic design of single-use fURS is same as reusable scopes. Previously single use fiberoptic scopes such as PolyScope (Lumenis, Israel. Polydiagnost, Germany), SemiFlex Scope (Maxiflex, New Orleans, LA, USA), and FlexorVue (Cook Medical, Indiana, USA) were available. Nowadays, only single-use digital flexible scopes are becoming popular. Most commonly used single-use flexible digital scopes are LithoVue (Boston Scientific, Massachusetts, USA), Uscope (Zhuhai Pusen Medical Technology Co, Ltd., Zhuhai, China), and Indoscope (Biorad Medisys Pvt. Ltd., India). Other single-use digital scopes available are NeoFlex-Ureteroscope (Neoscope Inc., California, USA), WISCOPE URS (innoMedicus, Switzerland), and ShaoGan (YouCare Technology Co. Ltd., Wuhan, China). The commonly used single-use flexible digital ureteroscopes are as follows:
- *LithoVue (Boston Scientific, Massachusetts, USA)* (**Fig. 4**): It has a new enhancement: A new fluid-resistant sealing process that shields the

handle electronics from fluid, called ClearSeal Technology. This makes the LithoVue single-use ureteroscope more reliable against image loss during procedures and reduces potential disruptions during surgery.

- *Uscope (Zhuhai Pusen Medical Technology Co, Ltd., Zhuhai, China) (**Fig. 5**)*: It is lightweight, weighing 147 g. The company has recently launched a prototype 7.5 Fr single-use digital scope, which would be slimmest digital scope. Some studies have been done to compare this scope with LithoVue scope have found comparable results based on visibility and maneuverability.

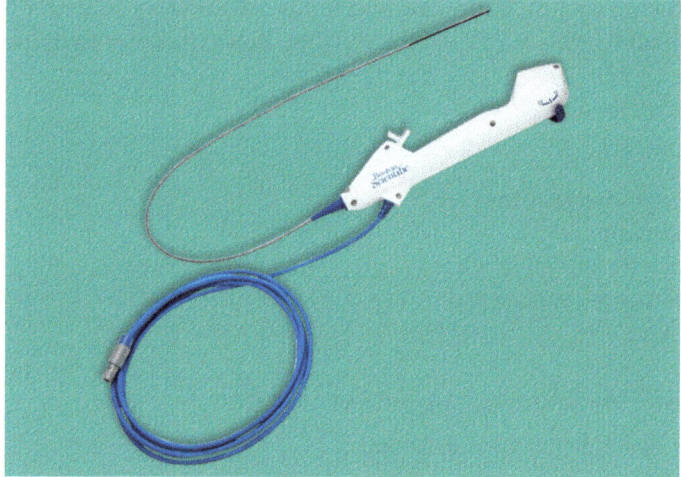

Figure 4: LithoVue.

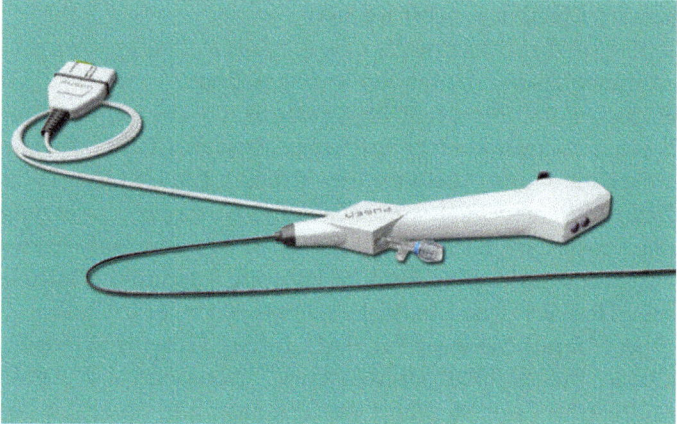

Figure 5: Uscope.

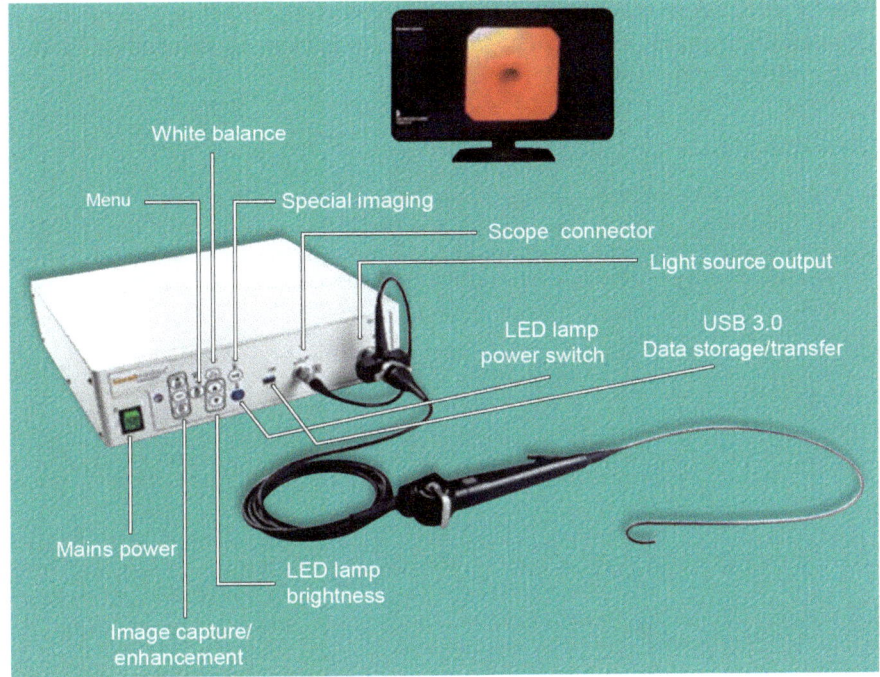

Figure 6: Indoscope.

- *Indoscope (Biorad Medisys Pvt. Ltd., India) (**Fig. 6**)*: The scope comes with usage lock for 21 hours as company does not strictly consider this scope as single-use scope. It can be reused by sterilizing it by Sterrad and ethylene oxide (ETO).

All the above described single-use flexible digital scopes have digital CMOS-based sensor chip at their tip. LithoVue scope needs manufacturer specific monitor as well as processing unit. Uscope as well as Indoscope require only video processing unit with any monitor.

Some facts about single use FURS
- All single, limited use FURS are digital and hence image quality is better
- Indovasive advocates reuse of scopes, however, sterilization by chemical sterilization (Cidex, Perasafe, etc.) is not commented by company. Such scopes are to be sterilized by either ETO or Plasma sterilization.
- All scopes are light weight and easy to handle
- All are available in both logic and antilogic variety
- Many publications have shown that single use FURS are cost effective and especially so when they are re-used
- Studies have also shown that biomedical waste created by single use ureteroscopes does not increase carbon footprint of environment.

- Better deflection, smaller fiber laser (200 micron), and single use FURS has enabled many lower calyx stones to be broken in situ rather than relocation to other calyces

REFERENCES

1. Marshall VF. Fiber optics in urology. J Urol. 1964;91:110-4.
2. Karl Storz. Uretero-renoscopes Flex-X2 and Flex-X (9th edition. 2012. pp. 202-4). [online] Available from: http://epc.karlstorz.com/epc/Starter.jsp?locale=eN&practiceArea=UrO&product=&sid=SID-e02F3390-37621460. [Last accessed February 2021].

CHAPTER 9

Laparoscopy and Robotics Instruments

LAPAROSCOPIC INSTRUMENTS

Introduction and Brief History

The first laparoscopic nephrectomy was performed by Clayman in 1991.[1] The first laparoscopic donor nephrectomy was performed by Ratner[2] Rane and colleagues are credited with the first urologic laparoendoscopic single-site (LESS) surgery.[3]

In this chapter, we describe the various instruments required for laparoscopic and robotic surgery. The instruments are described with emphasis on their specifications and uses.

The laparoscopic instruments will be described as follows:
- Armamentarium required for urologic laparoscopy
- Video-imaging armamentarium
- Access-related instruments
- Trocars
- Laparoscopic dissecting and retracting instruments
- Laparoscopic telescopes
- Clips applicator and staplers

ARMAMENTARIUM

Proper instruments are the "key" to successful completion of the procedure. Prior to initiating the procedure the surgeon should prepare a checklist as well as make sure that all the required instruments are arranged in a systematic manner on the operating room trolley. The instruments will vary as per the case, however, the general outline of armamentarium required for laparoscopy includes the following:
- Camera unit
- Connector cables from camera to monitor
- Video monitor
- Light source
- Light transmission fiberoptic cable

- Insufflators
- Carbon dioxide cylinder
- Carbon dioxide pressure regulator valve
- Tubing and Luer lock adapter for carbon dioxide to patient
- Suction irrigation apparatus
- Cautery machine with cables and foot control
- Extension cord
- Telescope
- Trocars and cannulas
- Veress needle
- Atraumatic graspers
- Toothed grasper
- Curved dissector
- Clip applicator with suitable clips
- Dissection hook
- Laparoscopic scissors
- Suction irrigation cannula
- Laparoscopic needle holder

The trolley is arranged in systematic fashion, and the telescope white balanced before starting the surgery. Preferably the assistant should be trained in this aspect rather than leaving this part for the nursing assistants to perform. The surgical principles remain the same in arranging the trolley as in open surgery. Sharp instruments should be kept away from the field, telescopes and cameras are placed in the center of the trolley and properly secured.

A rescue tray at all times should be kept ready on the table. The rescue tray includes:

- The rescue stitch which is prepared with a hem-o-lok^{TM} clip attached to the tail of the needle (Rescue stitch). Typically, a rescue stitch is a stitch on a CT-1 needle with a hem-o-lok^{TM} clip attached to the tail end of the suture. A knot is thrown over the hem-o-lok clip to prevent its slippage.
- A hemostatic agent such as surgicel^{TM}
- A cartridge of vascular clip such as hem-o-lok^{TM} clip
- A gauze which can be easily inserted through the port and has a radiopaque marker
- Two needle holders
- Satinsky clamp

The rescue stitch should be placed in a readily visible part of the operating room (OR) and used in the event of life-threatening bleeding.

VIDEO AND IMAGING

- Laparoscopic camera is one of the very important instruments and should be of good quality (**Figs. 1 and 2**).

CHAPTER 9: Laparoscopy and Robotics Instruments | 93

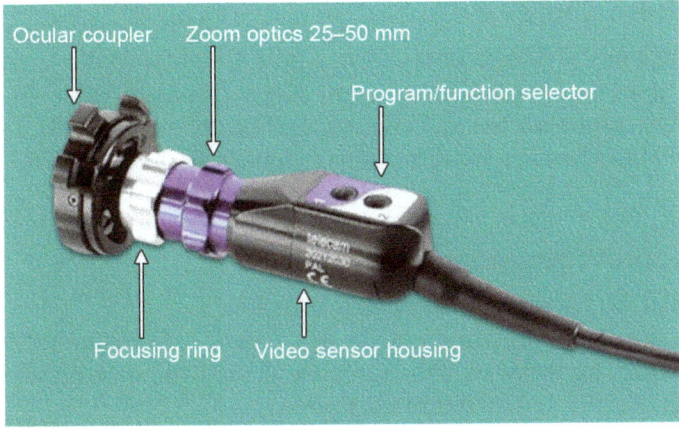

Figure 1: Laparoscopic camera.

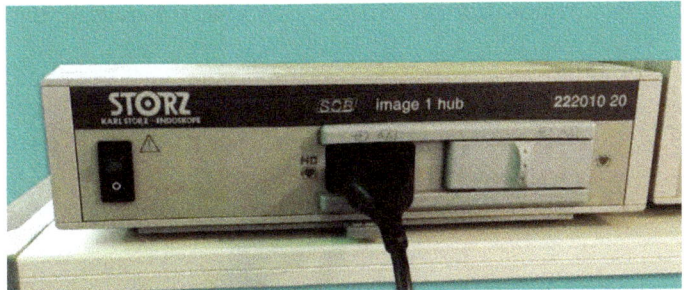

Figure 2: Storz Camera Hub.

- *Charge-coupling device (CCD) (Chip)* is an electronic memory that records the intensity of light as a variable charge.
- Their charges equate to shades of red, green, and blue when used with color filters. Three chip camera uses three CCDs, one for each of the red, green, and blue colors.
    - There is a zoom lens that focuses the image on the chip, and a CCD chip that "sees" an image taken by telescope.
- The chip has light-sensitive photoreceptors that generate pixels by transforming the incoming photons into electronic charges.
- The electronic charges are then transferred from the pixels into a storage element on the chip.
- The CCD then converts optical image into an electrical signal that is sent through the camera cable to camera control unit (CCU).
- Camera control unit—usually located on the trolley along with the monitor.

Video Output (Fig. 3)

The different types of video outputs are composite, S-video (older technology but better than composite), component video (separate cable for RGB, supports high resolution but still analog), and finally digital (DVI). DVI has digital signal transmission, no distortion or signal loss, and supports highest resolution.

Laparoscopic Video Monitor

- The size of the screen varies from 8 to 21 inches.
- The macula of the surgeon should be at a distance of five times the width of the screen, for instance, if the screen is 32 inch, the surgeon should be standing (32 × 5 = 160 inch) from the screen.

Video Resolution and Pixels (Table 1)

Generally, a video resolution is referred to the height of the pixels. For example, 1,080p, means that the quantity of pixels displayed by height

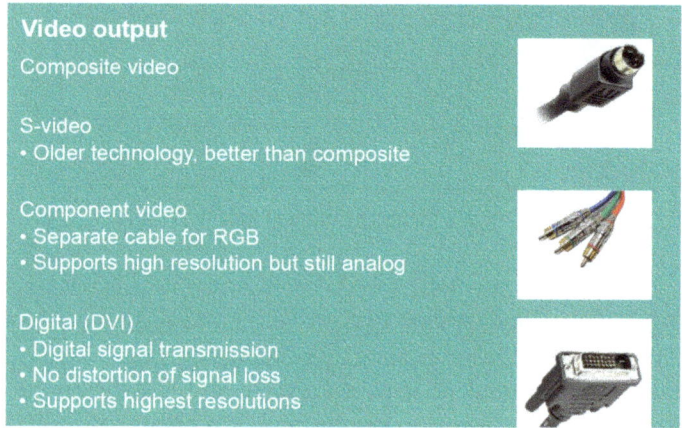

Video output

Composite video

S-video
- Older technology, better than composite

Component video
- Separate cable for RGB
- Supports high resolution but still analog

Digital (DVI)
- Digital signal transmission
- No distortion of signal loss
- Supports highest resolutions

(RGB: red, green, and blue)

Figure 3: Video output.

Table 1: Video resolution and pixels.

Resolution	Measurements (In pixels)	Pixel count
4K (UHD)	3,840 × 2,160	8,294,400
1,080p (full HD)	1,920 × 1,080	2,073,600
720p (HD Ready)	1,280 × 720	921,600
480p (SD)	640 × 480	307,000

is 1,080p, while the quantity of pixels displayed by width is 1,920p (1,920p × 1,080p).

Standard definition (SD): The quality of SD resolution (640 × 480) refers to the standard for most of channels and screens. The resolution refers to a pixel height of 480 in a single image.

SD video can be identified with 480i or 720 × 480

The letters "i" and "p" after the numbers 720, 1,080 letters refer to the method in which the video has been recorded where "i" stands for "interlaced" and "p" stands for "progressive" or "non-interlaced."

Interlacing video is a technique for doubling the perceived frame rate of a video display without consuming extra bandwidth. In interlacing, the eyes in reality gauge every alternative line of a picture frame. However, the eyes while perceiving the full image in motion, start filling in the gaps making a complete picture out of it.

Progressive scanning is a technique of displaying or transmitting moving images in which all the lines of each frame are drawn in sequence, without alteration. Progressive method delivers a better resolution in general, as the motion appears more fluid.

High definition (HD): It is the new resolution standard and refers to a pixel height of either 720 or 1,080 pixels. HD delivers more details per pixel, so the image is much clearer and sharper.

High definition has two variants—720 (HD Ready) or 1,080 (full HD) pixels tall. While it is available in both progressive and interlaced scanning, the progressive variant produces a superior quality image than interlacing.

4K or ultra HD: 4K is actually 2,160 × 3,840 pixels, but by "4K" we refer not to the height of the pixels but the width of the pixels (3840p from which the name "4K" is derived). There are two variants of 4K:
1. 3,840 × 2,160 pixels (used by TV broadcasters, and online media channels)
2. 4,096 × 2,160 pixels (mostly used in the movie industry)

8K: Super Hi-Vision System (SHV): Resolution in pixels is 7,680 × 4,320. At this level of resolution, the human eyes cannot notice the pixels and the displayed images look very clear as no dots are visible to the eyes.
- Three-dimensional (3D) video technology (**Fig. 4**):
  o Standard laparoscopy has two-dimensional (2D) images, so determining spatial distances due to the absence of shadows, stereovision, and parallax movement is difficult.
  o Initially, two 5-mm CCD lenses were integrated into one endoscope to create a double image on the monitor. These two images were then combined into a 3D picture by shutter glasses.
  o At present, 3D system takes two images from different angles and then digitally reconstructs a 3D image.
  o Polarized glasses permit visualization of a 3D image.
  o 3D HD video technology is available for 0° and 30° endoscopes.

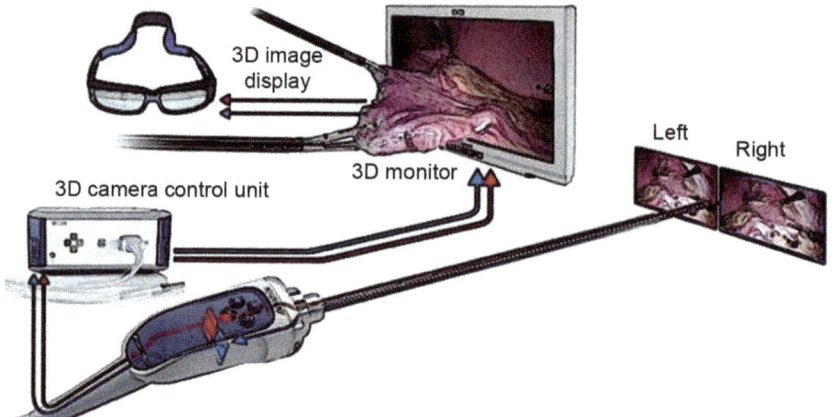

Figure 4: Three dimensional video technology.

ACCESS DEVICES

The access devices will vary with the approach (transperitoneal or preperitoneal). Proper peritoneal access is crucial for successful completion of surgery. Pneumoperitoneum can be achieved either with closed or open technique. The open technique is known as "Hassan's technique." The advantages of the open technique include theoretical less chance of bowel injury; however, if the fascial incision exceeds the diameter of the port, it may cause gas leak.

Insufflators

It is a quadri-manometric equipment that is used to create and maintain space and distension within the area of interest with the desired gas at the preset pressure.

Types of Insufflators

- *Classification 1*:
  - Analog—with mechanical valves
  - Digital—with electronically managed microprocessor-based valves
- *Classification 2*:
  - Low flow (20 L/min)
  - High flow (45 L/min)
- *Classification 3*:
  - They can also be classified depending if the insufflator insufflates during flow phase or pause phase.
- *Flow rates for insufflator*:
  - *Low-flow rate (Veress needle mode)*: 1 L/min (safety mechanism to prevent air embolism if inadvertent Veress cannulation into a vein) flow rate required for air embolism is 2 L/min.

- Medium-flow rates approximately 8–10 L/min (procedures where no much suction is required) maximum suction through a 5-mm suction cannula is 18 L/min.
- Low-flow rate (1 L/min) should be maintained when initial Veress needle is inserted. This helps in preventing air embolism.
- *Medium-flow rates (8–10 L/min)*: This should be used when not much suction is required.
- High-flow rates should be used when a lot of suction is used.
- Ideal reading and aerodynamics:
  - Ideal conditions in adult peritoneal capacity is a preset pressure of 12–15 mm Hg.

INSUFFLATION DEVICES

- *Veress needle (Fig. 5)*: The Veress needle is available either as a disposable or reusable needle. These are manufactured by Storz, Wolf as well as a few.

Indian manufacturers: Disposable Veress needles are manufactured by Autosuture and Ethicon.

Veress needle is available in three lengths—80 mm, 100 mm, and 120 mm. The length is measured from the tip to the hub. The longer one is useful in obese patients (150 mm). It is 14 gauge in diameter. The reusable needle is larger in diameter (3 mm).

The Veress needle has three parts (**Fig. 6**) which are as follows:
1. *The hub*: The hub of the Veress needle has an indicator which suggests the position of the needle (preperitoneal or peritoneal), a green indicator indicates the tip of the needle is in a negative milieu (peritoneum), a red indicator indicates the tip is in a preperitoneal space or is in the mesenteric fat or the needle is blocked (this feature is seen in Ethicon needle, not seen in Autosuture). This is a safety mechanism, once the

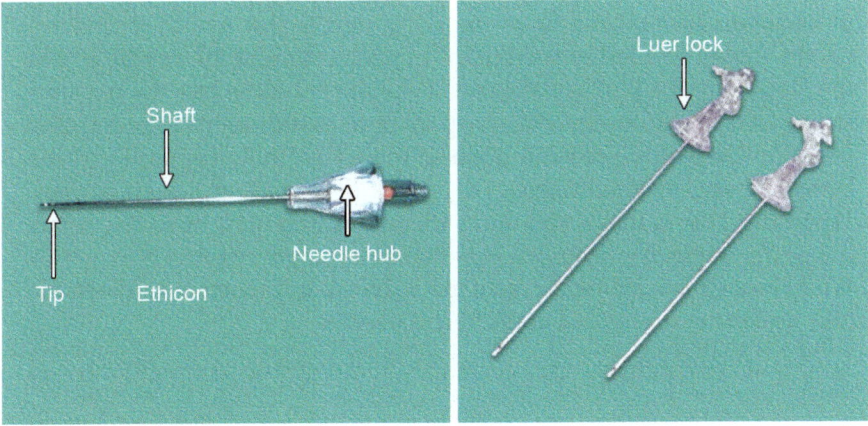

Figure 5: The Autosuture and Ethicon Veress needles.

98 | **SECTION 1:** Instruments

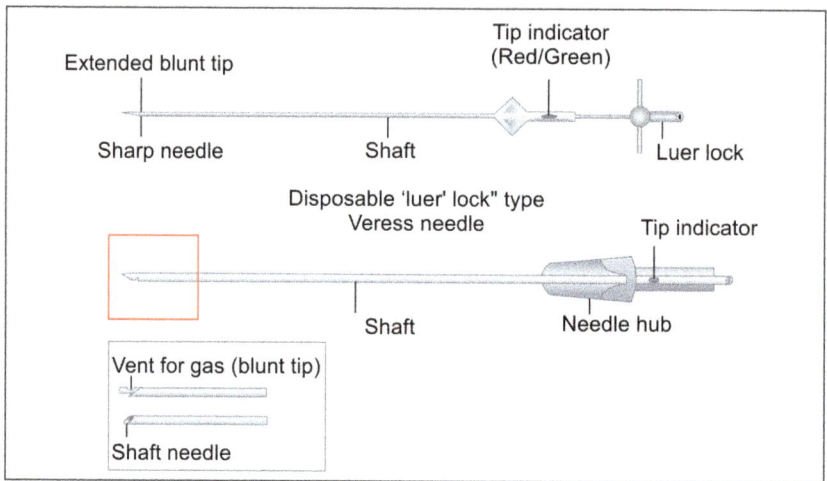

Figure 6: Parts of the Veress needle.

inner component completely protrudes beyond the stylet, the green indicator will show up, indicating it is in a hollow cavity, even with a minimal resistance (partially in), it will show up as a red indicator. The floating ball (red or green) at the center of the hub, will float when the tip of the needle is in the peritoneum. The hub has a Luer lock arrangement, which helps to attach syringe, thereby confirming the presence of needle in peritoneal cavity, on aspiration of air, it confirms presence of needle in the desired cavity. The floating ball remains suspended in the cylindrical portion of the hub, as the needle enters the peritoneal space, the ball falls to the base of the cylindrical space of the hub.

2. *The shaft*: It is metallic and is radiopaque. The shaft provides a conduit for passage of gas for insufflations.
3. *The tip*: The tip has two components. The inner component is blunt and projects just beyond the tip of the sharp needle (for 3 mm). The sharp needle (outer beveled sheath) helps in penetration of the needle across the fascia into the peritoneal cavity, once the needle enters the negative milieu of the peritoneum, the sharp tip retracts, this helps in preventing injury to the intraperitoneal organs. The lateral hole (opposite to the bevel) on the needle enables CO_2 to be delivered intra-abdominally. When the hole is inside the outer sheath, insufflations does not occur, hence theoretically preventing subcutaneous emphysema.

While inserting, it should be held like a dart. It is important to check the patency and the spring action of the Veress needle.

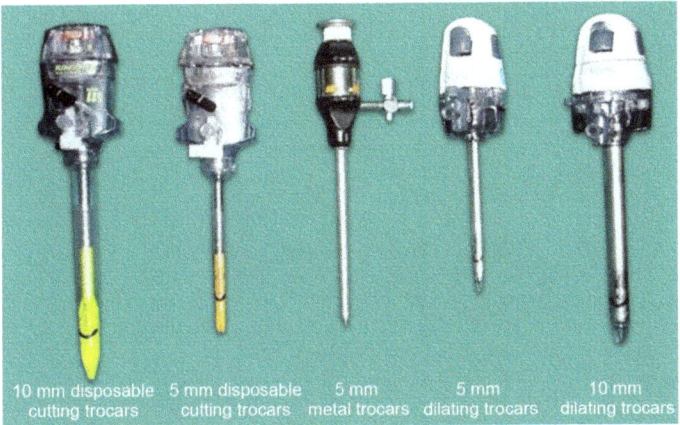

Figure 7: The trocars classification.

TROCARS (FIG. 7)

The trocars offer a conduit for entry and exit of instruments during the surgery. The trocars are available in various sizes ranging from 2 to 15 mm. The operating surgeon needs to understand the instruments which need to be passed through a suitably sized port.

The trocars can be classified in the following ways:
- *Classification 1*:
  o Disposable (plastic)
  o Nondisposable (metal) **(Fig. 14)**.
- *Classification 2*:
  o Bladed trocars
  o Nonbladed trocars
  They can also be classified depending on size—commonly used are 5 mm, 11 mm, and 12 mm.

Special types of trocar are as follows:
- *Miniport (Ethicon) (Fig. 8B)*: The port has two parts—an outer hollow sheath which acts a port, the Veress needle can be inserted through the outer sheath.
- Hybrid trocars (Autosuture) (both 5 mm and 11 mm channel) **(Fig. 8A)**. It has two channels one for 10 mm and second for 5 mm.
- *Newer smudge port (Ethicon)*: The specially designed valve prevents smudge and fogging of the telescope.

The trocar assembly (disposable) consists of the following **(Fig. 9)**:
The parts are: Cannula, obturator, and reducer

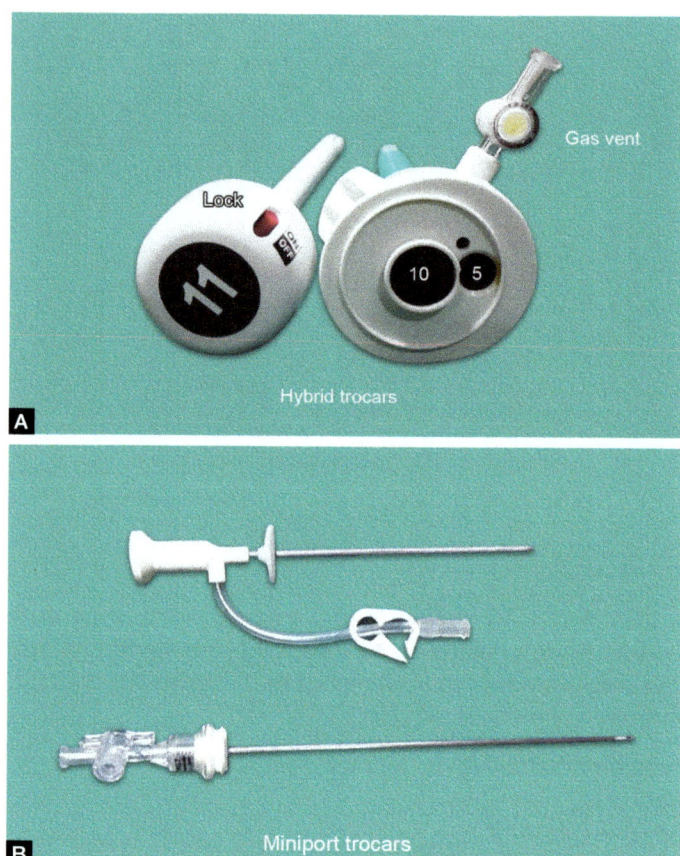

Figures 8A and B: The port has two parts—an outer hollow sheath which acts a port, the Veress needle can be inserted through the outer sheath.

Cannula: Cannula is made from plastic or metal. It has a shaft and housing. The shaft length is measured from the beveled length to housing. The shaft length and size is available as 75 mm (short) (only in 5 mm), 100 mm (standard) (12 mm and 5 mm), and 150 mm (extra-long) (12 mm and 5 mm). The cannula tip can be either straight or oblique. The parts of housing include valve and a gas vent with stop cock. The gas vent is distal to the valve. The valves in disposable trocars are nonflap, while in reusable trocars they are of a trumpet (flap) configuration. The housing also features a knob for attaching the reducer. The valves of cannula provide internal air seals, which allow instruments to move in and out within the cannula without the loss of pneumoperitoneum. These valves can be oblique, transverse, or in piston configuration. The valves can be manually or automatically retractable during instrument passage after removing the reducer.

Reducers (**Fig. 9**): It is used to reduce the size of the port from 11 mm, 12 mm, 10 to 5 mm, so that pneumoperitoneum is maintained whenever the surgeon

CHAPTER 9: Laparoscopy and Robotics Instruments | 101

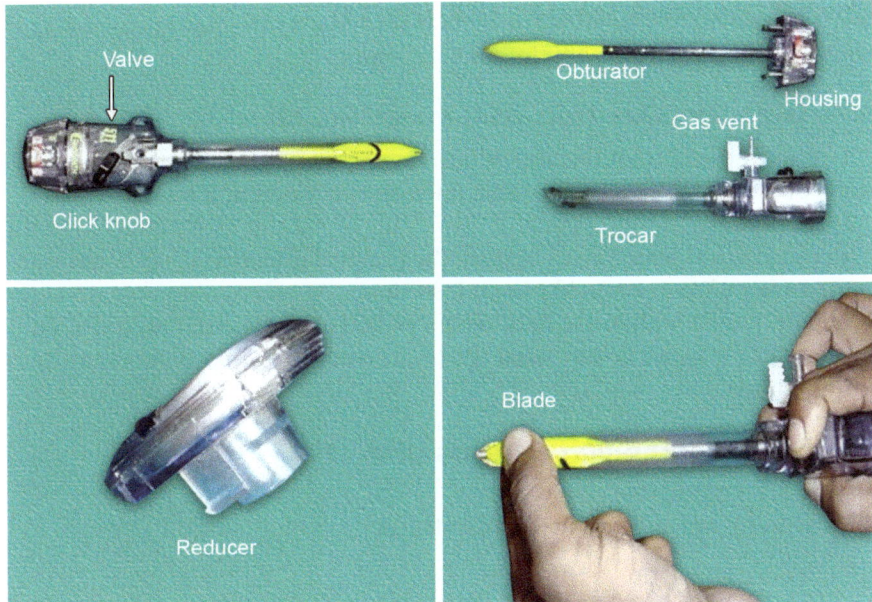

Figure 9: Parts of laparoscopic trocars.

changes the instrument from larger diameter to smaller diameter. The reducer sheaths are available either as (hollow rods) or can be used as attachments which can be fixed on the housing of the trocars.

Universal Reducer

The reducers help to use a instrument regardless of size of port without gas leak is available for 5 mm port.

Obturator

The obturator can be bladed or nonbladed. The obturator can be optiview (transparent at tip of trocar) or nonoptiview. The obturator has a knob/lock for attachment to the cannula, while it has lateral knob for fixation of the telescope. All cannulas have an end hole through which an appropriate size telescope can be passed. The obturator of disposable trocars has a sharp blade which retracts as soon as the trocar passes through the abdominal wall. The blade protrudes on resistance to tough tissue and retracts (unlocked) in negative milieu. The bladed trocars can be used as nonbladed provided you do not load the blade.

Visiport® (Covidien LP, USA) (Fig. 10)

It uses a firing blade under visual control.

Optiview® (Johnson & Johnson, USA) (Fig. 11)
Bladeless optical tip which eliminates blind entry.

The AirSeal® (SurgiQuest Inc., USA) Trocar (Fig. 12)
- It works by creating and maintaining a gas pressure barrier in the proximal end of the trocar for a more stable pneumoperitoneum. It has a valveless trocar design.
- No mechanical structure to impede the removal of material, and nothing to smudge a laparoscope during reinsertion.
- It has a double-walled cannula, which enables the system to deliver CO_2 through four nares in the distal tip, unobstructed by instruments inside the cannula.

EndoTIP® (Karl Storz GmbH, Germany) (Fig. 13)
- Optically controllable access
- The tissue is not cut through but displaced.

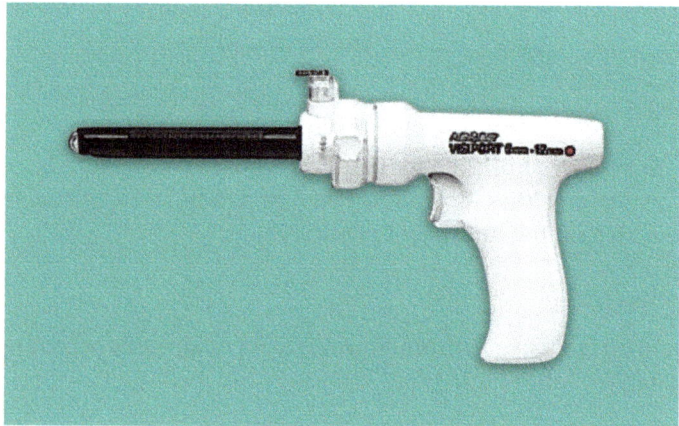

Figure 10: Visiport.

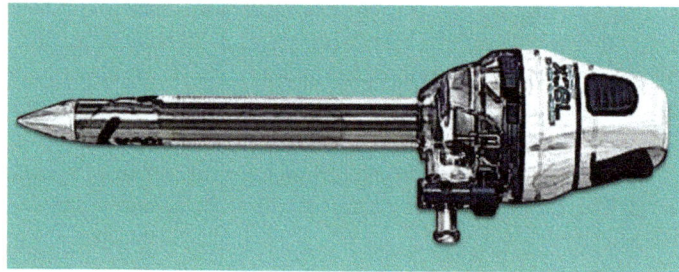

Figure 11: Optiview.

CHAPTER 9: Laparoscopy and Robotics Instruments | 103

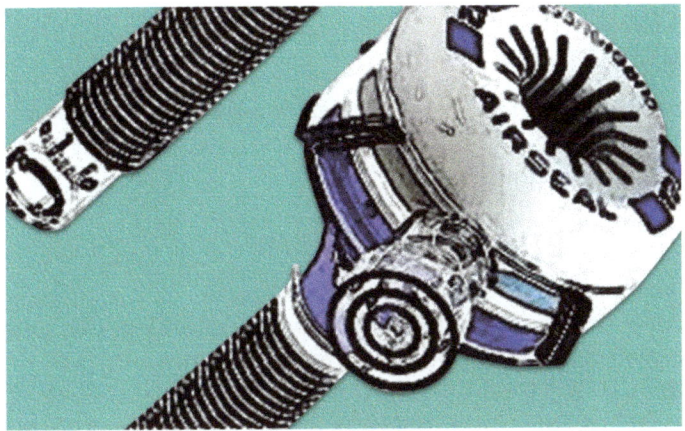

Figure 12: The AirSeal.

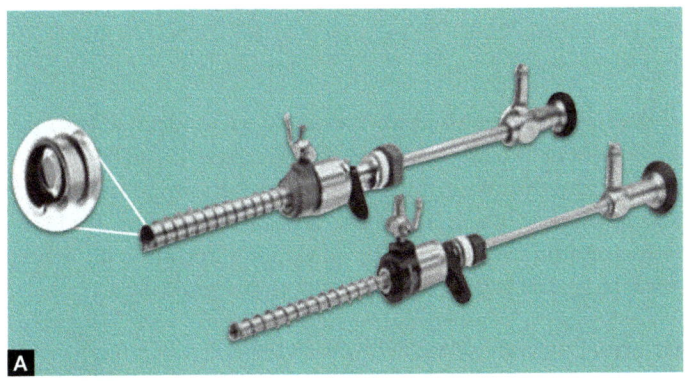

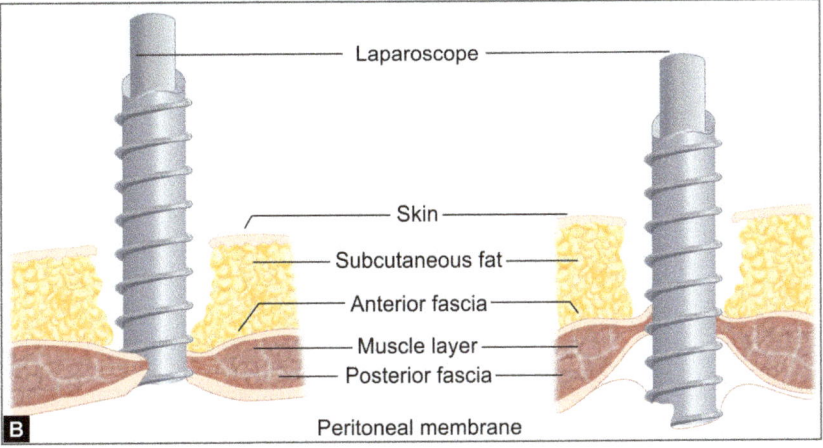

Figures 13A and B: EndoTIP Port.

Reusable Trocars

Hassan Trocar

The Hassan's cannula offers the advantage of reduced risk of injury to the bowels. It is especially useful in a patient who has previously undergone intra-abdominal procedures.

Parts of the cannula:
This cannula consists of three pieces:
1. A cone-shaped sleeve
2. A metal or plastic sheath with a trumpet or flap valve (**Fig. 14**). The sheath has two struts for affixing fascial sutures. These sutures are then wrapped tightly around the struts. Thereby firmly seating the cone-shaped sleeve into the laparoscopic port. This creates an effective seal to maintain pneumoperitoneum.
3. Blunt-tipped obturator

INSTRUMENTS USED FOR THE RETROPERITONEAL APPROACH

Dr Gaur is credited with the description of new device/technique for retroperitoneal surgery.[4] The retroperitoneal space is developed initially with the finger till the thoracolumbar fascia, once this is pierced either with a finger or an instrument, the space is created with a custom-made dissector or a glove and inflated with a rubber catheter. Alternatively, a balloon is available which helps in creation of the retroperitoneal space.

Retracting and Dissecting Instruments

The retractors are either disposable or nondisposable. The nondisposable instruments can be dismantled, so that they can be cleaned and reused.

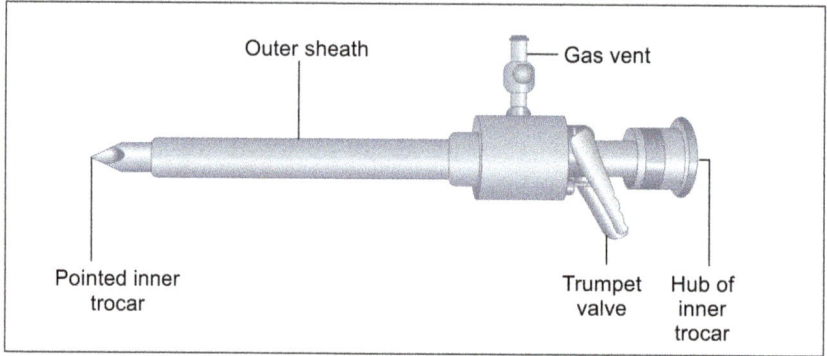

Figure 14: Metal cannula.

The parts of the instruments are as follows (**Fig. 15**):
- Handle
- Insulated outer tube
- Inner tube which is part of the tip of the instrument

The design and mechanism of action for the handle, outer sheath, and inner sheath differ with manufacturers.
- *Insulated outer tube*: The outer tube may be insulated or noninsulated. Insulation covering may be of silicon or plastic. The insulation coat is likely to be breached during cleaning and may be dangerous as this may lead to inadvertent injury during the course of surgery. The surgeon should make sure that the insulation cover is not breached prior to commencing the surgery. The outer tube also has a vent for cleaning and sterilizing. This helps to clean the instrument without dismantling the instrument. This feature is not seen in Wolf outer sheath. Extra-long outer sheath is 42 cm in length.
- *Insert of the instrument (**Fig. 16**)*: The insert of the instrument can be a scissor, grasper, or forceps, Maryland, Allis, etc. As shown in the figure, the forceps or the grasper will be a single-action mechanism or a double-action mechanism. The jaws of the single-action grasper open less than double-action grasper. The single-action graspers exert more force between the jaws than the double action. The double action is used for retraction while single action is for grasping. The insert is locked by rotating the distal end and clicking on the lock.

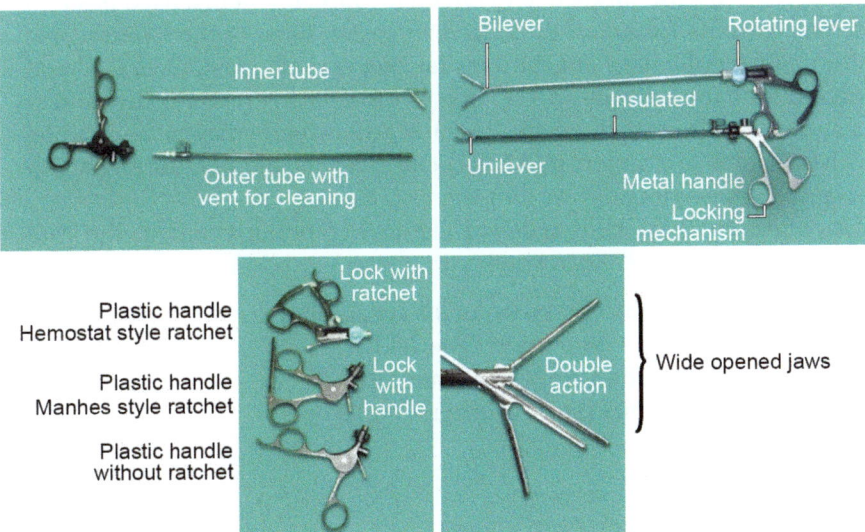

Figure 15: Parts of retracting and dissecting instruments.

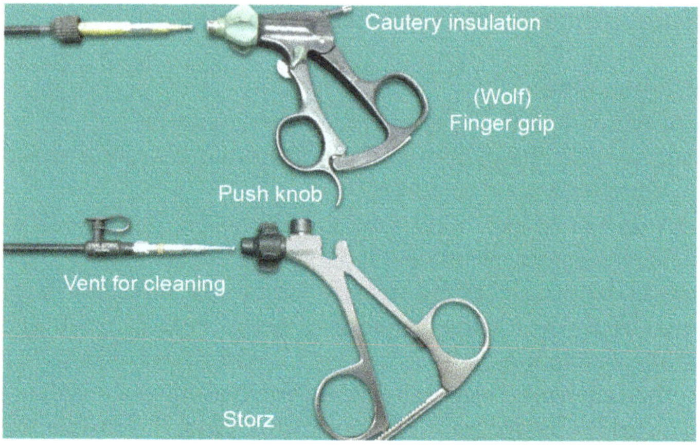

Figure 16: The difference between Storz and Wolf instrument.

- *Instrument handle*: This can be plastic or metal. The parts of the handle are as follows:
  - Finger grip
  - Rotating knob
  - Release button to release the inner and outer sheath
  - Cautery attachment

Handle: The handle of the "handheld" laparoscopic instruments has either a locking or nonlocking mechanism. The handle also has a pillar for attaching the cautery cable. The locking mechanism includes a "ratchet" mechanism for locking (Storz) or a button mechanism (Wolf) (**Fig. 16**). The locking mechanism helps the surgeon to maintain the instrument in a fixed position and hence avoids fatigue in prolonged surgeries. Most of the laparoscopic instruments handle have attachments for unipolar electrosurgical lead and many have rotator mechanism to rotate the tip of the instrument. The cautery attachment is oblique to the shaft. The latter arrangement may cause clashing which is avoided in a cautery pillar placed in a coaxial manner. The finger grip has special grooves for adjusting fingers.

The Press knob on the handle is a feature of Storz instrument. The Wolf instruments do not have Press knob.

Types of ratchet for retracting instruments are as follows:
- Manhes style ratchet (Storz catalogue, 33,122)
- Hemostat style ratchet (Storz catalogue, 33,123)
- Disengageable ratchet (Storz catalogue, 33,126)

Fan Retractor

The parts of a fan retractor are as follows:
- Outer tube—5 Fr and 10 Fr
- The inner tube has a grip and fans which get retracted inside the outer tube in resting position. It has 9 fan blades.

Needle Holders (Fig. 17)

The needle holder has either a pistol grip or straight grip. The grip is always single action as it offers a firm grip of the needle. The tip of the needle holder may be curved (right curve or left curve) or straight. The needle holders vary in length (33 cm). The pediatric needle holder is shorter in length (23 cm). In-line grip needle holders are ergonomically better than pistol grip needle holder.

Parts of the Needle Driver

Generally, they cannot be dismantled, laparoscopic needle holders are always locking. The lock can be thumb lock or finger lock. The needle driver can be single-toothed.

The parts are as follows:
- *Tip*: Curved (right or left) and straight
- *Shaft*: It has a cleaning vent.
- *Handle*: The handle can be pistol grip or an in-line grip.

KOH Macro needle holders: This is manufactured by Storz GmBH. It can be disassembled into the following parts namely.
- The handle
- Working insert
- Outer tube. The inserts are made of tungsten carbide.

LAPAROSCOPIC SCISSORS (FIGS. 18A AND B)

The type of scissors used varies according to the purpose of use and the surgeon comfort. The laparoscopic scissors can be used as a cold shears or hot shears.

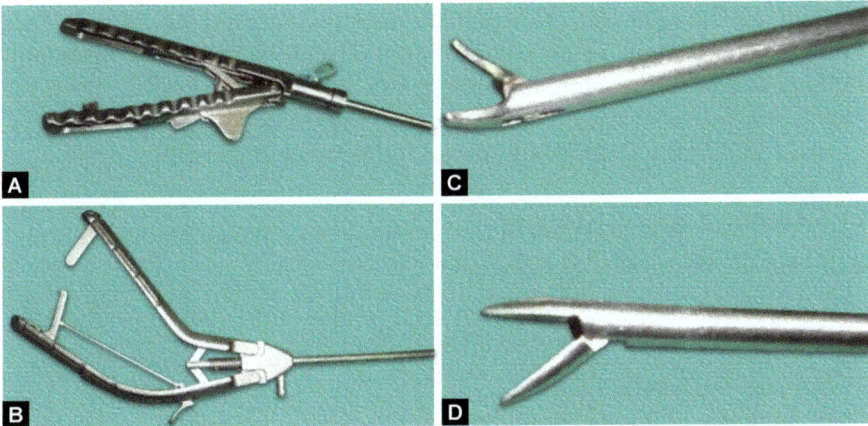

Figures 17A to D: Parts of a needle holder: (A) Handle grip; (B) Pistol grip; (C) Curved grip; (D) Straight grip.

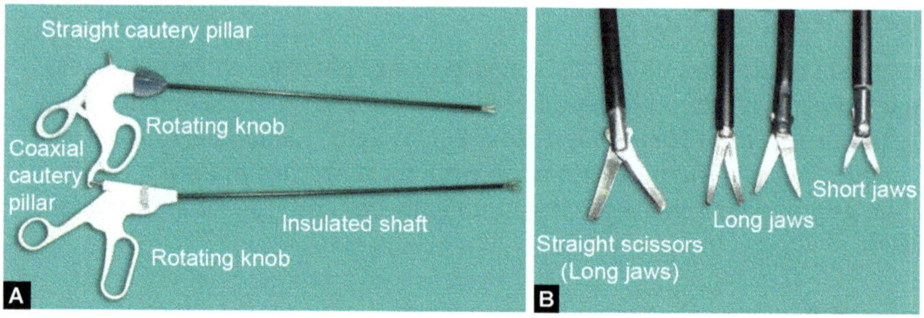

Figures 18A and B: Types of laparoscopic scissors.

Parts of the Scissors

In reusable scissors, the parts mimic those of retracting instruments, in the sense, it can be dismantled into insert, outer tube, and handle. The disposable scissors is integrated. These instruments are 30 cm in length.

They can be classified as:
- Disposable
- Non disposable

Laparoscopic scissors can also be classified as:
- *Straight scissors*: They are available either as short jaws or long jaw scissors. The longer straight variety is useful when performing donor nephrectomy to achieve optimal length of the vessels. The short straight scissors can be used as an aid during suturing.
- *Curved shears*: They can be used as dissectors. These are useful in spatulation of the ureter, during ureteric reimplantation, or pyeloplasty. During spatulation of a pyeloplasty, the ureter can be rotated in line with the instrument, the left hand is used for spatulation of the left ureter and scissors in the right hand for spatulation of the right-sided ureter. Long straight scissors can be used during partial nephrectomy as it delivers long cuts, hence restricting warm ischemia time.
- *Roticulator scissors*: The tip of the scissors rotates on its axis, this helps in spatulation during pyeloplasty and ureteric reimplantation.

Clip Applicators and Staplers

The clip applicators can be classified as:
- Preloaded (e.g., LigaMX™ and Allport™)
- Nonpreloaded with additional cartridge (e.g., Hem-o-lok™)

They can be also classified as:
- Multiload (e.g., Allport™ and LigaMX™)
- Single load (e.g., titanium clips)

They also can be classified as:
- Disposable
- Multiple use

The clips that were initially used were of multiple use and single load, the disadvantages were additional time required for every load, clips used to accidentally fall off while passing through the trocars and they lacked a rotating handle. All these shortcomings are overcome with multiload clips.

The advantages of multiload clips are:
- 360° rotating shafts
- Clips do not fall off while passing through the trocars
- Saves time while loading

They can also be classified as:
- Noninterlocking titanium clips 200 (white), 300 (green), and 400 (yellow)
- Polymer clips (hem-o-lok clips)—green (medium), (violet) large medium, and (gold) extra-large.

The color code is for the clip applicator and color code knob is located on the clip applicator. The clip applicator assembly includes the applicator and the clips. The varieties of clips available commonly use dare hem-o-lok™ and Ligaclip™. The other clips available are Ligaclip™ and LigaMX™.

Hem-o-lok Clip Applicators (Teleflex Medical Inc.)

This is a nonabsorbable polymer clip. There were concerns with the application of the hem-o-lok clips in donor nephrectomy. A Food and Drug Administration (FDA) warning (www.fda.gov/Medwatch/report.htm) has contraindicated the use of hem-o-lok clips in laparoscopic donor nephrectomy. The hem-o-lok clips are made of polymer and are radiolucent. They are available as a cartridge of six clips. They are interlocking clips and are held securely with the help of a knob and lock mechanism. The hem-o-lok clips are available in three sizes namely XL—gold, L—purple, and S—white (**Fig. 19**). A multi-institutional working group compiled a retrospective review of laparoscopic procedures in nine institutions. The procedures reviewed included 899 radical nephrectomies, 112 simple nephrectomies, 198 nephroureterectomies, and 486 donor nephrectomies. No clips failed in this series.[5]

Hem-o-lok Clip Applicator (Fig. 20)

This device is autoclavable and reusable. It cannot be dismantled. The parts of hem-o-lok clip applicators are:
- *Handle*: The handle has a palm grip and a thumb grip. The finger grip moves while the palm is fixed and provides support.
- *Rotator*: This features the color code of the clips to be applied. It helps in rotating the jaws. The shaft connects the handle to the tip and the jaws. The shaft has a vent for cleaning and sterilization.

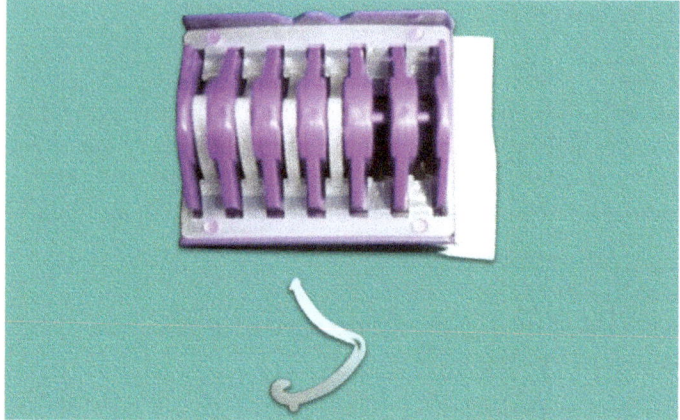

Figure 19: L-size clip color code is purple.

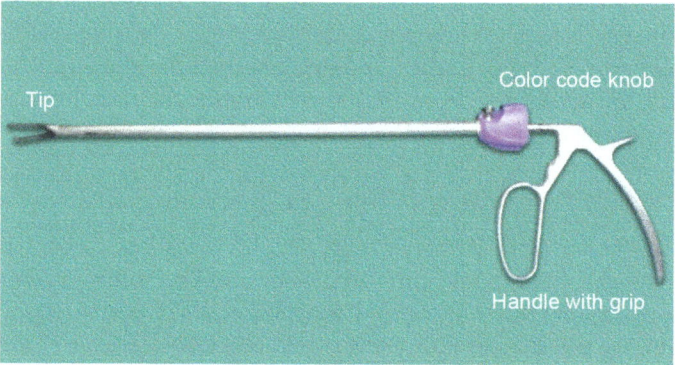

Figure 20: Clip applicator for hem-o-lok clip.

- *Tip/Jaw*: The jaw features a knob which corresponds to the knob on the clip. The jaws make an angle of approximately 5–10° to the shaft. This helps in application of the clips to the lumbar, gonadal, and adrenal vein.

How to Load the Clips?
Rules
- The clip applicator should be held at 90° to the handle of the clip.
- This should ensure that the knob fits into the corresponding notch on the tip of the jaw and the handle of the clip fits into the groove.

Hem-o-lok™ Clip: Rules for Application (Fig. 21)
- Always circumferentially dissect the vessel in concern prior to application.
- Hear the click of the knob after application of the clip.
- Always see the knob of the clip prior to application.

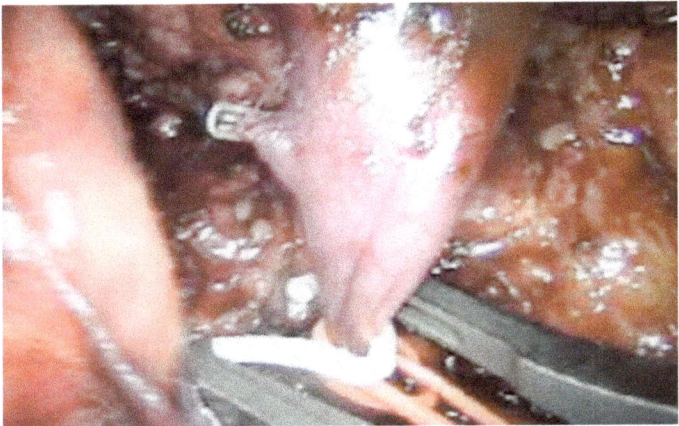
Figure 21: Always see the knob of hem-o-lok clip prior to application.

- Always apply two clips on the patient side.
- At least leave 2 mm cuff beyond the cut end of the clip.[5]

Hem-o-lok clips can be removed as follows:
- Hem-o-lok™ clip remover
- The clip can be cut open with harmonic scalpel.
- It can also be removed using scissors or two jaws of robotic needle holder.

Interlocking metal clips (also called as biting clips) (Allport™ Ethicon Endo-Surgery Inc., Cincinnati OH, LigaMX™, Ligaclip) (Ethicon Endo-Surgery Inc., OH), Endoclip (Autosuture, US surgical, Norwalk, CT). These clips are radiopaque and are interlocking, they are useful in securing smaller vessels such as the adrenal vein and the lumbar veins. They can be removed on the backbench and hence are useful in donor nephrectomy. These clips come preloaded and have clips in the set of 12–20. LigaMX™ (15 clips multiload). All these have a one-time use/one-patient use feature.

The typical preloaded clip applicator has the following components:
- *Handle*: The handle features an indicator which indicates the amount of clips consumed (the indicator color changes from white to orange as the clips get consumed). The finger grip gets locked once all the clips in the preloaded cartridge are consumed.
- *Shaft*: The length of the shaft is 32 cm (LigaMX™).
- *Tip*: The tip of a preloaded clip applicator has two metal jaws. Both the jaws move. Once the clip is deployed through the shaft, the clip is simultaneously further deployed in between the jaws. The jaws are capable of movement on a 360° axis.

Types of Interlocking Clips (Fig. 22)
- *Ligaclip™ AllPort*: This is manufactured by Ethicon Endo-Surgery, it is compatible with port size of 5 mm. It is available in a cartridge of

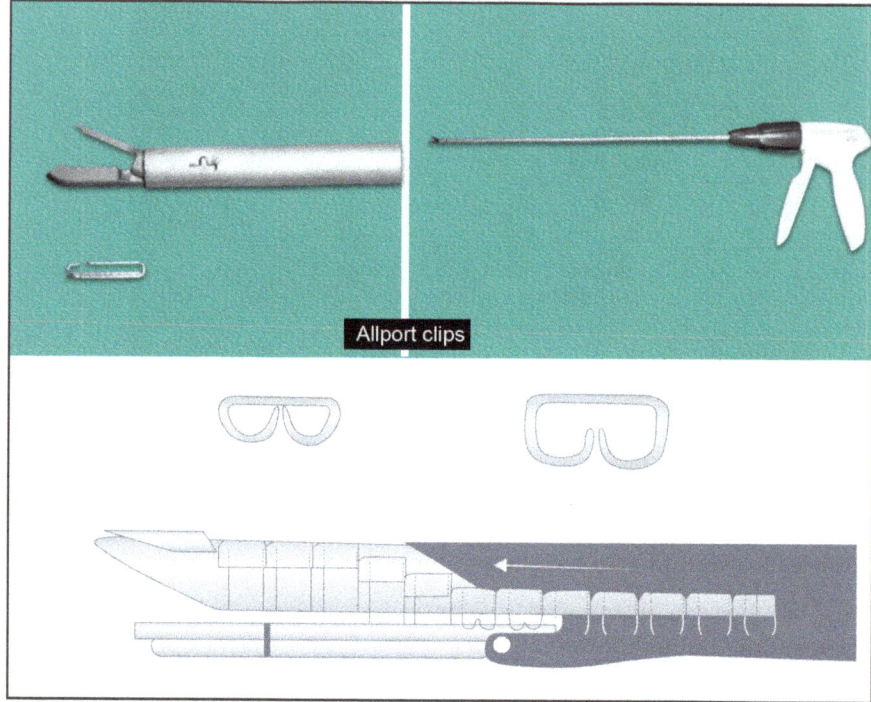

Figure 22: The Allport clips showing the way the clips are housed in a multiload applicator.

20–30 clips. It is available as medium, medium large, or large sizes. The clip loading is automatic.

- *Ligaclip^{TM} right angle*: It is manufactured by Ethicon Endo-Surgery, it is compatible with port size of 10 mm. It is available in a cartridge of 20 clips. It is available as medium-large sizes. The clip loading is automatic.
- *Ligaclip^{TM} MCA*: It is manufactured by Ethicon Endo-Surgery, it is compatible with port size of 12 mm. It is available in a cartridge of 20 clips. It is available as large size. The clip loading is automatic.
- *Endoclip^{TM}*: It is manufactured by Autosuture. It is compatible with port size of 5 mm. It is available in a cartridge of 20 clips. It is available as medium-large size. The clip loading is with separate lever.
- *Endoclip^{TM} II*: It is manufactured by Autosuture. It is compatible with port size of 10 mm. It is available in a cartridge of 20 clips. It is available as medium-large and large size. The clip loading is automatic.
- *Endoclip^{TM} multiclip applier*: It is manufactured by Autosuture. It is compatible with port size of 10 mm. It is available in a cartridge of eight clips. It is available as medium-large and large size. The clip loading is automatic.

LAPAROSCOPIC STAPLERS[6]

Broadly, the staplers can be classified as:
- Circular
- Linear
- Linear cutting
- Ligating

The linear staplers can be further classified as:
- *Cutting*: Six parallel rows of staples are fired. Once this is fired, a knife follows which leaves three staplers on either side. Always the staple line extends beyond the cut edge to avoid leaving any nonsecured edge. The knife cannot be redeployed without reloading the stapler.
- *Noncutting staplers*: These staplers simply fire four rows of staples and are helpful in right-sided donor nephrectomies for gaining extra length of the vein and repairing bladder injuries.

  The staplers can also be classified by length of staple line 30 mm/35 mm, 45 mm, and 60 mm. Further they can be classified depending on whether the firing end is articulating or otherwise. All the staplers have a rotating shaft. A stapling device has the following main components (**Fig. 23**):
    - *Cartridge*: They are further classified depending on length of the cartridge (30 mm, 45 mm, and 60 mm).
    - Cartridges are color-coded. White cartridge is for vascular stapling and blue is for other tissues. White is meant for compression of tissues to <1 mm, whereas blue is meant for tissue compression to <1.5 mm.
    - *Shaft*: Shaft can be straight or articulating.
    - *Handle*: It has two or three parts depending on the make, it has an additional button which during use will first insert suturing staples and later between the staple lines it will incise and cut.

  Recently, power staplers are available which are automated and use the battery energy for above actions.

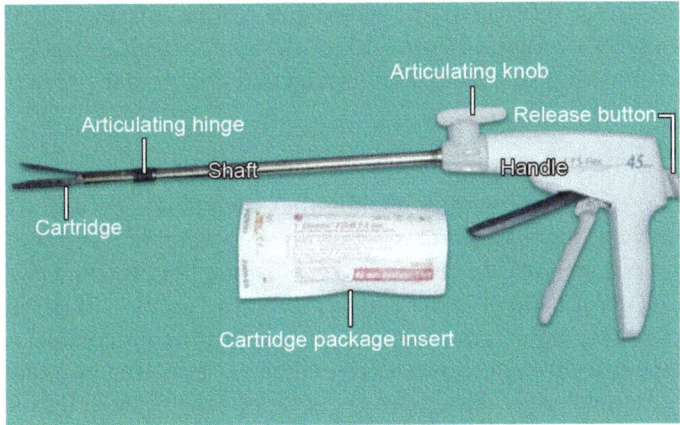

Figure 23: Parts of a stapler.

MISCELLANEOUS INSTRUMENTS

- *Stone removal forcep*: It is an instrument with working length of 42 cm with 5 mm diameter. It has spatulated end which is curved and measures 6 cm in length. It has rounded nontraumatic tip. It is useful for delivering stone during laparoscopic pyelolithotomy, nephrolithotomy as well as during hilar dissection, single-port transvesical prostatectomy.
- *Laparoscopic Satinsky forceps*: It is 10 mm in diameter and has 40 cm length. Jaw length is 7 cm. It also has cleaning port for instrument cleaning. It is available as single-action or double-action, i.e., either only one or both the jaws are mobile.
- *Probeplus II (Ethicon Endo-Surgery, OH)*: This instrument is used for laparoscopic stone surgery. The components of this instrument include:
  - *Handle*: The handle has two buttons—one for suction and one for irrigation. It also has a corresponding tubing for suction and irrigation ports. The handle also has a monopolar cautery attachment. The hub of the handle has a red button for detaching the shaft/probe. The probe rotates on its own axis.

    The probe has an outer covering and inner insert. The outer covering features a knob for rotating the probe and a cannula which helps in performing suction and irrigation at the distal end.

    The inner insert is available in two types:
    - *Needle tip*: Used for incising the pelvis and the ureter
    - *Spatula tip*: Used for dislodging the calculus. The insert can be retracted in and out and helps in precise control.
- Bull dog clip applier:

  The parts of the instrument are:
  - *Handle*: It has a finger grip and a thumb grip. In addition, it also has a knob (lock) for applying and releasing the bulldog clamp.
  - The shaft is self-rotating and has a cleaning vent. The tip of the applier has a knob which gets fixed with the socket of the bulldog clamp.
  - *Laparoscopic telescopes*: The telescopes can be classified depending on angle of view, size (5 mm, 10 mm), rigid or flexitip, and length of telescope (long and short) and coaxial and noncoaxial.

ANGLE OF VIEW (FIG. 24)

Three varieties of telescopes are available. They include 0°, 30°, and 45°.
- *0° lens*: It is a straight lens and typically used in operations on the pelvis. These operations include those on the prostate, bladder, and the lower ureter. The color code of these lens is green. The method of sterilization is autoclavable. Light transmission is through fiberoptic cables. Image transmission is through rod lens (H_2). They are available as 10 mm and 5 mm. Although longer telescopes are available, the usual length is 33 cm (working length) (total 39 cm: eyepiece to tip).

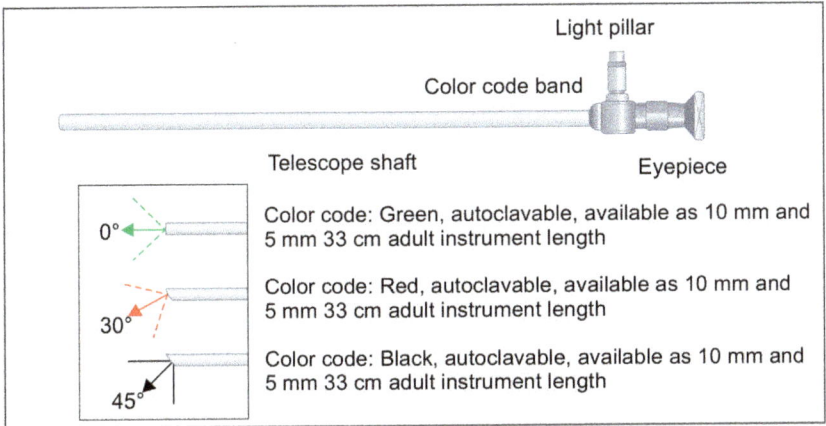

Figure 24: Laparoscopes: Angle of view.

- *30° lens*: This lens which has a color code red is used, the length is 33 cm. They are sterilized with an autoclave. The lens is typically used in surgeries on the kidney as the lens helps in visualizing the posterior aspect of renal hilum.
- *45° lens*: The use of these telescopes is not common color code is black, 33 cm in length.

SPECIAL LAPAROSCOPES

- *Coaxial cable laparoscopes*: The Olympus Endoeye™ has a coaxial light cable. It is particularly useful in single-site surgery as the light pillar of the routinely used camera produces a "nutcracker" effect because of clashing of instruments. The coaxial light cable helps in preventing clashing. A few variations in this laparoscope are available which include laparoscopes with an extender and a flexible tip laparoscope, both these variations are helpful in preventing crowding and clashing of instruments.
- *Endocameleon*: This telescope has a feature of having an interchangeable angle of view (0–120). The angle of view can be decided according to the procedure to be done and surgeon preference.
- *3D laparoscopes*: These laparoscopes give a 3D vision. The surgical field has to be viewed with 3D glasses.
- *Needloscopes*: They can be introduced through a miniport or a Veress needle.

NEWER INSTRUMENTS

Instruments with Increased Degree of Freedom

A limitation in laparoscopy is the reduction in the range of motion due to the fixed trocar position, which determines the angle of the instrument to the working field. The incision point reduces the degree of freedom (DOF) of any instrument to only four—yaw, pitch, rotation, and insertion (**Figs. 25 and 26**).

This drawback can be partially overcome by use of angulated instrument tips, such as a right angle dissector, and adequate trocar arrangement. Several laparoscopic instruments have been developed which provide six or seven DOF.

Dextérité Surgical System DEX® (France)

The instrument handle is a grip-type handle, which is connected by a mechanical joint to the instrument shaft.
- Hand held for haptic feedback
- Motorized instruments
- Motor-assisted rotation of the needle

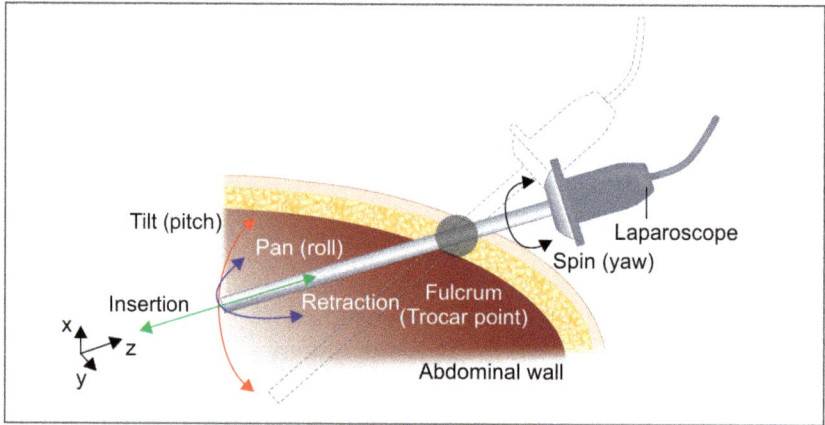

Figure 25: Laparoscope with co-axial cable.

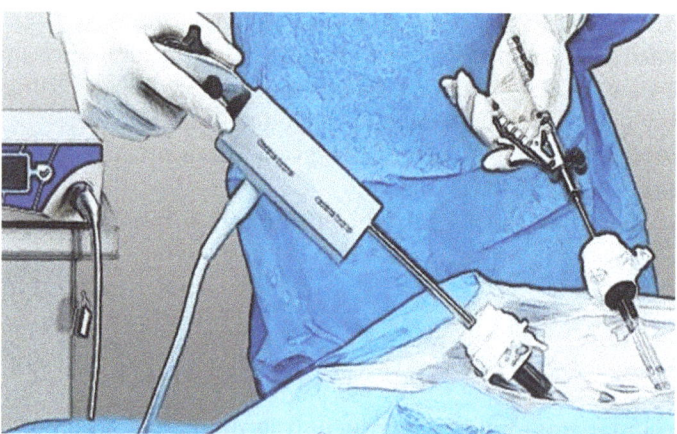

Figure 26: Dextérité surgical system DEX® (France).

Ergonomic and Articulate Handle for Postural Comfort

7° of freedom: 3D distal mobility

Other articulating instruments available are: Artisential articulating laparoscopic instrument(s) (LIVSMED, South Korea), HandX™ by Human Xtensions (Israel), FlexDex system (Olympus), Radius Surgical System (2007) [Tuebingen Scientific (Germany)], and The Autonomy® and LaparoAngle® [Cambridge Endo (USA)].

NEW PLATFORMS FOR LAPAROSCOPY

Ergonomic Chair

Two ergonomic chairs are available.

Ergonomic Body Support (Fig. 27)

It consists of a platform with foot pedal, a semi-standing support, a remote control, and a chest support.

ETHOS™ Platform (Fig. 28)

- The surgeon has two adjustable armrests and footrests with integrated foot switches which enable electrically motorized movements of the chair.
- The sitting position and armrests reduce the fulcrum effect of laparoscopy.

ROBOTICS SURGERY IN UROLOGY

The use of robotic-assisted laparoscopic surgery has increased exponentially over the past few decades. There are many theoretical advantages of the

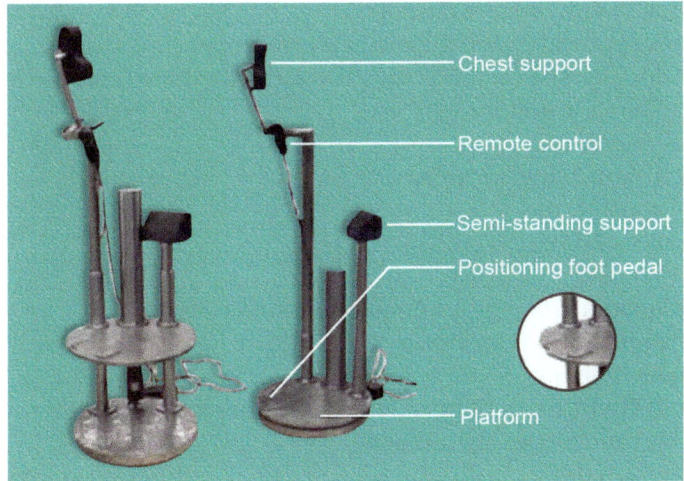

Figure 27: Ergonomic body support.

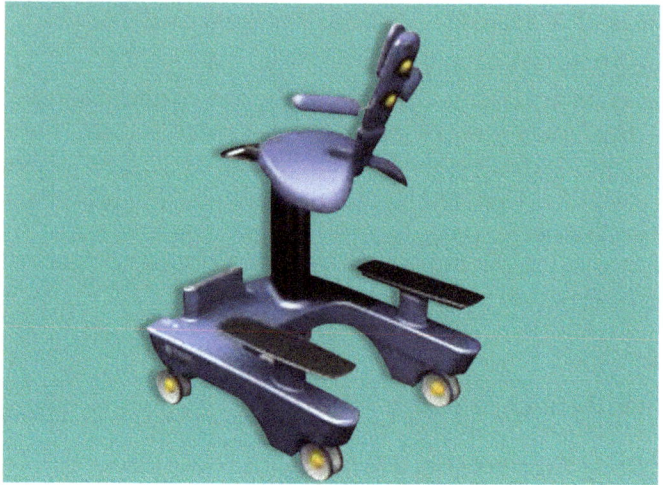

Figure 28: ETHOS™ platform.

robotic surgical system which include 3D, HD vision improved dexterity, and tremor filtration.

Short History of Robotic Devices

- *1980*: DARPA (Defense Advanced Research Projects Agency) remote (battlefield) surgery research program
- *1996*: ARTEMIS: System used in porcine model. Open console and three single arms.
- 1999- Zeus: Computer Motion Inc. (USA) developed the voice-controlled camera arm AESOP, and the ZEUS system, enabling long-distance manipulation. Intuitive surgical acquired computer motion in 2004.
- *1999*: First da Vinci system introduced
- *2000*: FDA approval da Vinci 2000 for laparoscopy
- *2003*: Major upgrade: Addition of fourth arm, HD vision, and Tile Pro
- *2006*: da Vinci S introduced
- *2009*: da Vinci Si
  - Finger-based clutch mechanism
  - Dual console
  - Enhanced HD vision (1080i)
- *2014*: da Vinci Xi
  - Multiquadrant boom—multiquadrant surgical access
  - 30° camera toggles up/down
  - Camera hopping
  - Inbuilt Firefly technology (fluorescence filter for isocyanine green)
  - Thinner and longer instruments
  - Robotic stapler
- *da Vinci X*: This system is a version between Si and Xi.

Equipment and Supplies

The basic requirement for the operating room is that it should be large enough to accommodate all the components of the robot. The various items which need to be procured beyond those available in the operating room are: Reusable robotic accessories such as sterile drapes, scopes (0° and 30°), light guide cables, specific 8-mm robotic instrument compatible trocars. The hospital needs to decide the inventory prior to commencement of cases. The other equipment which are needed are a suction/irrigator, scope warmer, a surgeon chair with an optimal height so that the surgeon can see comfortably in the console, video equipment for recording. To say it in short, robotics is "labor intensive." A dedicated team is essential. A constantly changing team might hamper the program from an efficacy and result standpoint.

The components of the robot include a patient cart, a vision cart, and the console. The surgeon sits on the console and controls the masters. The currently available robot is known as the *da Vinci Si and da Vinci Xi*. The previous two generations were *da Vinci* and *da Vinci S*.

The patient cart has the following components: The central pillar and the patient safety manipulator (PSM). The arms work on the principle of remote center technology where in the arms move around a fixed point in space and provide the expected dexterity and precision.

Robotic Instrumentation (Fig. 29)

- *Robotic trocars*: These are reusable and are available with reducers. The shaft of the trocars has a black band which is known as the "remote center." After insertion of the port, the band should lie on the inner surface of the peritoneum. This band acts as a remote point in space around which the robotic arms move. The robotic ports can be sterilized with autoclave or plasma sterilization. The robotic trocars are available as 8-mm and 5-mm trocars.
- *Robotic drapes*: These are one-time use drapes which have adapter to be installed on the robotic arms.
- *Robotic working instruments*: They are robotic shears, robotic needle holder, robotic Maryland (bipolar forceps), robotic scissors, robotic hook, all these instruments have a limited use depending on whether they are training instruments, or pediatric use instruments.

The parts of typical robotic instrument are as follows. The only contraindication for its use are its use on cartilage, bone, and hard objects.

These instruments are called as EndoWrist instrument™. The five main components are as follows:
1. The release lever (A)
2. The instrument shaft (B)
3. The wrist (C)
4. Tip or end effector (D)
5. Instrument housing (E)

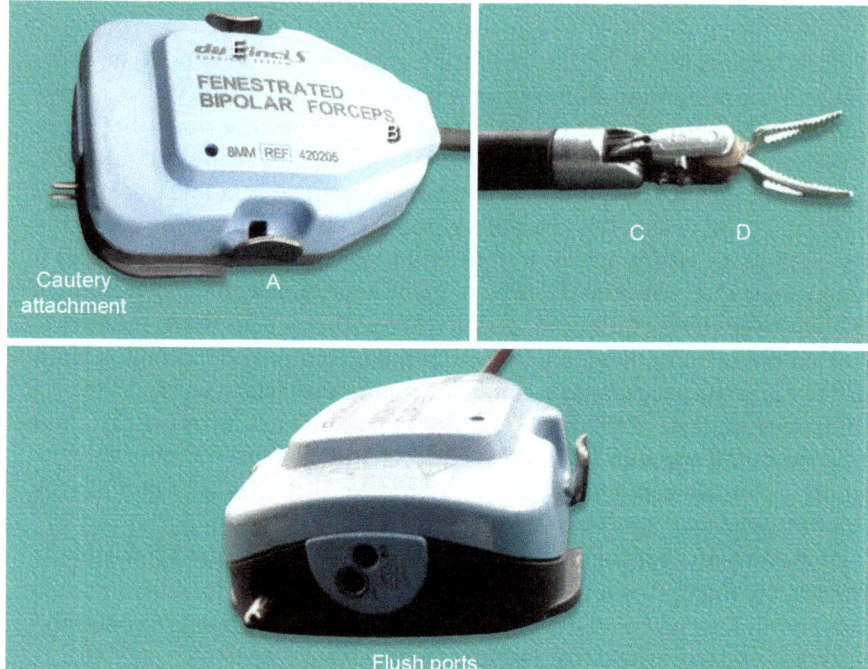

Figure 29: The release lever (A), the instrument shaft (B), the wrist (C), tip or end effector (D), and instrument housing (E).

Instrument Housing (E)

The da Vinci S, Si instruments can be differentiated by their length, housing color, and graphics. The maximum total length of the shaft is 52 cm. The da Vinci S and Si have a blue housing. Red housing is for training instrument. Light gray for da Vinci. The S instrument are 5 cm long. The housing on the profile has two flush ports (Si) and three flush ports (S). The emergency release grip is seen on the housing for release of stuck instruments. The housing also has ESU connection probe.

Once the robot is draped, it is brought near the patient and attached to the laparoscopic/robotic ports. This process is called as "docking."

Robotic Systems for Single-port/Single-site Surgery: Recent Advances

SP 1098 Platform (da Vinci) (Fig. 30)

- It has 3D/HD flexible telescope and three flexible instruments (6 mm) on a single arm.
- Introduced through umbilical incision (2.5 cm), the flexible instruments have a snake style wrist which separates to achieve triangulation.

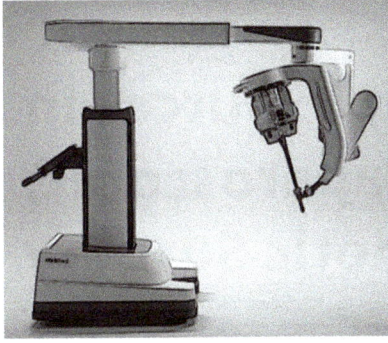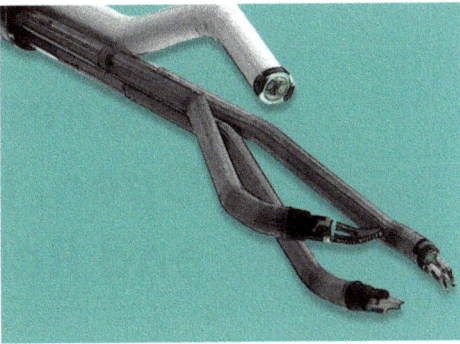

Figure 30: SP 1098 Platform (da Vinci).

- Device is controlled by use of EndoWrist technology at its distal joint and an additional elbow joint which facilitates intracorporeal re-establishment of triangulation without requiring crossing of the instruments.

Alternative and Upcoming Robotic Systems

Telelap Alf-X (Senhance), Medtronic: (MiroSurge), Avatera: (Germany), Revo-I: (South Korea), Medicaroid: (Japan), Verb Surgical, SPORT-Surgical System (Titan) (for single-port LESS).

Newer devices coming up are in experimental stages for LESS such as ARAKNES (Array of Robots Augmenting the Kinematics of Endoluminal Surgery), IREP (Insertable Robotic Effectors Platform), University of Nebraska Robot System, Waseda-University Device.

Another set of platform which is being developed is Bedside-based device for robot assisted single-port surgery and laparoscopy such as SURGIBOT [Spider System (Transenterix)] and LODEM (flexible locally operated end-effector manipulator) (Japan).

REFERENCES

1. Clayman RV, Kavoussi LR, Soper JN, Dierks SM, Meretyk S, Darcy MD, et al. Laparoscopic nephrectomy: Initial case report. J Urol. 1991;146(2):278-82.
2. Ratner LE, Ciseck LJ, Moore RG, Cigarroa FG, Kaufman HS, Kavoussi LR. Laparoscopic live donor nephrectomy. Transplantation.1995;60(9):1047-9.
3. Rané A, Rao P, Rao P. Single-port-access nephrectomy and other laparoscopic urologic procedures using a novel laparoscopic port (R-port). Urology. 2008;72(2):260-3; discussion: 263-4.
4. Gaur DD. Laparoscopic operative retroperitoneoscopy: use of a new device. J Urol. 1992;148(4):1137-9.
5. Ponsky L, Cherullo E, Moinzadeh A, Desai M, Kaouk J, Haber GP, et al. The Hem-o-lok clip is safe for laparoscopic nephrectomy: a multi-institutional review. Urology.2008;71(4):593-6.
6. Mcguire J, Wright IC, Leverment JN. Surgical staplers: A review. J R Coll Surg Edinb. 1997;42(1):1-9.

CHAPTER 10

Energy Sources in Open, Laparoscopic, and Robotic Surgery

"Heat cures when everything else fails"
—Hippocrates

INTRODUCTION

Surgery can be defined as the art of tissue dissection and tissue reapproximation. A variety of energy sources have been used in tissue dissection to provide energy for cutting and hemostasis. Unfortunately, many surgeons poorly understand the biophysics of these sources. For most of us, pressing the cautery pedal is like taking a leap of faith without knowing the science behind it.

Let us in the coming few pages try to understand the energy sources available in market today for different kinds of procedure.

DEFINITIONS[1]

Electrosurgery

It is the use of radiofrequency (RF) alternating current to raise the cellular temperature to vaporize or coagulate tissue.

Electrocautery is not same as electrosurgery. Electrocautery uses direct current, whereas electrosurgery uses alternating current and in electrosurgery patient is a part electrical circuit.[1]

Cautery (Kauterion = Hot Iron)

Destruction or denaturation of tissue by passive transfer of heat or application of caustic substance.
- Current = Flow of electrons during a period of time, measured in amperes
- Circuit = Pathway for the uninterrupted flow of electrons
- Voltage = Force pushing current through the resistance, measured in volts
- Impedance/resistance = Obstacle to the flow of current, measured in ohms (impedance = resistance)

CLASSIFICATION

- Based on the type of generator used:
  - Electrosurgical
  - Further subclassified into:
    - *Simple generator*: Monopolar/bipolar cautery
    - *Advanced bipolar systems*:
      - LigaSure
      - PK system
      - EnSeal
    - Ultrasonic
    - Integrated ultrasound and advance bipolar generators
    - Argon beam coagulator (ABC)
    - Lasers
    - *Others*: RF, microwave, cryo
    - Based on their use in urologic surgeries:
      - *Open surgery*: Monopolar, bipolar, vessel sealing (LigaSure and EnSeal), ultrasonic, and ABC
      - *Laparoscopic surgery*: Monopolar, bipolar, vessel sealing (LigaSure, EnSeal, and PK), ultrasonic, ABC, laser
      - *Robotic surgery*: Monopolar, bipolar, ultrasonic, and PK

Electrosurgical Generator

Frequency Spectrum (Fig. 1)

A typical electrosurgical generator takes our household current of 60 cycles/s and raises the frequency to 200,000 cycles/s. Such high frequencies are radiofrequencies, when current passes at such high frequency through the human body no neuromuscular stimulation occurs and patient does not get an electric shock.

Monopolar Generator[1]

They are the most commonly available electrosurgical units in all operating rooms (**Fig. 2**).

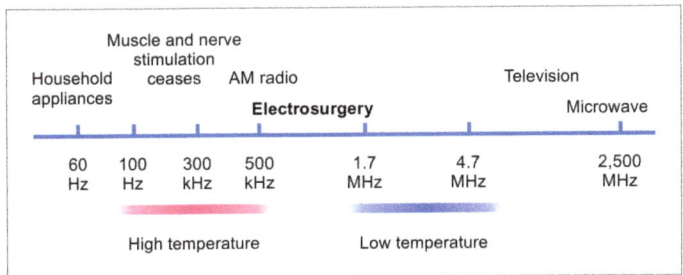

(AM: amplitude modulation)

Figure 1: Frequency spectrum.

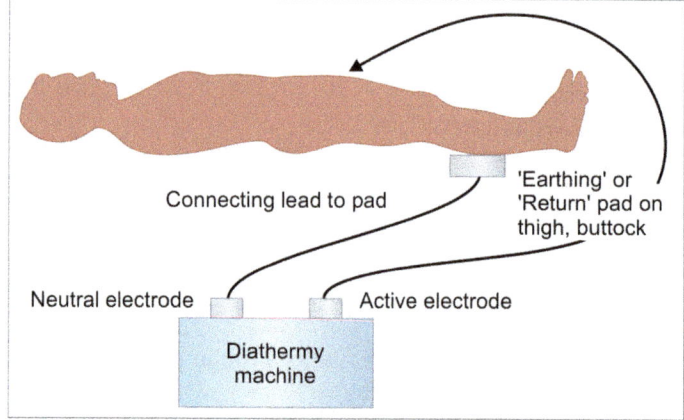

Figure 2: Monopolar circuit.

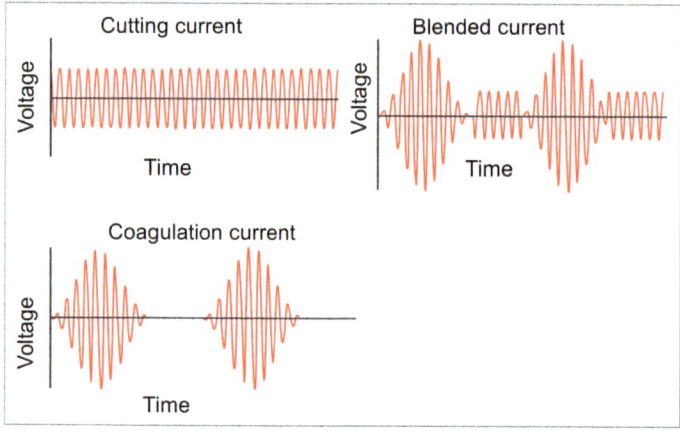

Figure 3: Waveform.

Monopolar circuit: Generator—active electrode—patient—patient return electrode.

Various waveforms generated by electrosurgical generators (**Fig. 3**) are:[1]
- *Cut*: Waveform is constant, heat is generated rapidly leading to tissue vaporization or cutting.
- *Coagulation*: Waveform is interrupted, less heat is produced, and no tissue vaporization occurs instead coagulation occurs.
- *Blend current*: It is modification of duty cycle. Using a lower duty cycle, less heat is produced and less heat produces coagulation. Conversely, higher duty cycle produces lot of heat that vaporizes tissue.

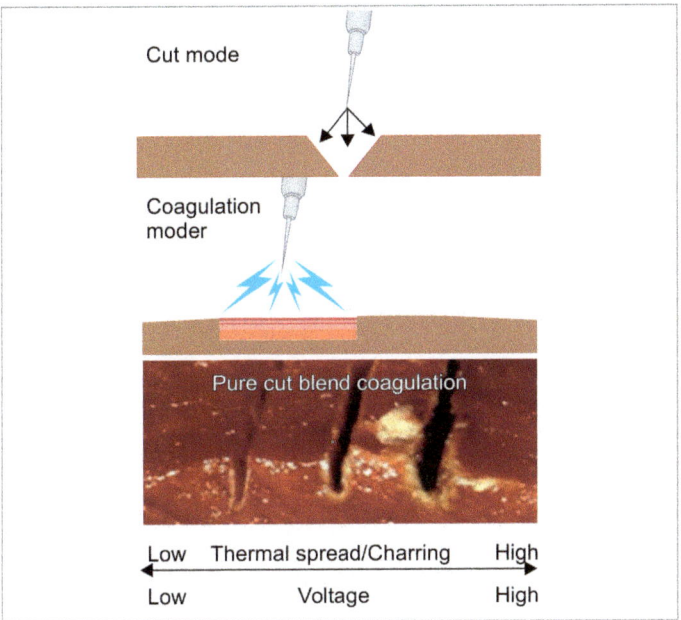

Figure 4: Electrosurgical tissue effect.

ELECTROSURGICAL TISSUE EFFECTS (FIG. 4)

Electrosurgical Cutting

By using this mode, surgeon can cut like a knife, as the intense heat produced vaporizes tissue. When the electrode is held slightly away from the tissue maximum current concentration and maximum cutting can be achieved.

Fulguration

In this mode, charring occurs involving a wider area. In fulguration mode, the duty cycle (on time) is only 6%, this leads to heating up of tissue and coagulation rather than vaporization.

Desiccation

When an electrode directly touches tissue less heat is generated as a result, the cell do not vaporize and instead dry up and form coagulum.

Surgeons can cut with coagulation current and coagulate with cutting current. Cutting current will penetrate deeper and coagulation current will have lateral spread. When coagulating with the cutting current you require less voltage and cutting with cut current also requires less voltage. The above facts have a bearing when you are using electrosurgery in laparoscopic surgery.

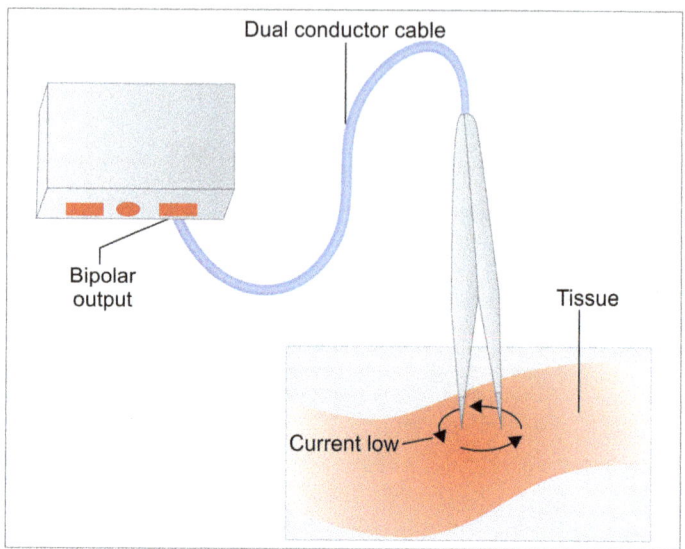

Figure 5: Bipolar circuit.

Bipolar[1]

In this form of electrosurgery, the active and the return electrode are the part of the bipolar device and no patient plate is required. The current passes from one prong of bipolar device to the other through the tissue in between and circuit is completed (**Fig. 5**).

ADVANCE BIPOLAR SYSTEMS

- *LigaSure (**Fig. 6**):* It is advanced bipolar energy source available in surgical armamentarium today. It is combines pressure and energy to create a seal. It consists of a specialized generator system that reliably seals vessels, tissue bundles, and can be used as tool for surgical ligation of tissues in open and laparoscopic surgery.

  LigaSure uses higher current and lower voltage (180 V) along with optimal pressure delivery by the instruments in order to fuse the vessel walls and to create a permanent seal. It has a feedback control mechanism, which gives an alarm once the tissue is adequately sealed. Vessels up to 7 mm can be reliably sealed using this device. It has minimal thermal spread and the seal site is often translucent, this allows the surgeon to look for hemostasis prior to cutting the tissue.

  Sealed blood vessel can withstand a rise in blood pressure equal to three times, the systolic pressure. Sealing tissue and blood vessels with this device is as effective as suture ligation or clip application.

  LigaSure devices are available for open (LigaSure precise) as well as laparoscopic surgery (LigaSure vs. LigaSure lap). LigaSure is as of now not available for robotic platform.

CHAPTER 10: Energy Sources in Open, Laparoscopic, and Robotic Surgery | 127

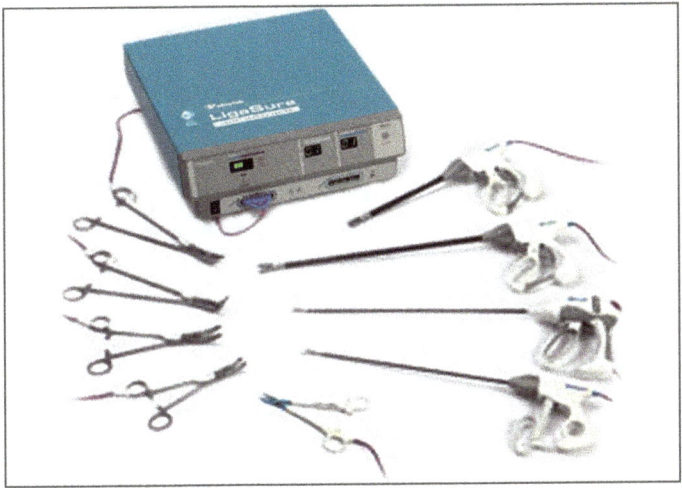

Figure 6: LigaSure.

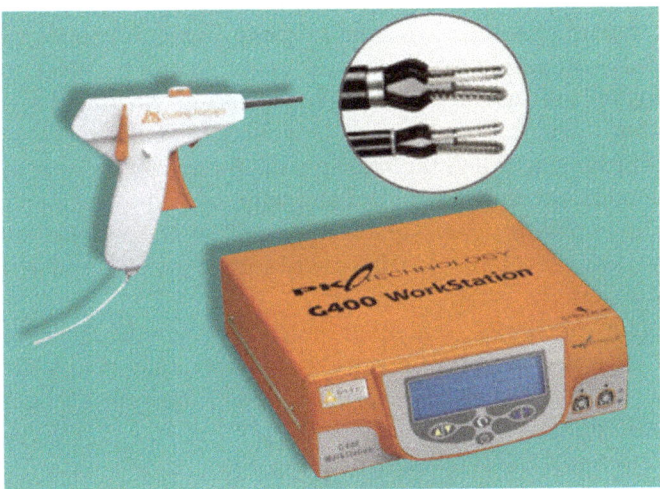

Figure 7: PK system.

- ○ Reliable, consistent permanent vessel wall fusion
- ○ Minimal thermal spread
- ○ Reduced sticking and charring
- ○ Seal strength than other energy-based techniques
- ○ Seal strength comparable to existing mechanical-based techniques
- *The Gyrus PK tissue management system (Gyrus Medical, Inc., Minneapolis, Minnesota)* (**Fig. 7**): Gyrus PK system uses bipolar RF energy to seal, transect, coagulate, dissect, vaporize, resect, and mobilize tissue all with the precision and control from one workstation. It is based on principle of vapor pulse coagulation (VPC). On application of the energy, tissue fluid

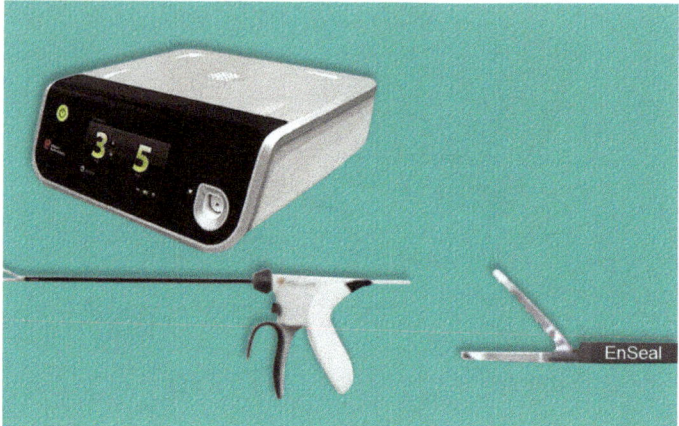

Figure 8: EnSeal.

boils producing steam which forms vapor pockets, these vapor pockets coalesce to form vapor zones. This heating of the tissue causes denaturing of vessel wall protein and coagulum formation, which occludes the vessel lumen, pulse-off periods allow tissue for cooling and moisture to return to the targeted area, greatly reducing hot spots and coagulum formation. This system provides enhanced hemostasis, uniform coagulation, minimal sticking, and less thermal spread. The Gyrus PK system has its own generator, which works in tandem with its own instruments. It has application in open surgery, laparoscopy, and robotic surgery. Separated instruments are developed for all types of surgeries but the generator can remain the same.

For open surgery PK, seal open forceps is available, for laparoscopy cutting forceps, dissecting forceps, hook and spatula are available. Recently, the PK dissecting forceps for robotic surgery was launched but not in common use till now.

- EnSeal^{TM} (SurgRx, Inc., Palo Alto, CA) (**Fig. 8**).

Ethicon Endosurgery Generator

The EnSeal tissue sealing system uses an advanced bipolar technology to seal the tissue within the blades of the instrument. It uses the patented I blade technology, which offers strong uniform compression along the tissue sealing line. EnSeal uses a smart electrode technology, which includes numerous conductive particles embedded in a plate, which is temperature-sensitive. Each of these particles acts like a discrete thermostatic switch to regulate the quantity of current that passes into the tissues in contact, thereby generating heat within it. Once the tissue starts heating above a critical level, these nanoparticles interrupt the flow of current and when the temperature dips below, the desired level they again reactivate the current, this cycle is continued till desired temperature is reached (temperature is regulated to a set level of 100°C). The procedure continues until the entire tissue segment is uniformly heated and fused without charring or sticking. Less heat is needed to accomplish fusion, since the tissue volume is minimized through compression; energy is focused about the captured segment; and the vessel walls are fused through compression and protein denaturation. It can seal vessels up to 7 mm with a seal strength of seven times the systolic pressure and has one-step actuation for both cutting and sealing. EnSeal was United States (US) Food and Drug Administration (FDA) approved in 2003.

EnSeal has instruments for open surgery (e.g., super jaw tissue sealer)[2] as well as laparoscopic surgery (straight and curved tissue sealer) but not for robotic arm. It has an articulating tissue sealer (G2 articulating tissue sealer)[2] which can have application in single port surgery.

Ultrasonic Generators (Fig. 9)

Physics of Ultrasound

Ultrasound is longitudinal wave, whose frequency is above the audible range. High power ultrasound can be harnessed to produce surgical cutting, coagulation, and dissection of tissues. This involves mechanical propagation of sound (pressure) waves from a power source via a medium to an active blade element.

Ultrasonic dissectors are of two types:
1. *Low power*: These operate at a low frequency and cleaves water-containing tissues by cavitations. The organized structures with low water content are sparse, e.g., arteries, bile ducts, etc. For example, (ultrasonic cavitational aspirators) bring liver surgery and neurosurgery (Cusa, Selector). They do not achieve coagulation.

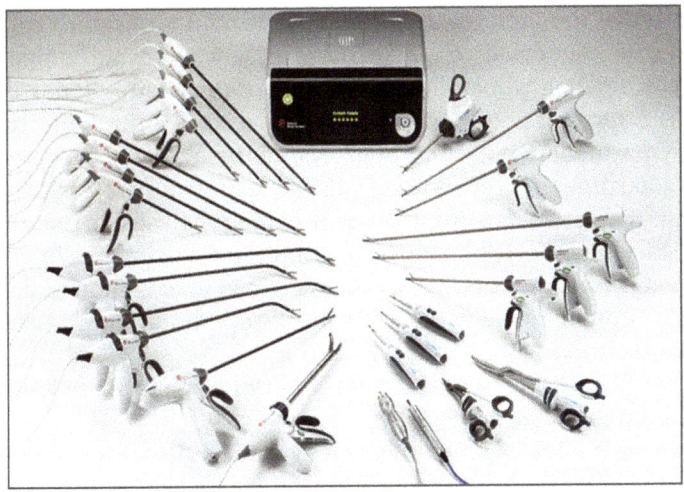

Figure 9: Ultrasonic generator.

2. *High power*: These systems operate at high frequency of 55.5 kHz, which cleave loose areolar tissues by frictional heating and, therefore, cut and coagulate the edges simultaneously. In laparoscopic surgery, high power ultrasonic systems are utilized extensively. Ultrasurgical devices consist of a generator, hand piece, and blade. The ultrasonic transducer is housed in the hand piece, a collection of piezoelectric crystals sandwiched under pressure between metal cylinders. The transducer is attached to a mount, which is then connected to the blade extender and blade. The harmonic scalpel cools the hand piece with air. AutoSonix and SonoSurg systems have a large diameter hand piece made of heat-dissipating materials to remove the heat and stop heat buildup.

Once activated, the electrical energy is passed to hand piece, piezoelectric ceramic disks in hand piece become excited, this electrical energy is transferred into mechanical energy. Mechanical energy is amplified at nodes in shaft of the instrument and reaches a maximum amplitude of 55,500 cycle/s at blade tip, when in contact with tissue pressure causes coaptation of vessels, H+ bonds are broken and cell protein is denatured forming sticky coagulum.

Ultrasonic hook or spatula blade can coagulate blood vessels within the 2 mm diameter range quite easily and also the scissors can coagulate vessels up to 5 mm in diameter. Heat generated using the harmonic is limited to temperature below 80°C. This leads to reduced tissue charring and desiccation and also minimizes the zone of thermal injury. Ultrasonic surgery causes slower coagulation than that observed with either electrosurgery or laser surgery, but is as effective.

Incisions made with the ultrasonically activated scalped or cold steel scalpel heal almost identically and, therefore, are superior to electrosurgically made incisions.

Due to the vibration from the active blade, the coagulated tissue does not stick to the active element, this is a unique feature of ultrasonic coagulator as compared to other sources. Also there is less charring compared to other sources, leading to better visualization of the tissue planes thereby improving the surgical precision. It also has a second cutting mechanism, which is the particular "power cutting" offered by a relatively sharp blade vibrating 55,500 times per second over a distance of 80 μm. Excessive heating of ultrasonic dissectors causing collateral damage is well documented in clinical practice, therefore, one must be careful while using this instrument as a dissector. Ultrasonic surgical dissection allows coagulation and cutting with less instrument exchanges (reduction in operating time), decreased smoke, and no current.

Ultrasonic dissectors are available for both open (harmonic focus) and laparoscopic surgery (harmonic ACE).

Now harmonic ACE^{TM} curved shears is available for da Vinci S/Si system.

Salient Features

- Mechanical energy at 55,500 vibrations/s
- Disrupts hydrogen bonds and forms a coagulum
- Temperature by harmonic scalpel—80°C
- Temperature through electrocoagulation—200–300°C
- Minimal collateral damage
- Multifunctional instruments
- Less tissue sticking
- Less smoke formation
- No stray energy
- No neuromuscular stimulation
- No electrical energy to or through the patient

Factors Affecting Cutting and Coagulation in Ultrasonic Devices

- Tissue tension
- Blade sharpness
- Time
- Power level
- Grip force

It can be sterilized by autoclaving/ethylene oxide (EtO)/Sterrad.

Integrated Ultrasound and Advanced Bipolar Generators

The Thunderbeat™ (Olympus)[3] was the first device to integrate the ultrasonic and advanced bipolar generator. Both the generators can be used interchangeably. Ethicon has also come up with an integrated generator ETHICON ENDO-SURGERY™ compatible with all harmonic and EnSeal devices. The sealing capabilities of this device is necessarily same as ultrasonic or advanced bipolar depending on the generator used.

Comparison of Various Energy Sources

Device	Safety: Minimal thermal spread	Vessel sealing efficacy on vessels ≤7 mm	Efficiency: Treatment time	Consistency: Independent of user	Utility: Multiple uses
Harmonic scalpel	1 mm	Poor	Excellent	Poor	Excellent
Gyrus PK	2–6 mm	Poor	Excellent	Fair	Fair
LigaSure V	2–3 mm	Excellent	Good	Excellent	Fair
EnSeal	1 mm	Excellent	Poor	Excellent	Poor

ARGON BEAM COAGULATOR[1]

The ABC uses RF electrical energy, which is delivered to tissue through a jet of argon gas. It provides noncontact, monopolar, and electrothermal hemostasis. Argon is inert and noncombustible. Easily ionizes, making it more conductive and safe medium for electric current to pass. The depth of penetration is less and less smoke is produced.

It is particularly useful in repair of solid organ injury and finds its utility in cases of partial nephrectomy in urological spectrum of surgeries. Drawback of ABCs in laparoscopy is that it increases the intra-abdominal pressures dangerously and may cause fatal gas embolism (**Fig. 10**).

Properties of Argon
- Inert
- Noncombustible
- Easily ionized by RF energy
- Creates bridge between electrode and the tissue
- Displaces nitrogen and oxygen
- Advantages of ABC
- Decrease smoke and odor
- Decreases blood loss, rebleeding, and tissue damage
- Flexible

Light amplification through stimulated emission of radiation (LASER): All the discussion about lasers in urology revolves around prostatectomies. Lasers have been used in laparoscopy. Lasers described for laparoscopic use have been CO_2, diode, KTP, holmium, thulium. Though the use is still not widespread, there have been many animal studies and few clinical trials. CO_2 laser has been used in open surgeries like wide local excision for carcinoma penis, head, and neck surgeons used it for excision of head and neck malignancies.

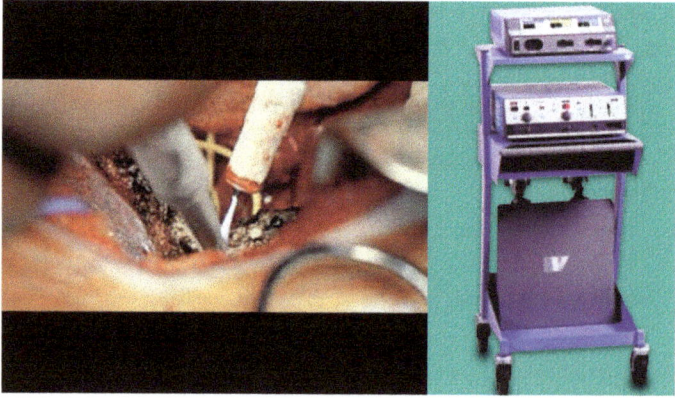

Figure 10: Argon beam coagulator.

In laparoscopy, CO_2 laser has been used in gynecological practice to treat endometriosis, etc.

Lot of experimental work in animal models has been done demonstrating utility of laser in laparoscopic partial nephrectomy. Clinical studies have also demonstrated use of thulium and holmium lasers for laparoscopic partial nephrectomy.

A study by KUN Pang et al. demonstrated use for thulium laser for resection of distal ureter with bladder cuff in case of transitional cell carcinoma (TCC) kidney. An Italian study has demonstrated use of thulium laser for partial nephrectomy. On the whole, use of lasers in laparoscopic surgeries is yet to find its distinct place, but as the search for a better cutting and coagulating energy source continues, more studies on lasers in laparoscopy are going to tell us if lasers in laparoscopy are here to stay.

Note: Details about physics of laser can be found elsewhere in the book.

Radiofrequency Ablation

It consists of a probe, which may be a simple needle, or in form of prongs. The probe is mounted on a RF generator. The generator sends RF waves through the needle, RF energy causes atoms in the cells to vibrate that will create friction. This generates heat (as much as 100°C) and leads to coagulative necrosis. The use of RF ablation as energy source is limited.

Gill et al. have studied animal models of laparoscopic and percutaneous RF ablation of part of kidney. The application of RF ablation is more studied in malignancy, e.g., ablation of small renal masses and carcinoma prostate. It is as of now less likely to be used as a hemostatic agent.

Microwave Ablation

Like RF ablation, microwave ablation is also being used for tumor ablation rather than as a hemostatic agent for surgery. It is an alternate way of producing thermal coagulation of tissue, microwaves induce ultrahigh speed (2,450 MHz) alternating field current, resulting in rotation of water molecule. This heats up the tissue causing coagulative necrosis. Majority of experience comes from its use in hepatocellular carcinoma. It is being used in management of small renal masses and carcinoma prostate. It can be used laparoscopically as well as image guided.

Cryotherapy

The cell destruction by rapidly cooling the cell and the thawing is the principle of cryotherapy. It can be used laparoscopically as well as under image guidance. It is being used in management of small renal masses and carcinoma prostate. As of now it cannot be used for cutting and coagulating tissue in open and minimal access surgery.

SAFETY CONSIDERATION[1]

- *Patient pad placement*: Patient plate should be in contact over a large surface area at least 100 cm^2. One should avoid bony prominences; soft pads are better than metallic plates as they give uniform area of contact. The pads should be placed near the area of interest.
- *Demodulated current*: Modern generators filter demodulated current so that only electrical current of 250–2,000 kHz is delivered. Demodulated currents occur in common practice when an active electrode is activated off metal after which touched toward the metal, like the common practice of "buzzing a hemostat." Demodulated currents produce neuromuscular activity. The flickering movements in laparoscopic surgery may be caused by demodulation of current to diaphragm and adjoining muscles.
- During minimally invasive surgery:[1]
  - *Direct application*: Direct application of active electrode to an unintended area causes tissue injury.
  - *Direct coupling*: When the activated active electrode touches a nearby metallic instrument it energizes it and this stray energy may find its way to the patient plate causing injury. Like if a monopolar hook touches a laparoscopic telescope, if the telescope is in turn in contact with bowel. The energized telescope will cause thermal injury to the bowel (**Fig. 11**).
  - *Insulation failure*: Breaks in the insulation can cause energy to stray and cause tissue injury. For example, if a portion of monopolar hook has an insulation break and this area comes in contact with bowel, it will cause the current to leak and may lead to bowel injury (**Fig. 12**).
  - *Capacitative coupling*: Capacitance is the charge generated when an insulator separates two conductors. This charge has a tendency to

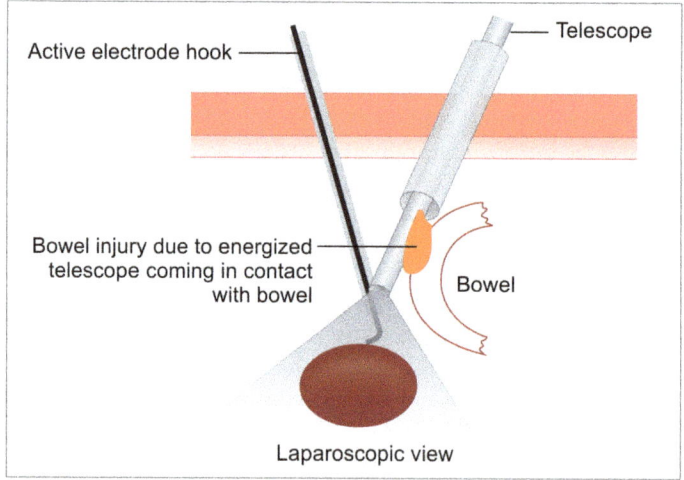

Figure 11: Direct coupling of current.

CHAPTER 10: Energy Sources in Open, Laparoscopic, and Robotic Surgery | 135

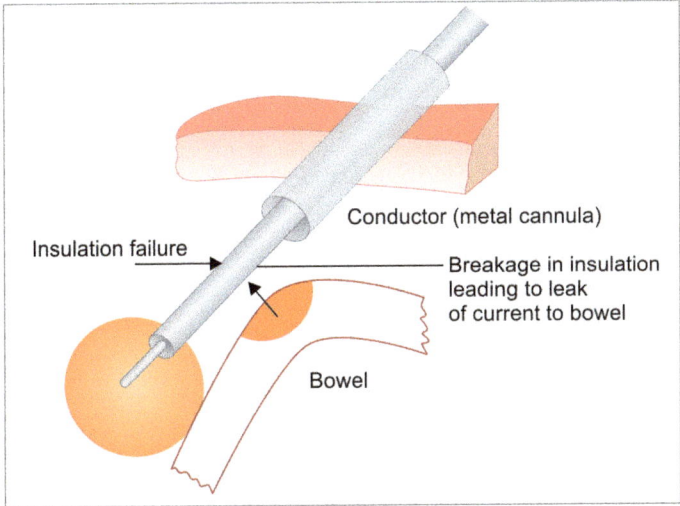

Figure 12: Insulation failure.

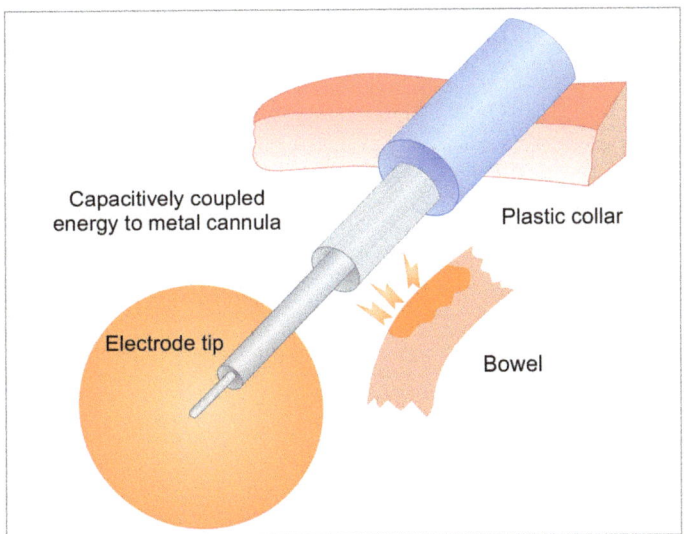

Figure 13: Capacitative coupling.

complete circuit and cause surrounding organ injury. For example, hybrid cannula with suction and hook have a metallic hook covered by an insulator which is fixed within a metallic suction cannula. The insulator between to metallic conductor acts as a capacitor and when it comes in contact with adjacent bowel the stray energy may be leaked causing a bowel injury (**Fig. 13**).

REFERENCES

1. Association of Surgeons in Training. . Prinicpals in electrosurgery. [online] Available from: www.asit.org/assets/documents/Prinicpals_in_electrosurgery.pdf. [Last Accessed February, 2021].
2. Ethicon. Enseal G2 tissuesealers. [online] Available from: http://www.ethicon.com/healthcare-professionals/products/advanced-energy/ enseal/enseal-g2-tissue-sealers. [Last Accessed February, 2021].
3. Olympus. Products. [online] Available from: http://medical.olympusamerica.com/products/thunderbeat-1. [Last Accessed February, 2021].

CHAPTER 11

Accessories

URETERIC CATHETER

Material
The material is polyethylene with radiopaque coating, a Luer lock/simple adapter is provided at proximal end of the catheter for attaching the syringe. Markings—single marking at every centimeter. The marking is as follows:
- 5 cm—single mark
- 10 cm—two marks
- 15 cm—three marks
- 20 cm—four marks
- 25 cm—five marks
- 30 cm—one bold mark
- 35 cm—two marks
- 40 cm—three marks
- 45 cm—four marks
- 50 cm—five marks

No marking beyond 50 cm. The length generally is 70 cm.

Types of Ureteric Catheter
The ureteric catheters are classified depending on the tip configuration:
- *Open-end catheter* (**Figs. 1A and C**)[1]: Single opening at the tip, no side openings. It is used for drainage and performing pyelography. It can be passed over glide wire across obstruction or kink.
- *Close-end catheter*[2]: This always comes with a stylet. It has a round blunt tip and two holes on the side.
- *Cone-tipped ureteric catheter*[3] (**Fig. 1D**): Available in different sizes. The size is described as the size of tip and the catheter. The tip is pointed and a hole just proximal to the tip. This is used for bulb ureterogram. Generally, available as 5 Fr and 14 Fr (bulb) and 4 Fr and 8 Fr (bulb) (cook). This has to be back loaded if it is 14 Fr, smaller bulb can be passed without back loading through a larger cystoscope sheath.

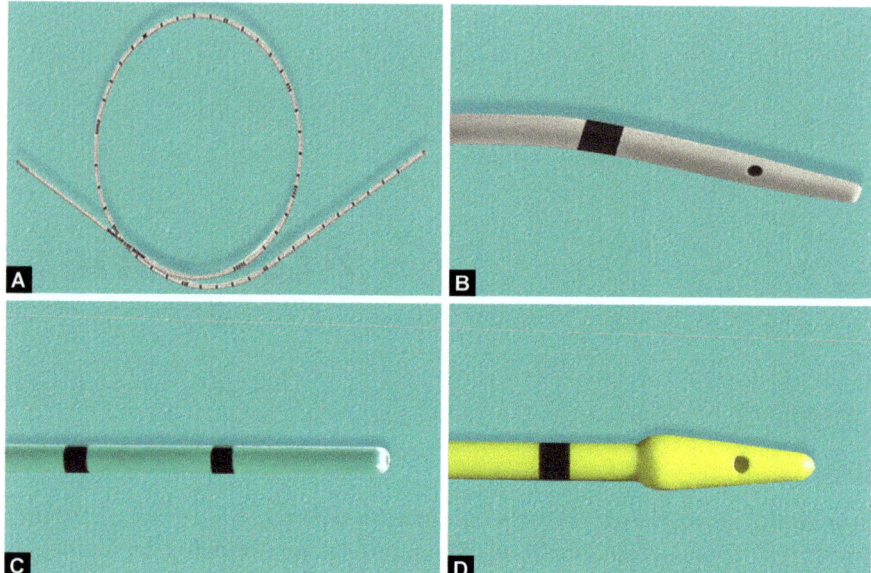

Figures 1A to D: (A) Ureteric catheter with markings; (B) Angle tipped ureteric catheter; (C) Open end ureteric catheter; (D) Cone tipped ureteric catheter.

- *Angled tip ureteral catheter (Coude)*[4] (**Fig. 1B**): This was used for negotiating an awkward ureteric orifice and kinks in the ureter. With the guidewire in use, these have become obsolete. They can be angled at either 20° or 40°.
- *Whistle tip catheter*[5]: It is oblique (like a whistle) open end catheter. It is used for performing a retrograde ureterogram.
- *Balloon ureteric catheter*: It has a separate channel where the balloon can be inflated.
- *Pig tail ureteric catheter*[6]: Available as 70 cm and 90 cm. It has a single curl at the kidney end. This can be kept as self-retaining ureteric catheter.
- *EchoTip open-end ureteral catheter*[7] (**Figs. 2A and B**): Used for drainage and irrigation. The EchoTip® band enhances ultrasonic and fluoroscopic visualization of the catheter tip location.
- *Double lumen ureteric catheter* (**Figs. 3A to C**): It is 10 Fr in size and has two channels, one opening at the tip and one on the side (**Figs. 3A to C**). The openings are approximately 1 cm apart. This is used for passing additional safety catheter or performing a contrast study without removing the preplaced wire. It is 50 cm long. The placement lumen diameter is 0.038 inch (0.97 mm), while the injection lumen diameter is 0.050 inch (1.26 mm). A variant in the form of flexitip is also available. This catheter eliminates the need for multiple catheterizations. The flexitip is intended for a traumatic catheterization into the ureter (adapted from cook catalog supplement, 1996).

CHAPTER 11: Accessories | 139

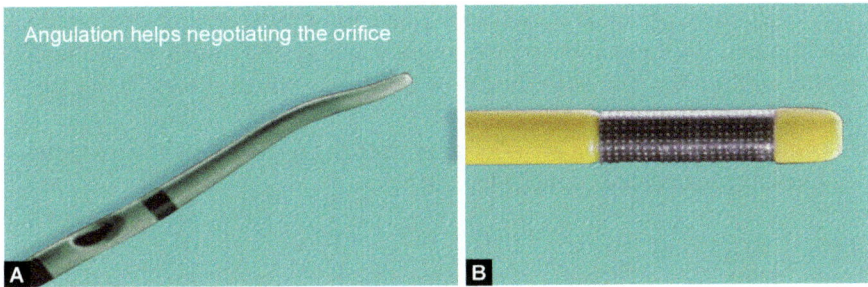

Figures 2A and B: (A) Angled-tipped ureteral catheter; (B) Echo-tipped ureteral catheter.

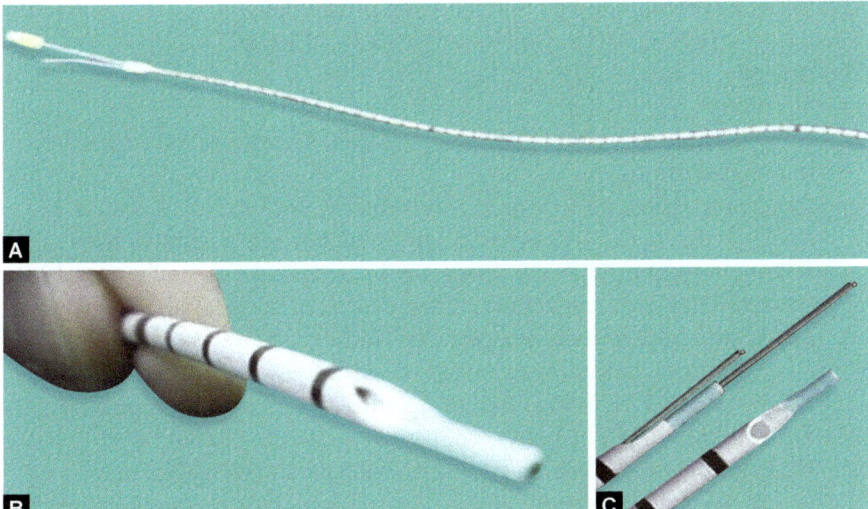

Figures 3A to C: (A) Hosing the two channels; (B) Showing two channels; and (C) Showing two guidewires.

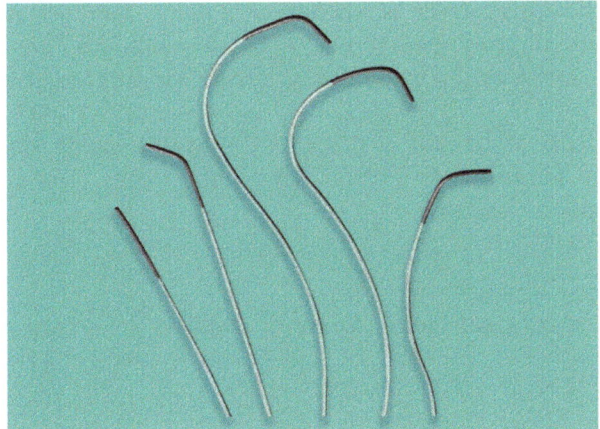

Figure 3D: Torqueable tip ureteral access catheter.

- *Spiral tip ureteral access catheter*[8]: Used for drainage and retrograde pyelogram. The spiral tip aids in negotiation of a tortuous or partially obstructed ureter. The large side port below the spiral allows passage of a guidewire.
- *Torqueable tip ureteral access*: Catheter used for negotiation of a tortuous or partially obstructed ureter (**Fig. 3D**).

GUIDEWIRES

They are used for access or dilatation of tract. There are different types of guidewire—straight tip, flexible tip, stiff, hydrophilic, etc.

Guidewires can be classified by the following properties:
- *Size*: Size—0.018–0.038 inches, length usually—150 cm
- Tip design
  - Straight tip
  - Angled tips negotiate awkward located ureteral orifices (i.e., in median lobe hypertrophy)
  - J tips are beneficial in preventing ureteral perforation, because the leading edge of the wire is an "elbow," which is less traumatic than the relatively sharper end of a straight wire. They are especially useful in patients who have impacted ureteral calculi or ureteral tortuosity. It is also useful in percutaneous nephrolithotomy (PCNL).
- Surface coating—characteristics (**Figs. 4A and B**)
  - Most standard *stainless steel* guidewires are coated with polytetrafluoroethylene (PTFE).
  - Hydrophilic-coated wire—glidewire. Its *superelastic nitinol alloy* core tapers gradually at the tip and is covered in polyurethane with a thin hydrophilic coating.
  - *Shaft rigidity*: *Three main parts of guidewire*: A spring guide, an inner core wire, and a mandrel.

Typically, the spring guide is a round wire tightly wrapped around the inner metal core and mandrel. The core provides strength and stability to the wire, whereas the spring guide acts as a track for the smooth passage of instruments.

The inner core is usually welded to the spring guide (fixed core); however, some wires have nonfixed (movable) cores. The tip can be flexible for 8 cm.

Types

- *Stainless steel core guidewire (fix core)*: Stainless steel core with PTFE coating.

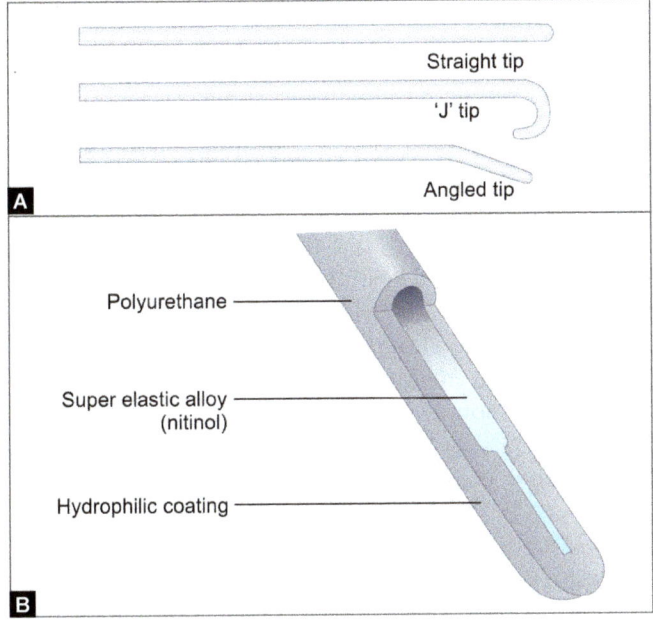

Figures 4A and B: (A) Types of guidewire; (B) Parts of guidewire.

It is used for dilatation of tract or stent placement.
- ○ Advantage—more stable and does not slip out
- ○ Disadvantage—more prone to get kinked and outer coating may come out if there is a kink, high chances of perforation (ureteric), or submucosal passage
- Nitinol core hydrophilic guidewire—(glidewire)
  - ○ Core—nitinol core for flexibility
  - ○ Coating—polyurethane coating for smooth soft surface has tungsten added for radiopacity
  - ○ Hydrophilic material—(M polymer) which causes water to stick on surface to make it smooth and slippery
  - ○ Diameters (inch)—0.018, 0.025, 0.035, and 0.038
  - ○ Lengths (cm)—80, 150, 180, and 260
  - ○ Advantage
  - ○ Smooth and atraumatic so used to pass across stones, stricture, kinks, etc.
  - ○ Smooth coating so wire does not kink—disadvantage
  - ○ Very slippery can come out easily
- *Amplatz fixed core guidewire (Boston Scientific)*: This is a super stiff guidewire[9]—stainless steel core with PTFE coating, more stiff wire.

Used for PCNL tract dilatation, ureteral sheath, or stent placement. It can be stiff, extra stiff, or ultrastiff. Extra stiffness is given by the larger flat mandrel.
- *Zebra guidewire*[10]: Nitinol core with smooth PTFE coating with blue and white stripes, lubricious (Uro-Glide)™ coating. Platinum distal tip for better fluoroscopic visualization. It had advantages of both guidewire and glidewire and disadvantage of none. It has advantage of a radiopaque tip, so tip is like a glidewire and shaft like a guidewire. It is kink resistant, better handling qualities, and flexible tip.
- *Sensor wire (Boston Scientific) (Hybrid wire)*: Nitinol core, distal 5 cm has hydrophilic coating, it has a floppy tip, flat wire outer core, and rest of the wire has a smooth PTFE coating. It has tungsten-filled radiopaque tip for fluoroscopic visualization.
- *Road runner wire (Cook Medical)*: It has nitinol core, platinum tip, hydrophilic polymer coating. It is available as standard shaft or stiff shaft.
- *Bi-wire—double floppy tip*[11]: Flexible tips at both ends. Hydrophilic coating with nitinol core. One flexible tip used to pass atraumatically in ureter and other flexible tip causes less damage to endoscopes on rail loading it over wire.

DOUBLE J STENT (FIG. 5A)

Double J (DJ) stent can be classified on basis of:
- Length
- Size
- Material
- Miscellaneous

Classification on Basis of Length

Length of stent is the straight part of stent and not from tip to tip.

For tortuous ureter, larger length is necessary. Generally, length is variable between 12 cm and 30 cm.

Different ways to measure length of DJ are as follows:
- Formula for deciding the length of the stent:
  - *Pediatric age group*: Age + 10 (in cm)
  - *Adults*: Height from 149.5 to 178.5 cm—DJ length of 22–26 cm
- On plain X-ray, kidney, ureter, and bladder (KUB) (of actual size) length of DJ required is equal to length measured from xiphisternum to pubic symphysis.
- In an intravenous pyelogram (IVP) plate (of actual size), length of the DJ required is equal to distance between vesicoureteric junction (VUJ) and pelviureteric junction (PUJ).

Classification on Basis of Size

Size is measured at the shaft and represents at the outer diameter of stent. It generally varies from 3 to 8 Fr.

Classification on Basis of Material Used

- Polymers:
  - Polyurethane
  - Silicone
  - C-Flex—(Cook Urological)
  - Sof-Flex (Cook Urological)
  - Percuflex (Boston Scientific)
- Metallic (Resonance and Memokath)
- Biodegradable

Types of Stents

- *Polyurethane stents*[12]: It has good tensile strength and can be passed over guidewire and does not collapse on extrinsic pressure easily. Rigidity causes more stent-related discomfort and can damage ureter. More prone to encrustation and colonization, should not be left for >6 months ideally should be removed within 3 months.
- *Silicone stent*: It has high biodurability and biocompatibility but it has poor tensile strength and susceptible for extrinsic compression. Poor strength requires low inner diameter to outer diameter ratio which leads to smaller lumen. It has poor drainage efficiency as compared to polyurethane. The poor coil retention leads to spontaneous migration.
- *Percuflex, C-Flex, Sof-Flex*[13]: These are made of proprietary copolymers softer and less bladder irritation. More biocompatible and can be left for longer time. These have higher inner diameter/outer diameter ratio and hence have bigger lumen. This property is permitted by these copolymers with higher strengths. These stents have hydrophilic polymer coating for smooth surface and easy insertion.[14]
- *Metallic stent (Resonance stent) (Cook Medical)*[15]: It is made of special metallic material, unlike other stent, it is not hollow and is solid cylindrical stent. Preferably used for extrinsic compression of ureter. Resistant to encrustation can be left for 12 months.
- *Memokath—nitinol (Nickel/Titanium alloy*[16]*)*: It expands to predetermined size at warm temperature 65°C. Resistant to encrustation and can be left for longer duration, used for variable length of strictures, benign, and malignant.

Steps of Memokath Deployment

- Measure the stricture and mark it on skin with radiopaque markers
- Park a guidewire across

- Use access sheath with dilator to go beyond the stricture
- Remove the dilator
- Pass Memokath deployment system from within the access sheath
- Withdraw the sheath below the stricture
- After ensuring the appropriate level of stent, put sterile normal saline (NS) at 65°C
- Stent expands and is held in place by expanded cranial end
- Unscrew the rest of the assembly and remove the sheath
- *Drug-eluting stents*: They are coated with varying chemicals to decrease encrustation or biofilm formation. Still under trial.
  - Heparin—provides antiadhesive surface which resists encrustation and biofilm formation
  - Hydrogel-coated, PTFE-coated, antimicrobial triclosan, antibody-coated, phospholipid polymer-coated, titanium nitric oxide-coated
- *Biodegradable/Bioabsorbable stent*: Polyglycolide, poly D, L-lactide, poly L lactide, and uriprene are biodegradable polymeric. Complete stent absorption occurs over a varied period. Data are inadequate for human use. Stent polymers are not radiopaque and the radiopacity is afforded by metallic salts of barium or bismuth. Stents are available with more than one coil at end which may make its use possible as multilength stent.

Miscellaneous Stents

- *Dangler stents*[17] are usual DJ with additional nylon or prolene wire loops dangling out of the stent end. This helps in its removal without cystoscopy.
- *Endopyelotomy stent* (**Fig. 5B**)[18-20]: Used after endopyelotomy or endourological management of upper ureteric stricture or PUJ obstruction, to maintain the lumen of the upper ureter and PUJ. Proximal end is wide with narrow distal end-like usual stent.

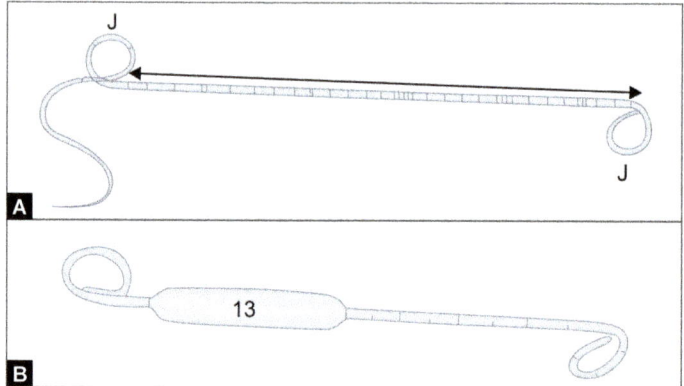

Figures 5A and B: Double J stents: (A) The length of the stent is measured excluded the 'J'; (B) Endopyelotomy stent.

Tubes and Urethral Catheters

A urinary catheter is a tube placed in the body to collect urine from the bladder. Urinary catheters are available in variety of sizes (8–26 Fr), materials (latex, silicone, and Teflon™), and types (Foley, straight, and coudé tip). Size is usually measured in French catheter scale or "French units" (Fr) or Charrière (Ch) which measures the outside diameter of catheters (1 Fr is equivalent to 0.33 mm, or 1/77" of diameter). French also indicates the circumference in millimeter, i.e., 16 Fr catheter has 16 mm circumference (circumference = p d = 3.14 × diameter = 3 × diameter).

Catheters can be classified as:
- Single-use (nonindwelling)
- Indwelling (Foley) catheters

Types of Urethral Catheters

Depending on retention mechanism
- Simple catheter (nonindwelling):
  - Simple rubber catheter (K90 = 14 Fr, K91 = 10 Fr, Teimann, female catheter, Nelaton catheter). K90, K91 are now available as r90 and r91
  - Metallic catheters, etc.
- Self-retaining catheters:
  - Foley catheter
  - Gibbons catheter
  - Malecot catheter
  - Pigtail catheter

DESCRIPTION OF INDIVIDUAL CATHETERS

Red Rubber Catheter (Robinson Catheter)

Made up of India rubber for single use to empty bladder, it has two eyelets (two opposing eyes), which provide high flow of urine. It is radiopaque due to lead oxide content.[21] Available in 8–22 Fr size.[22] Red rubber catheter used is declining as India rubber is irritant to urothelium.

Nelaton Catheter

Nelaton catheter is a simple tube with one hole at side (rounded tip ensure an easier insertion) or at tip ("open-ended" catheter), and a connecting piece at the opposite end to connect to a collecting bag. Most are made up of polyvinylchloride (PVC) and have some rigidity and radiopacity.

Foley Catheters

Foley catheter is a self-retaining catheter because of balloon mechanism at the end, balloon connected to a nozzle with a valve mechanism to the other end through a small tube running through the wall of catheter. Balloon capacity is mentioned on the side of nozzle end.[23]

Apart from the "all known" Foley catheter the other contributions that Foley is credited with are:
- Foley completely rotatable resectoscope
- A hydraulic cystolithotomy table
- Pressurized fluid delivery system
- A canister which would inflate any balloon catheter
- A urethral sphincter device

Types of Foley Catheters (Based on Type of Material Used)
- Simple latex Foley catheter
- Siliconized latex Foley catheters (Silicolatex)
- Silicone Foley catheters

Types Based on Use
- Simple Foley catheter
- Three-way hemostatic catheters
- Hematuria catheters

Different Types of End Holes and Catheter Tips

These are the types of catheter tips:
- *Straight tip*: This is the most common type.
- *The Delinotte tip (also called Mercier tip/Coudé tip)*: It is same as straight tip but with bent end for easy passage through prostate.
- *The Couvelaire tip (also called the whistle tip)*: Helps in easy passage of debris, clots from the bladder.
- Dufour tip (combination of coude and whistle tip)
- *The Tiemann tip*: Rigid slightly bent tip and bulbous end for easy passage through prostate

Siliconized Latex Foley Catheters

These catheters have a silicon coating over latex, latex is supposed to be irritant to the urothelium of the urinary tract leading to microulcerations and stricture. Some patients have allergy to latex too. To overcome above drawbacks silicon coating was done over latex as former is considered to be urothelium friendly. With time silicone layer may be damaged exposing underlying latex, restricting their use for 2-3 weeks only, needing removal or replacement after that.

Silicone Foley Catheters

Completely made of silicone and are costlier compared to siliconized latex catheter. These catheters are often transparent but they also come in white, blue, green, and other colors. Main advantage is that they are less irritant, resistant to wear and tear, less prone to encrustation, and are more rigid than siliconized latex catheters (easy passage in obstructive prostate gland).

The balloon when empty forms a slight thickening leading to slight increase in external diameter by French or two which may sometimes make passage difficult through stricture. Because of inert nature they can be placed in bladder for 6–8 weeks.

Three-way Hemostatic Catheters

Also called as three-way catheters, they are specialized Foley catheters, have an extra nozzle at the end connected to an extra tube in the wall of the catheter that opens distally to the balloon used for continuous irrigation. These catheters are often of a larger diameter (20–24 Fr) which allows large debris to pass through the catheter. Catheter is reinforced with steel or nylon spiral meshed inside the tube wall or some type of catheter are made up of more rigid type of material, to prevent collapse when suction is applied for removal of debris. Tip has a wide hole for removal of debris.

VARIOUS SIZE PARAMETERS AND COLOR CODING OF CATHETERS (TABLE 1 AND FIG. 6)

Each catheter has a color code at connecting piece or the filling opening of the balloon in Foley type catheter which denotes the external diameter of the catheter.

Three-way Foley Hematuria Catheters[24] (Fig. 7)

Large eyeholes in the hematuria catheters reduce the risk of clots blocking the eye and funnel strength is maximized to resist collapse during aspiration of clots.

TABLE 1: Color coding for Foley catheter.

Channel size	Balloon size	Color	Length (cm)
8 Fr	3 cc	Aquamarine	30
10 Fr	3 cc	Black	30
12 Fr	5–10 cc	White	40
14 Fr	5–10 cc	Green	40
16 Fr	5–10 cc	Orange	40
18 Fr	5–10 cc	Red	40
20 Fr	10–20 cc	Yellow	40
22 Fr	10–20 cc	Purple	40
24 Fr	10–20 cc	Blue	40

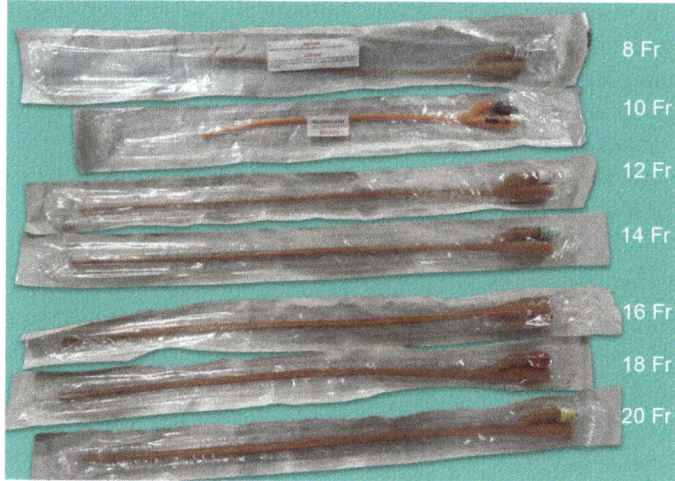

Figure 6: Various two-way Foley catheters with color coding.

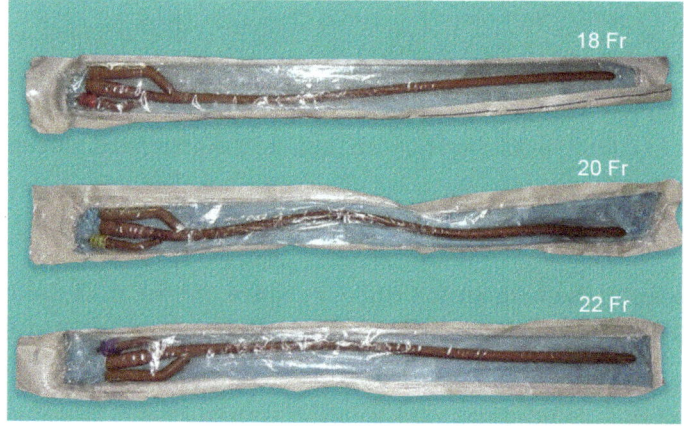

Figure 7: Three-way catheters with color codes.

Tiemann Catheter (Fig. 8)

Tip is bulbous, coude, and relatively rigid because of the gentle curve it is easy to pass through the urethra. Color code is same as Foley's.

Nephrostomy Tubes (Figs. 9A and B)

The nephrostomy tube helps to drain the kidney after the procedure, acts as a conduit to remove residual stones after a PCNL if they are detected on a postoperative film; in addition, the nephrostomy tubes also help to tamponade any bleeding.

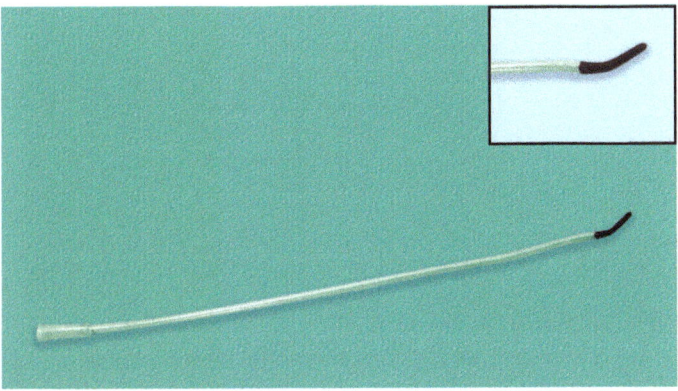

Figure 8: Tiemann catheter with characteristic distal end and proximal tip.

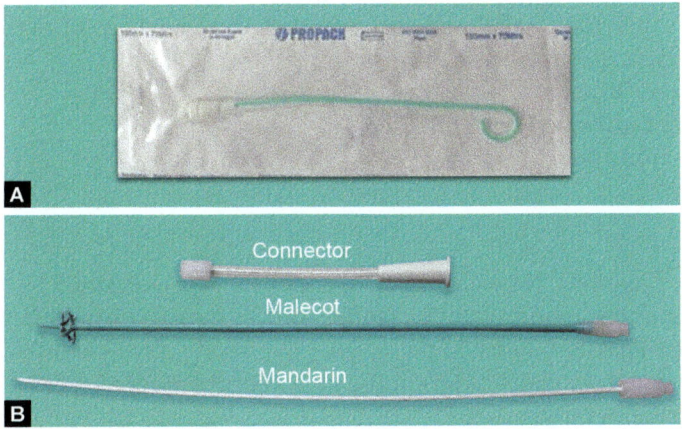

Figures 9A and B: (A) Pig tail catheter; (B) Malecot continuous drainage catheter with mandarin and connector.

The varieties of nephrostomy tubes available are:
- *Councilman catheter*: This is a modified Foleys catheter, with an end on hole. This type of nephrostomy drainage is useful if the nephrostomy tube requires frequent changes.
- *Kaye's tamponade balloon*: Originally, the catheter was designed to arrest post-PCNL bleeding. The tamponade is provided by the balloon and the central channel provides drainage.
- *Nelaton catheter* (**Fig. 10A**): The catheters range in size from 12 to 28 Fr. This is the preferred method of drainage after PCNL.
- *Foley catheters*: These are used for long-term drainage and in those patients which require repeat tube changes. Disadvantage is, it is not radiopaque.
- *Malecot catheter* (**Fig. 9B**): These catheters have a flower at the end of catheter as self-retaining mechanism which open when "mandarin" a sort

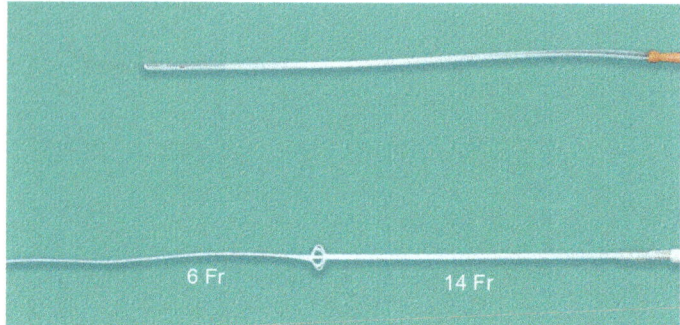

Figures 10A to C: (A) Nelaton catheter; (B) Re-entry catheter.

of stick inside the lumen of catheter is removed. "Mandarin" keeps the tip flat during insertion and removal. These catheters are less secure then Foley as they tend to fall out with firm pull. Not widely used as urethral catheters, mainly used as nephrostomy catheter.
- De Pezzer catheters
- Re-entry catheters (**Figs. 10B and C**)
- Circle nephrostomy tubes

BASKETS AND RETROPULSION DEVICES (FIG. 11)

- NCircle™ basket[25] (Cook Medical, Spencer, IN)—peculiarities
  It is a tipless manipulator for stone removal. It made up of nitinol sizes, 1.5 Fr, 2.2 Fr, 3.0 Fr, and 4.5 Fr.
  The length available is 65 cm (flexible nephroscope) and 115 [flexible ureteroscope (FURS)].
  It does not occupy much space and hence can be opened in small calyx. Once the basket is opened the diameter is either 2 cm or 1 cm in size.
- NCompass™ basket[26] (Cook Medical, Spencer, IN)—peculiarities
  Multiwire geometry, made of nitinol, tipless, available in two sizes, 1.7 Fr, 2.4 Fr, length 115 cm, basket diameter after opening—1 cm and 1.5 cm. It does not occupy much space and hence can be opened in small calyx. It has 12-16 tightly weaned wires for intact removal of multiple fragments.
- Ngage™ basket[26] (Cook Medical, Spencer, IN)—peculiarities
  Stone extractor (ureter or calyx) engages, reposition, and releases the stone as required. Available as 1.7 Fr and 2.2 Fr and 115 cm in length, open diameter is 8 mm or 11 mm. The basket configuration on opening is triangular in shape.
- NForce™ (Cook Medical, Spencer, IN)[27]
  Nitinol helical stone extractor (nitinol helical stone extractor)

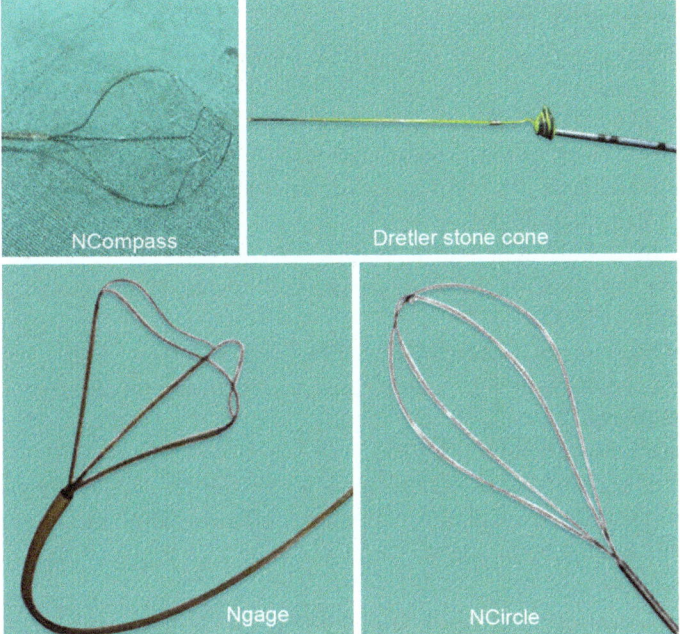

Figure 11: Different types of baskets and retropulsion devices.

- Graspit™ (Boston Scientific)[28]
- Captura™ helical stone extractor (Cook Medical)[29] Sheath 1.7–4.5 Fr, a similar basket from Boston Scientific is called as Gemini™ helical stone extractor.[29,30]
- Segura Hemisphere stone retrieval basket[31] (Boston Scientific, Natick, MA)

Peculiarities
- Zero tip nontraumatic. Nitinol
- Working length, 120 cm or 90 cm
- Sheath size, 2.4 Fr, 3.0 Fr, or 4.5 Fr
- Basket diameter is 16 mm or 20 mm
- Sheath material of polyimide or PTFE
- They are available as 4, 3, and 6 wire basket.

Two Types
- *Round wire*: To prevent ureteral trauma, they have 4 wire configured.
- *Flat wire*: Maintain basket configuration even during difficult stone manipulation. They are 3 or 6 wire configured (Boston Scientific catalogue).

Retropulsion Devices

These devices are used for preventing retropulsion of stone into the pelvicalyceal system:
- NTrap basket[32] (Cook Medical, Spencer, IN)
    - It is used as an antiretropulsion device.
    - Basket configuration (7 mm umbrella configuration on opening)
    - It is 2.8 Fr and 145 cm
- Stone cone[33] (Boston Scientific, Natick MA)
- Made of nitinol and is available as either 7 mm or 10 mm coil with 3 Fr shaft made of PTFE.
- COAx Stone control device[34] (Accordion Medical)
- Made of polyurethane film which conforms to the shape of the ureter and prevents migration
- Backstop[35] (Boston Scientific)

It is a thermosensitive polymer that is water soluble. It is deployed with access sheath like device and, thereafter, washed away with cold saline.

(see **Table 2** for specifications)

TABLE 2: Sizes/Length and other specifications for baskets and retropulsion devices.

Model	Available size (Fr)	Available basket size (mm)	Length (cm)	Features
Dimension (Bard)	2.4, 3.0	10, 13, 16	115	Articulating four wire, zero tip
Expand 212 (Bard)	3.0	11	90, 115	Articulating, 2-1-2-1, wire design filiform tip
Escape (Boston scientific)	1.9	11, 15	90, 120	4 wire cage with channel for 200 micron laser fiber
Optiflex (Boston scientific)	1.3	6, 7, 9, 11	90, 120	Rotates 360°, can entrap small fragments with preservation of vision
Zerotip (Boston scientific)	1.9, 2.4, 3.0	12, 16	90, 120	Zero tip helps entrapment near parenchyma
N Circle (Cook Medical)	2.4	10, 20	115	Triangular shape allows very large wire mass, tipless mass
NForce (Cook medical)	2.2, 3.2		115	3 wire
NGage (Cook Medical)	1.7, 2.2	8, 11	115	Allows repositioning

URETHRAL BALLOON DILATORS

The urethral balloon dilators are used to dilate the male and female urethra to treat stricture disease. They are intended for one-time use. They are 29 cm long and can be available with or without coudé tip. They are available either as 9.0 Fr or 7.0 Fr in size. The inflated balloon diameter is 8.7 mm in either sizes. The balloon length is 18 cm. The balloon can withstand 6 atmospheric pressure (90 psi). They are intended for one-time use. A 0.038 inch wire can pass through its lumen.

URETERIC DILATOR

Ureteral dilators are: Active and passive.

PASSIVE DILATORS: DOUBLE J STENTS

Active Dilators

- *Single step (Fig. 12A)*: Long-tapered ureteral dilator (Nottingham)—6/12 Fr or 6/14 Fr, tip is 6 Fr, and gradually diameter increases to 12 Fr or 14 Fr, it is made of polyethylene and is 60 cm long. Ureter can be dilated by single passage.
- *Serial Teflon ureteral dilator (Fig. 12B)*: 6 Fr, 8 Fr, 9 Fr, 10 Fr, 11 Fr, 12 Fr, 14 Fr, 16 Fr, and 18 Fr, they have to be passed one after the other to dilate the ureter.
- *Ureteral balloon dilator (Fig. 12C)*: It is around 65 cm in length and balloon is 4–5 mm in width on inflation and 4–6 cm in length. In collapsed state, it is 3–7 Fr depending on make. Available as passport, ascend, etc.

Access Sheath

Flexible ureterorenoscopy can be performed with or without an access sheath. Ureteral access sheath facilitates multiple passes into ureter, reduces operative time, minimize patient morbidity, and improves overall outcome of the procedure. It maintains low intrapelvic pressure (<20 cm water with pressurized irrigation up to 200 cm water) by allowing return of irrigant fluid through the sheath and around the ureteroscope (**Table 3**). Thus, if repeated passes of FURS or prolonged surgery is expected, then an access sheath is placed. Ureteral access sheaths are inserted over a super stiff working guidewire, either directly or after serial ureteric dilatation using ureteric balloon dilator or serial dilators. Among the available access sheaths, the Cook Flexor (**Figs. 13A and B**) sheath has been found to be more resistant to both buckling at the ureteral orifice and kinking after removal of the inner dilator.[4]

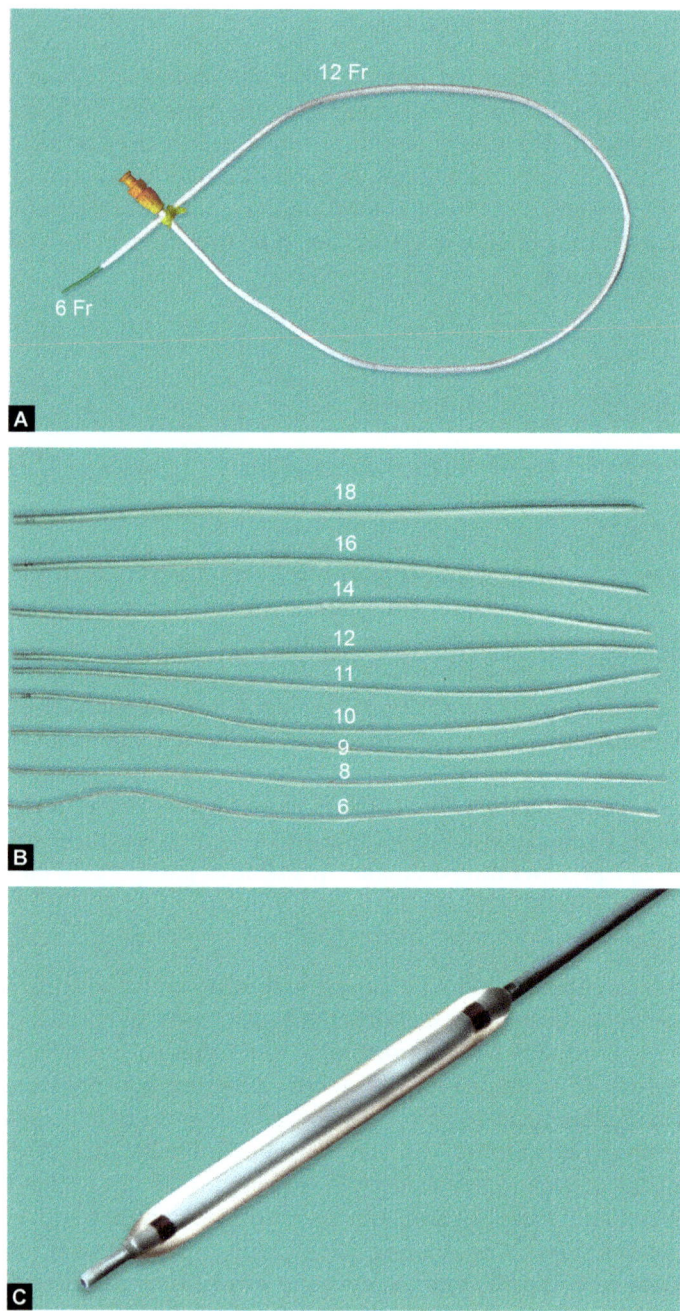

Figures 12A to C: The figure shows the accessories used during ureteroscopy: (A) Nottingham urethral dilator; (B) Serial Teflon ureteral dilator; and (C) Balloon ureteral dilator.

TABLE 3: Access sheaths specifications.

Company	Name	Inner diameter (Fr)	Outer diameter (Fr)	Length (cm)
Cook Urological	Cook Flexor	9.5/12/14	11.5/14/16	13/20/28/35/45/55
	Cook Flexor DL	9.5/12	11.5/14	13/20/28/35/45/55
Applied Medical Resources	Forte	10/12/14	12/14/16	20/28/35/45/55
ACMI Corporation	ACMI-Gyrus Uropass®	12	14	24/38/54
Bard	Aquaguide®	12/13	14/15	25/35/45/55

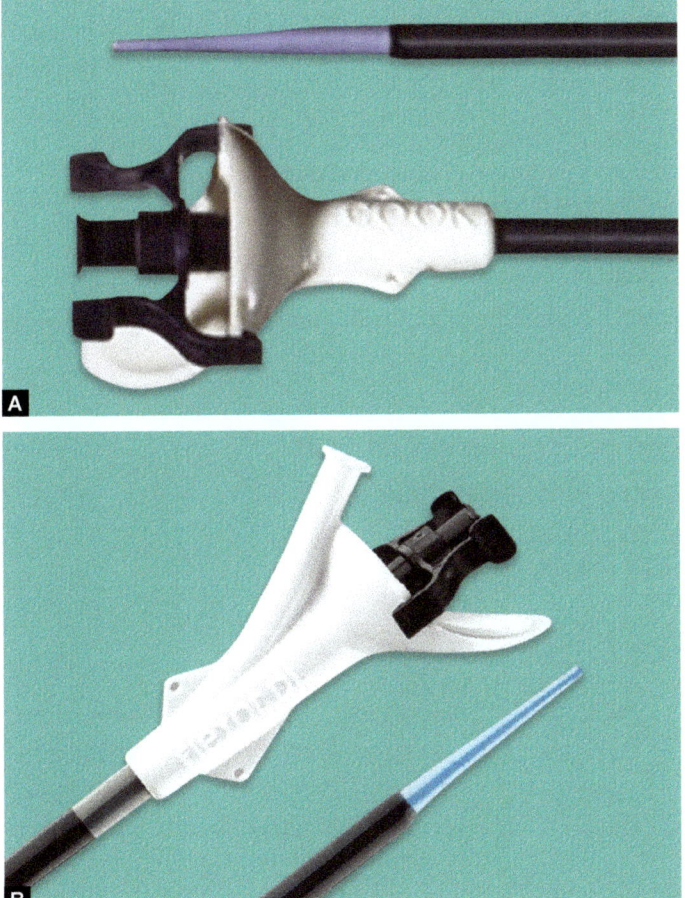

Figures 13A and B: (A) Cook Flexor access sheath; (B) Cook Flexor DL access sheath.

Parts

Access sheaths have an inner dilator and outer sheath. The dilator has a pointed conical tip with a channel for passage over guidewire. The proximal end of the dilator has a clipping mechanism to fix the dilator to the sheath. The sheath is cylindrical with a widened flange at the proximal end. The tip of the sheath has a circular radiopaque marker. The sheath is coated with a microthin layer of hydrophilic polymer to create a low friction surface. In dual channel access sheaths (e.g., Cook Flexor DL with 3 Fr secondary channel), there is a secondary channel for passage of guidewire, basket, or laser fiber (**Figs. 13A and B**).

Available Sizes

Access sheaths are available in various sizes with inner diameter ranging from 9.5 to 13 Fr, outer diameter ranging from 12 to 15 Fr, and length ranging from 13 cm (pediatric) to 55 cm.

Types

- Based on construction—reinforced and nonreinforced
- Based on length—female/male

Special Types

Dual lumen access sheaths, e.g., Cook Flexor DL picture of cross-section, material.

Comparison of Companies (Table 4)

Properties of an Ideal Access Sheath
- Kink resistant sheath
- Hydrophilic coating

TABLE 4: Comparison of different access sheaths.

Company	Name	Inner diameter (Fr)	Outer diameter (Fr)	Length (cm)
Cook Urological	Cook Flexor	9.5/12/14	11.5/14/16	13/20/28/35/45/55
	Cook Flexor DL	9.5/12	11.5/14	13/20/28/35/45/55
Applied Medical Resources	Forte	10/12/14	12/14/16	20/28/35/45/55
ACMI Corporation	ACMI-Gyrus Uropass®	12	14	24/38/54
Bard	Aquaguide®	12/13	14/15	25/35/45/55

- Unique hub design
- Radiopaque marker band
- Dual tapered tip

PERCUTANEOUS NEPHROLITHOTOMY ACCESSORIES (FIGS. 14A AND B)

The various accessories used during PCNL help in retrieving stones. The specifications of these accessories are as shown in **Figures 14A and B**. The accessories include:
- Various types of forceps—broadly the accessories can be classified as:
  - *Triflange*: Requires a larger space to open. Both the biflange and the triflange cannot be easily dismantled.
  - *Biflange*: Requires a smaller space to open.
  - *Alligator*: Requires in a smaller space, hence can be used in compact system.
- *Suction cannula*: Helps in evacuation of smaller fragments and thus, reducing the operative time.

The top figure shows the two varieties of suction cannulas available. The bottom figure shows the PCNL graspers in closed and open position. The figures denote the available sizes (6 Fr, 9 Fr, and 12 Fr) and the length of the instrument (360 mm).

*Alken needle with sheath (**Fig. 15**)*: 8 Fr needle which is passed over the wire. It does not have sharp cutting edges at the tip. The Alken sheath is 10 Fr, this

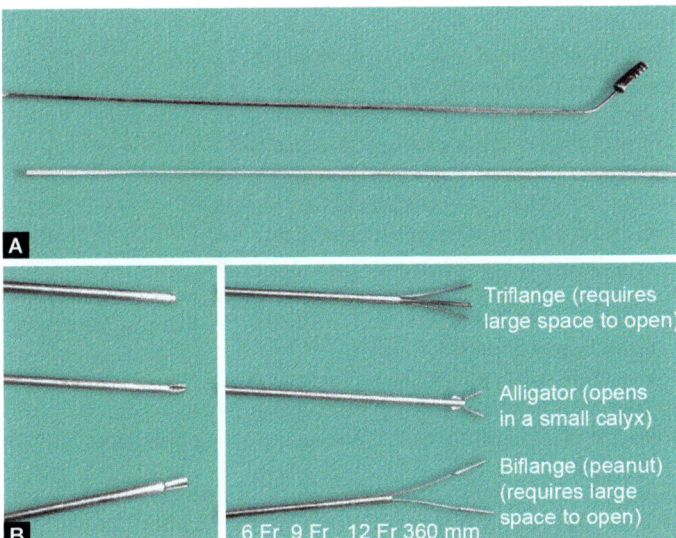

Figures 14A and B: (A) Suction cannula; (B) Various types of forceps used in percutaneous nephrolithotomy (PCNL).

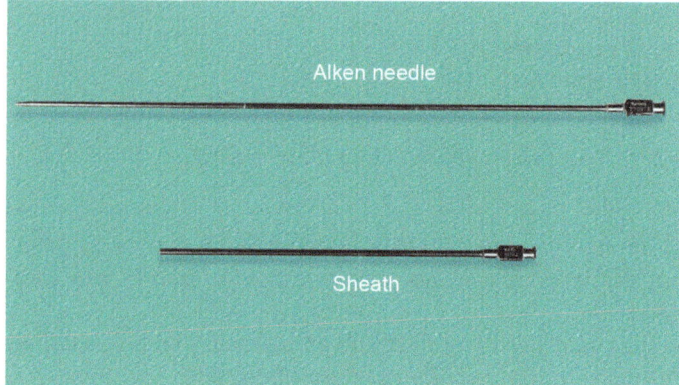

Figure 15: Alken needle.

snuggly fits over the needle. Alken needle length is 26 cm, sheath length is 15 cm. While introduction of the needle the sheath is preintroduced and the needle is passed over the wire. Once the needle reaches the pelvicalyceal system the sheath is advanced into PCS and the needle withdrawn. Sheath is useful to pass a safety guidewire. The guide rod goes through the sheath after which it is withdrawn and the dilatation be started.

The Alken needle is also useful to negotiate oblique (zig-zag) tracts or to negotiate through a tough fibrous tissue as it is made up of stainless steel. Alken sheath can also be used to insert antegrade DJ stent.

REFERENCES

1. Cook Urology 2010.
2. Cook Urology 2010. Domestic product catalogue. p. 23.
3. Cook Urology 2010. Domestic product catalogue. p. 15.
4. Cook Urology 2010. Domestic product catalogue. p. 18.
5. Cook Urology 2010. Domestic product catalogue. p. 22.
6. Cook Urology 2010. Domestic product catalogue. p. 25.
7. Cook Urology 2010. Domestic product catalogue. p. 20.
8. Cook Urology 2010. Domestic product catalogue. p. 14.
9. Cook Urology 2010. Domestic product catalogue. p. 10.
10. Boston Scientific. [online] Available from: http://www.bostonscientific.com/templatedata/imports/Microsite/Stone/ collateral/products_for_Ureteroscopy.pdf. [Last accessed February 2021].
11. Cook Urology 2010. Domestic product catalogue. p. 6.
12. Cook Urology 2010. Domestic product catalogue. p. 84.
13. Cook Urology 2010. Domestic product catalogue. p. 88 (Cook Urology 2010. Domestic product catalogue. p. 89).
14. Boston Scientific. [online] Available from: http://www.bostonscientific.com/templatedata/imports/Microsite/Stone/ collateral/percuflex-Brochure.pdf. [Last accessed February 2021].
15. Cook Urology 2010. Domestic product catalogue. p. 94.

16. Endotherapeutics. [online] Available from: http://www.endotherapeutics.com.au/memokath. [Last accessed February 2021].
17. Singh I. Indwelling JJ ureteral stents-A current perspective and review of literature. Indian J Surg. 2003;65(5):405-12.
18. Boston Scientific. [online] Available from: http://www.bostonscientific.com/templatedata/imports/Microsite/Stone/ collateral/retromax-Brochure.pdf. [Last accessed February 2021].
19. Ho CH, Chen SC, Chung SD, Lee YJ, Chen J, Yu HJ, et al. Determining the appropriate length of a double-pigtail ureteral stent by both stent configurations and related symptoms. J Endourol. 2008;22(7):1427-31.
20. Palmer JS, Palmer LS. A simple and reliable formula for determining the proper JJ stent length in the pediatric patient: Age + 10. Urology. 2007;70:264.
21. Mountain Medical Equipment. [online] Available from: http://www.mountainside-medical.com/products/red-rubber-catheters.html. [Last accessed February 2021].
22. Sportaid. [online] Available from: http://www.sportaid.com/bard-red-rubber-catheters-8-22-fr.html. [Last accessed February 2021].
23. Tatem AE, Klaaseen A, Lewis RW, Terris MK. Frederick Eugene Basil Foley: Fredric e.B Foley (1891–1966) his life and innovations. Urology. 2013;81(5):927-31.
24. Laborie. [online] Available from: http://www.genmedhealth.com/static/Foley_catheter. [Last accessed February 2021].
25. Cook Urology 2010. Domestic product catalogue. p. 60.
26. Cook Urology 2010. Domestic product catalogue. p. 58.
27. Cook Urology 2010. Domestic product catalogue. p. 61.
28. Boston Scientific. [online] Available from: http://www.lifebeatonline.com/templatedata/imports/collateral/Urology/broc_graspit_01_ur_us.pdf. [Last accessed February 2021].
29. Cook Urology 2010. Domestic product catalogue. p. 62.
30. Boston Scientific. [online] Available from: http://www.bostonscientific.com/templatedata/imports/collateral/Urology/ spec_gemini_04_us.pdf. [Last accessed February 2021].
31. Boston Scientific. [online] Available from: http://www.lifebeatonline.com/templatedata/imports/collateral/Urology/broc_ segura_01_ur_us.pdf. [Last accessed February 2021].
32. Cook Urology 2010. Domestic product catalogue. p. 60.
33. Boston Scientific. [online] Available from: http://www.bostonscientific.com/templatedata/imports/collateral/Urology/ broc_stonecone_01_ur_us.pdf. [Last accessed February 2021].
34. Percsys. [online] Available from: http://www.percsys.com/pdfs/Accordion%20coAx%20Stone%20control%20 Device%2090-0949-01%20rc%201-11.pdf. [Last accessed February 2021].
35. Boston Scientific. [online] Available from: http://www.bostonscientific.com/templatedata/imports/Microsite/Stone/ collateral/Backstop-Brochure.pdf. [Last accessed February 2021].

CHAPTER 12

Sterilization

DEFINITIONS

Disinfection and sterilization are necessary to ensure that medical and surgical instruments do not transmit infectious pathogens to patients. The method of sterilization varies from patient-to-patient. *Sterilization* is defined as the process by which an article, surface, or medium is freed of all living microorganisms either in the vegetative or spore state. *Disinfection* means the process that eliminates all pathogenic microorganisms (or in other words organisms capable of giving rise to infection), except bacterial spores, on inanimate objects. A few disinfectants will kill spores with prolonged exposure times (3-12 h); these are called chemical sterilants.[1] High-level disinfectants work at similar concentrations but with shorter exposure periods (e.g., 20 min for 2% glutaraldehyde), by killing all microorganisms, except large numbers of bacterial spore.[1] Intermediate-level disinfectants might destroy mycobacteria, vegetative bacteria, most viruses, and most fungi but do not necessarily kill bacterial spores.[1] Low-level disinfectants can kill most vegetative bacteria, some fungi, and some viruses in a shorter period of time (<10 min).[1]

Germicide is an agent that can kill microorganisms, particularly pathogenic organisms ("germs"). Germicides differ markedly, primarily in their antimicrobial spectrum and rapidity of action.[1]

Antiseptics are substances that prevent or arrest the growth or action of microorganisms by inhibiting their activity or by destroying them. Antiseptics are applied to living tissue and skin; disinfectants are antimicrobials applied only to inanimate objects. In general, antiseptics are used only on the skin and not for surface disinfection, and disinfectants are not used for skin antisepsis because they can injure skin and other tissues.[1]

Cleaning is the removal of visible soil (e.g., organic and inorganic material) from objects and surfaces and is usually performed manually or mechanically using water with detergents or enzymatic products.[1]

Decontamination refers to the process of removing pathogenic microorganisms from objects so they are safe to handle, use, or discard.[1]

APPROACH TO DISINFECTION AND STERILIZATION

Spaulding believed the nature of disinfection could be understood readily if instruments and items for patient care were categorized as critical and semicritical. He devised a classification system >40 years ago which is still in use in most of the international guidelines on sterilization and disinfection including the Centers for Disease Control and Prevention (CDC) guidelines.[2]

Spaulding Classification[2]

The items were classified as follows:
- *Critical items*: These were defined as those items which enter the body cavity, vascular system, or nonintact mucous membranes. All the surgical instruments are classified as critical. The goal should be to make objects sterile. The preferred method of sterilization is steam sterilization or low temperature sterilization, e.g., forceps and scalpel.
- *Semicritical items*: These are the items which directly or indirectly come in contact with intact mucous membrane or nonintact skin. The aim is to offer high level disinfection which will make the object free of microorganisms, except bacterial spores. However, it is always preferable to sterilize semicritical items whenever they are compatible with available sterilization, e.g., cystoscope.
- *Noncritical items*: These are the items which come in contact with skin but not mucous membrane such as blood pressure (BP) cuffs or crutches. The aim is low level disinfection by cleaning.

DIFFERENT METHODS OF STERILIZATION[1,3]

Steam Sterilization

- *Mechanism of action*: Moist heat causes irreversible coagulation and denaturation of enzymes and structural protein.
- *Advantages*: Nontoxic, easy to control and monitoring, rapidly microbicidal, least affected by organic/inorganic soils, rapid cycle time.
- *Disadvantages*: Heat-sensitive instruments cannot be sterilized and repeated sterilization with this technique will lead to loss of sharpness of cutting instruments.
- *Uses*: Critical and semicritical items that are heat- and moisture-resistant.

Facts Regarding/Steam Sterilization

All instruments (assembled endoscopes) should be opened or unlocked to allow the steam to reach all parts of the instrument. Temperature should be 121°C, with pressure of 106 kpa (15 lb/inch^2) for 30 minutes. 20–30 minutes should elapse to permit the sterilizer to cool sufficiently. This ensures complete sterilization.

Common Procedural Mistakes

- Not allowing sufficient time and hurrying up to get instruments/linen fast, thus not achieving enough pressure or exposure time for sterilization
- Tight packing of linen in drums does not allow enough steam to circulate.
- Autoclaved items stored for long time without lid lead to ineffective sterilization.

Following devices may be steam sterilized—rigid telescopes (autoclavable), working elements, trocars/sheaths, reusable thick tubing, 3 L saline bottles, insulated and noninsulated surgical instruments (forceps, scissors, suction tubes, etc.). Sharp instruments are not autoclaved as their sharpness is lost. Wherever possible this method should be used, as it is the cheapest and most reliable method of sterilization.

Dry heat sterilization is another way to sterilize needles and endoscope instruments. A convection oven with an insulated stainless steel chamber and perforated shelving to allow the circulation of hot air is recommended, but dry heat sterilization can be achieved with a simple oven as long as a thermometer is used to verify the temperature inside the oven. It has got advantages of being an effective procedure even for instruments that cannot be disassembled, protective for sharp instruments, leaving no chemical residue and eliminating wet pack problems in humid climates. The main disadvantage as compared to steam sterilization is requirement of more time, continuous source of electricity besides being contraindicated for plastic and rubber items. Generally, after the desired temperature is reached, timing begins. The following temperature/time ratios are recommended; 170°C 60 minutes, 160°C 120 minutes, 150°C 150 minutes, and 140°C 180 minutes depending upon the temperature selected, the total cycle time (preheating, sterilization time, and cool down) will range from about 2.5 hours at 170°C to >6 hours at 140°C.

Hydrogen Peroxide Gas Plasma Sterilization

Plasma sterilization: This method uses 1.8 mL of 58% hydrogen peroxide, which is vaporized, in a sterilization chamber. The vapor is converted into plasma through the use of radiofrequency (RF) energy. Plasma consists of highly charged particles and free radicals to sterilize instruments in about 1 hour without producing toxic residues or emissions. Commercially, marketed as Sterrad™ (**Fig. 1**).

- *Mechanism of action*: Destroys by combined use of hydrogen peroxide gas and generation of free radicals (hydroxyl and hydroperoxyl free radicals)
- *Advantages*: Nontoxic, cycle time from 35 to 60 minutes, simple to operate, most of the instruments can be sterilized.
- *Disadvantages*: Linens cannot be processed. It requires special unit for packaging. Plastics and corrosion sensitive metal cannot be processed.

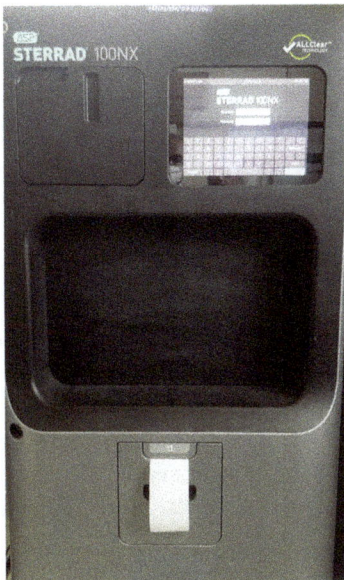

Figure 1: Sterrad.

- *Uses*: Compatible with most (>95%) medical devices and materials (laparoscopes, nephroscopes, semirigid and flexible ureteroscopes, cables, etc.).

It is useful to sterilize almost everything such as rigid telescopes, flexible fiberscopes, and semi-rigid fiberscopes, video cameras, fiber- and fluid light cables, surgical instruments, insulated (forceps, scissors, etc.), surgical instruments, noninsulated (forceps, scissors, etc.), high frequency, cords, etc.

Ethylene Oxide Sterilization

Ethylene oxide (EO or ETO) gas is commonly used to sterilize objects sensitive to temperatures greater than 60°C such as plastics, laparoscopes, endoscopic lens, wires, and electric items. ETO treatment is generally carried out between 30°C and 60°C with relative humidity above 30% and a gas concentration between 200 and 800 mg/L for at least 3 hours. ETO penetrates well, moving through paper, cloth, and some plastic films and is highly effective. ETO can kill all known viruses, bacteria, and fungi, including bacterial spores and is satisfactory for most medical materials, even with repeated use. However, it is highly flammable, and requires a longer time to sterilize than any heat treatment. The end products of the cycle are toxic and carcinogenic Aeration unit is required to remove the toxic gases or else, long time exposure to atmosphere is required. The process also requires a period of poststerilization aeration to remove toxic residues. ETO is the most common sterilization method, used for over 70% of total sterilizations, and for 50% of all disposable medical devices.

Problem: It is the best and relatively cheapest method of sterilization. But takes long time. Poststerilization aeration does not make it useful on day-to-day basis.

Mechanism of Action

Alkylation of protein, DNA, and RNA
- *Advantages*: Penetrates packaging materials, device lumens, user friendly, and compatible with most medical devices
- *Disadvantages*: Requires time for preparation, ethylene oxide (ETO) is toxic, a carcinogen, and flammable, lengthy cycle/aeration time
- *Uses*: Critical items (and sometimes semicritical items) that are moisture or heat sensitive and cannot be sterilized by steam sterilization

Instruments frequently gas sterilized in urology practice include: Fiberoptic endoscopes, surgical telescopes, laparoscope, plastic instruments (e.g., specula and syringes), anesthesia masks and circuits, rubber and plastic tubing (e.g., catheters), respirators, and inhalation therapy supplies.

Chemical Agents Used as Disinfectants/Sterilants

Alcohol (Ethyl Alcohol, Isopropyl Alcohol, 60–90% Solutions in Water)

- *Mechanism of action*: Denaturation of proteins
- *Advantages*: Easily available, no activation time
- *Disadvantages*: Lacks sporicidal action, damages the shellac mountings of lensed instruments, tends to swell and harden rubber and plastic, and flammable.
- *Uses*: To disinfect external surfaces of equipment (e.g., stethoscopes, ventilators, manual ventilation bags), and ultrasound instruments

Aldehyde Group of Chemical Disinfectants [Glutaraldehyde (2.4%) and Formaldehyde]

- *Mechanism of action*: Alkylation of sulfhydryl enzymes and amino acid (AA)
- *Advantage*: Relatively inexpensive and compatible with most of the instruments
- *Disadvantages*: Respiratory irritation from glutaraldehyde vapor, pungent, and irritating odor. Relatively slow mycobactericidal activity. Coagulates blood and fixes tissue to surfaces. Allergic contact dermatitis.
- *Uses*: Formaldehyde preparation of viral vaccines, to preserve specimens, and to disinfect fluid pathways in dialysis machines.

ALDEHYDE

Glutaraldehyde

- High level disinfectant for endoscopes, laparoscopic trocars

Glutaraldehyde (Cidex) Sterilization

Decontaminate, clean, and thoroughly dry all instruments and other items to be sterilized. Water from wet items will dilute the chemical solution, thereby reducing its effectiveness. Prepare the glutaraldehyde-containing solution (or other chemical solution) by following the manufacturer's instructions. After preparing the solution, put it in a clean container with a lid (**Fig. 2**). Always mark the container with the date the solution was prepared and the date it expires (usually 2 weeks). Open all hinged instruments and other items and disassemble those with sliding or multiple parts. The solution must contact all surfaces in order for sterilization to be achieved. Completely submerge all instruments and other items in the solution. All parts of the items should be under the surface of the solution. For sterilization, 10–12 hours of soakage is required. After that, instruments should be cleaned by sterile water, as glutaraldehyde is toxic to the endothelium.

Product Description
- 2.45% w/v glutaraldehyde with activator
- It is available in a 1 L, 2 L, and 5 L package. The use life is 14 days.

Facts

Cidex is commonly used for rapid sterilization. Instruments are soaked only for 20–30 minutes. This achieves only disinfection. Telescopes if soaked for 12 hours may cause damage of cement resulting in fogging of telescopes.

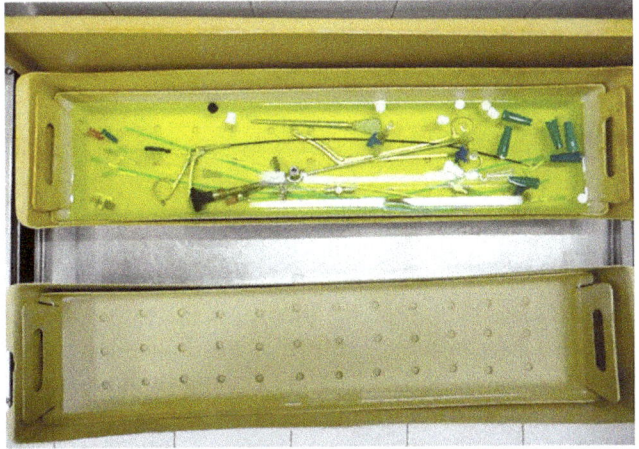

Figure 2: Cidex container with instruments.

Even other instrument's life may be reduced with long soakage. Thus, it is myth that Cidex sterilizes instruments, it only disinfects!!

For it to be effective, instruments should be cleaned thoroughly preferably by enzymatic solution; it is hardly ever done thus severely compromising even the disinfection process.

All instruments should be dissembled. Many of our scopes cannot be dissembled; all joints cannot be separated, thus further compromising disinfection process.

Instruments are taken in and out several times resulting into dilution thereby further reducing efficacy of solution.

Not covering by lid continuously and no monitoring of pH. Thus, not knowing about effectiveness of solution.

Thus, Cidex, the way in which it is commonly used is nothing but eyewash and far from sterilization.

FORMALDEHYDE

One of the curious applications of this agent, prevalent in surgical operation theaters in India, is in the form of tablets for the sterilization of delicate instruments that can be damaged by heat. These are available in the form of paraformaldehyde polymer of formaldehyde, as tablets of 1 g each. A literature search did not provide adequate information regarding the efficacy of this form of formaldehyde in sterilization. This form of sterilization is already discarded from almost all countries. One Indian study suggested that exposure of formaldehyde vapors for at least 24 hours in airtight compartment may result in sterilization. However, this recommendation is on personal experience and not evidence based.

Myths: Formalin tablets are kept in acrylic box containing scopes. No standardization about number. of tablets, duration of exposure, how many times the door of box is opened, when to change the tablets, etc. Thus, most common method of instrument sterilization adopted in private practice is the one, which is obsolete...!!

Orthophthalaldehyde (OPA)
- *Mechanism of action*: Interacts with AA, proteins to cause their breakdown.
- *Advantages*: Fast-acting high-level disinfectant. No activation required. Nonirritant. Excellent materials compatibility. Does not coagulate blood or fix tissues to surfaces. High stability over a wide pH range.
- *Disadvantages*: Stains skin, mucous membranes, clothing, and environmental surfaces. Repeated exposure may result in hypersensitivity in some patients with bladder cancer. More expensive than glutaraldehyde. Eye irritation. Slow sporicidal activity.
- *Uses*: High level disinfectant for endoscopes, anesthesia equipment, laparoscopic trocars. Pack size: 1 L and 5 L. The shelf-life is 2 years for

unopened bottle and 75 days for open bottle (provided they have not extended beyond expiry). Test strips are used to determine minimum effective concentration (MEC). The Cidex orthophthalaldehyd (OPA) strips are used to determine the use life (up to 14 days). OPA does not require activator.[4]

Per Acetic Acid

It is increasingly used nowadays in place of glutaraldehyde. Perasafe$^{(TM)}$ is 0.2 % peracetic acid.
It has a 5 minute disinfection cycle and a 10 minute sterilisation cycle.
- *Mechanism of action*: Oxidizing agent which denatures protein, disrupts cell wall, and oxidizes sulfhydryl group
- *Advantages*: Rapid sterilization cycle time. Low temperature (50–55°C) sterilization. Environmental friendly by-products (acetic acid, O_2, and H_2O). It is 100% biodegradabe. 80 g in 5 L is used. The life of the solution is 24 hours. In automated endoscope reprocessors, it can be used for 20 reprocesses.
- *Disadvantage*: Potential material incompatibility (e.g., aluminum anodized coating becomes dull)

Used for immersible instruments only. Only one scope or a small number of instruments can be processed in a cycle. Serious eye and skin damage (concentrated solution) with contact. Point-of-use system, no sterile storage.[5]

Uses

Automated machine used to sterilize medical instruments (laparoscopes and endoscopes), surgical instruments, and dental instruments.

Iodophors

- *Mechanism*: Disruption of protein and nucleic acid structure and synthesis by iodine
- *Advantages*: Nonstaining, easily available, and relatively inexpensive
- *Disadvantages*: High level disinfectant, adversely affect silicone tubing and hence should not be used on silicone catheters, cannot be used as hard surface disinfectants due to concentration differences.
- *Uses*: Used as antiseptics, disinfecting blood culture bottles and medical equipment such as thermometers and endoscopes.

STEPS OF STERILIZATION AND PROCESSING OF SURGICAL INSTRUMENTS

- *Precleaning*: Gross soil (blood and sputum) should be removed at point of use. If cleaning not possible, then submerge instruments in detergent/enzymatic cleaner to prevent organic matter from drying.

- *Disassembly*: Facilitates the access of cleaning agent to the device surfaces.
- *Cleaning*: Cleaning is the removal of foreign material (e.g., soil and organic material) from objects and is normally accomplished using water with detergents or enzymatic products. Thorough cleaning is required before high-level disinfection and sterilization because inorganic and organic materials that remain on the surfaces of instruments interfere with the effectiveness of these processes. Cleaning is done either manually or mechanically. With manual cleaning, the two essential components are friction and fluidics. Friction (e.g., rubbing/scrubbing the soiled area with a brush) (**Fig. 3**) and fluidics (i.e., fluids under pressure) (**Figs. 4A and B**) are used to remove soil and debris from internal channels. The most common types of mechanical or automatic cleaners are ultrasonic cleaners, washer-decontaminators, washer-disinfectors, and washer-sterilizers.
- *Packaging*: Once cleaned and dried, instruments requiring sterilization must be wrapped or placed in rigid containers and should be arranged in instrument trays/baskets. Options include peel open pouches, roll stock/reels, and sterilization wraps.
- *Loading*: In perforated trays for free circulation of sterilizing steam/agent to ensure proper exposure of all instruments
- *Sterilization process*: According to the type of instruments/devices to be sterilized
- *Storage*: Shelf-life varies according to the porosity of the packaging material and storage conditions. Heat-sealed (**Fig. 5**), plastic peel-down pouches in 3-Mil (3/1,000 inch) polyethylene overwrap have been reported to be sterile for as long as 9 months after sterilization, whereas the double-layer muslin covering can keep the contents sterile for a period of 1 month.

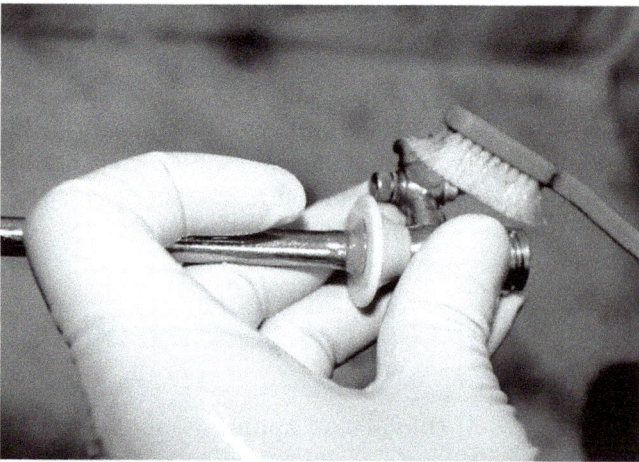

Figure 3: Manual cleaning-friction.

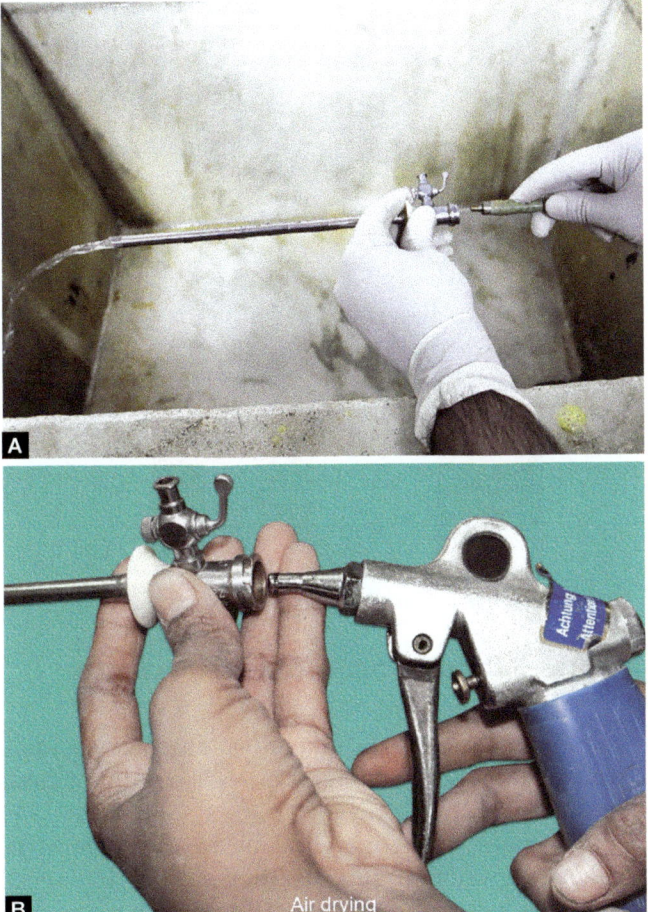

Figures 4A and B: (A) Manual cleaning fluidics; and (B) Air drying.

- *Monitoring*: It is done by using a combination of mechanical, chemical, and biological indicators to evaluate the sterilizing conditions and indirectly the microbiologic status of the processed items. Biological indicators are considered to be the ideal monitors of the sterilization process because they measure the sterilization process directly by using the most resistant microorganisms (i.e., *Bacillus* spores). Chemical monitors are either heat- or chemical-sensitive inks that change color when one or more sterilization parameters (e.g., steam-time, temperature; ETO-time) are present and they should be preferably placed on the inside of the pack too.

Sterilization of Individual Instruments

The various instructions for sterilization vary with manufacturers. The following are general guidelines for various instruments and assembly:

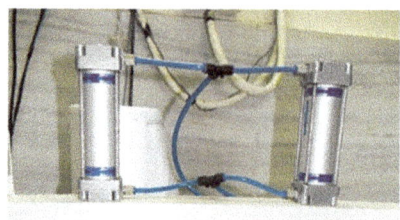
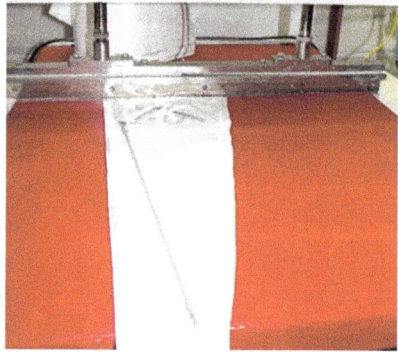

Figure 5: Packaging for sterilization.

TURP Instruments—Spaulding-high Level Disinfection or Sterilization

- *Predisinfection*: Separate the cable from the working element immediately after use, remove the telescope immerse the various parts of the assembly in a disinfectant solution.
- *Cleaning*: The working element should be separated from the high-frequency cord and rinsed with tap water. The basic principle after cleaning is to ensure that the hollow tubes are dry. This can be accomplished with a brush and dry cotton swab. In this assembly, the telescope channel and the electrode channel should be cleaned thoroughly. Special care should be taken to avoid damage of the insulation.
- *Disinfection*: The parts are again placed in a disinfectant solution (glutaraldehyde), following which the instruments are again rinsed and dried.

Sterilization

- Telescope—autoclavable, plasma, and ETO
- Working element—autoclavable and plasma sterilization
- High-frequency cord, ETO, and Sterrad (glutaraldehyde)
- Sheath—autoclavable and plasma sterilization
- Loops, plasma sterilization, and ETO
- Light cable—Sterrad and ETO

The color code knob and the plastic ring tend to get worn off with repeated uses, either with gas or steam sterilization.

Sterilization of Ureteroscopes-semicritical Item—Recommended High Level Disinfection

- *Decontamination*: Allow the instrument to soak in a disinfectant and cleaning solution. This helps to get rid of the microorganisms and detach the residual clots and debris over the instrument. Prior to cleaning, the light cable should be detached from the instrument.
- *Cleaning*: This can be done by holding the instrument under running tap water and with the help of a pressure injector or a brush. The parts in the ureteroscope which should be especially taken care of are the eyepiece, objective lens, light cable entry point. Thereafter, the instrument should be meticulously dried.
- *Sterilization:* Steam or gas sterilization

Sterilization of Accessories

- *Decontamination*: These instruments after sterilization should be kept immediately in a disinfectant or cleaning solution.
- *Cleaning*: This step is critical because any residual debris renders the ensuing steps useless. However, one should ensure that the insulation and other protective coatings do not come off. The accessories can be cleaned with an ultrasound cleaner. Care should be particularly taken to keep all the hinges and joint open, instruments being completely immersed, the channels can be flushed with cleaning gun. Thereafter, the channels should be dried inside and out.

Sterilization

- Baskets—ETO and plasma (cannot be autoclaved)
- Dilator sets—ETO and plasma
- Alken dilators—autoclavable, ETO, and plasma
- Percutaneous nephrolithotomy (PCNL) forceps—autoclavable, ETO, and plasma
- Energy probes—autoclavable, ETO, and plasma
- Ultrasonography (USG) probe—autoclaved

Sterilization of Laparoscopic Instruments

- Insulated instruments—autoclave
- Ports—metal-autoclavable, Sterrad, or ETO
- Scissors—blunts the sharpness in autoclave
- Retracting instruments—autoclave

- Camera-Sterrad, some cameras glutaraldehyde
- Nephroscopes—autoclavable (Hopkins 2). All Hopkins 2 telescopes are autoclavable
- Ureteroscopes—autoclavable
- Flexible ureteroscope—ETO and H_2O_2 (glutaraldehyde)

Salient Features for Sterilization of Cystoscopes and Telescopes

Autoclavable telescopes can be sterilized with autoclaving. If a nonautoclavable telescope (used in the past) is autoclaved, the metals and the glass items would expand unequally, as the temperature would decrease and the external surface cooled the metals would shrink to its normal size. This phenomenon was described on the basis of the principle of coefficient of expansion. In the older version of telescopes, the coefficient of expansion would vary and they would expand and shrink at different rates, thus the rod lens would expand but the metal sheath covering would not expand thus leading to breakage. This shortcoming is overcome with the advent of autoclavable telescopes.

Telescopes can be sterilized in glutaraldehyde. The telescopes need to be kept for over 12 hours for the same. Prolonged insertion can at times leads to fogging. The surgeon should specifically look for cracks on the sheath prior to insertion in glutaraldehyde. The other methods of sterilization include hydrogen peroxide and ETO sterilization.

Tips and Tricks in Sterilizing

Since cystoscope accessories except the telescope are made up of metal, they can be autoclaved. The plastic rings for color coding get damaged during the sterilization. The sheaths can be disinfected (high level) with glutaraldehyde, or can be sterilized by hydrogen peroxide. Before placing the instrument in formalin chamber, it is necessary to clean the inner and outer wall with water, following this they should be completely dried, in order to prevent corrosive action of formaldehyde with water. Prolonged insertion of the instrument in water particularly in hard water results in deposition of crystals. The crystals lead to malfunction of the inlet/outlet taps. The taps can be periodically dismantled and cleaned to prevent this. Formaldehyde reacts with water and forms formic acid, which gives black discoloration to the instrument. The summary of sterilization methods is listed in **Table 1**.

TABLE 1: Summary of sterilization methods.

	Autoclave	Plasma sterilization	ETO
TURP instruments	See text	See text	See text
Telescope	Yes	Yes	Yes
Working element	Yes	Yes	Yes
Loops	No	Yes	Yes
High frequency cord	No	Yes	Yes
Light cable	No	Yes	Yes
PCNL instruments	See text	See text	See text
Amplatz dilator	No	Yes	Yes
Metallic dilator	Yes	Yes	Yes
PCNL forceps	Yes	Yes	Yes
Energy probe	No	Yes	Yes
Laparoscopic instruments			
Metal ports	Yes	Yes	Yes
Scissors	No	Yes	Yes

(ETO: ethylene oxide; TURP: transurethral resection of the prostate; PCNL: percutaneous nephrolithotomy)

REFERENCES

1. Centers for Disease Control and Prevention. (2008). Guideline for Disinfection and Sterilization in Healthcare Facilities. [online] Available from: https://www.cdc.gov/infectioncontrol/pdf/guidelines/disinfection-guidelines-H.pdf. [Last accessed February 2021].
2. Spaulding EH. Chemical disinfection of medical and surgical materials. In: Lawrence C, Block SS (Eds). Disinfection, Sterilization, and Preservation. Philadelphia: Lea and Febiger; 1968. pp. 517-31.
3. Rutala WA, Weber DJ. Disinfection of endoscopes: review of new chemical sterilants used for high-level disinfection. Infect Control Hosp Epidemiol. 1999;20:69-76.
4. Russell AD. Bacterial resistance to disinfectants: present knowledge and future problems. J Hosp Infect. 1998;43:S57-68.
5. Rutala WA, Weber DJ. Clinical effectiveness of low-temperature sterilization technologies. Infect Control Hosp Epidemiol. 1998;19:798-804.

CHAPTER 13

Open Urology Instruments

OPEN SURGERY RETRACTORS

Bookwalter Retractor (Fig. 1)

Bookwalter retractor includes:
- Table post
- Horizontal bar
- 1″ postcoupling
- Medium oval ring
- 2″ × 6″ Malleable retractors (2 ea.) 51 mm × 152 mm
- 2″ × 3″ Kelly retractors (2 ea.) 51 mm × 76 mm
- 2″ × 4″ Kelly retractor 51 mm × 101 mm
- Balfour retractor
- Ratchet mechanisms (2 ea.)
- Tilt Ratchet mechanisms (6 ea.)
- Segmented ring
- 1 1/2″ × 6″ Malleable retractor 38 mm × 152 mm
- 3″ × 6″ Malleable retractor 76 mm × 152 mm

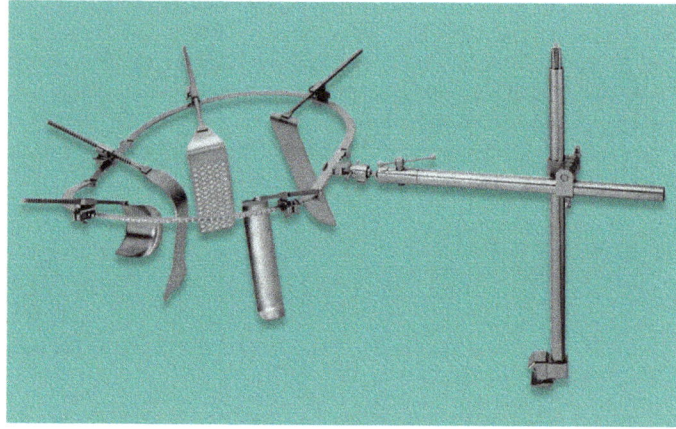

Figure 1: Bookwalter retractor.

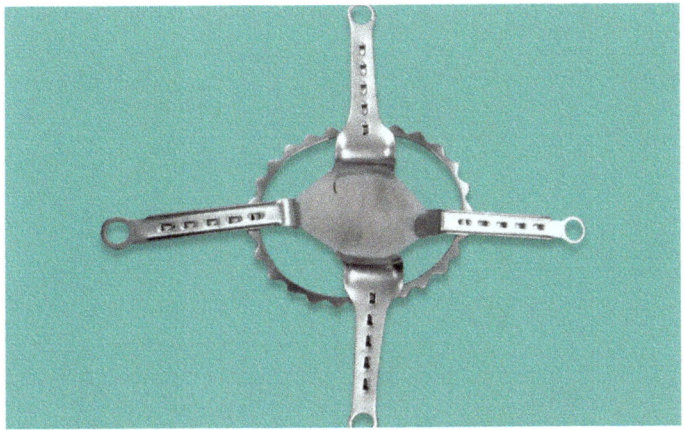

Figure 2: Denis Brown abdominal retractor.

- 2″ × 5″ Kelly retractor 51 mm × 127 mm
- 2″ × 6″ Kelly retractor 51 mm × 152 mm
- Horizontal flex bar
- Harrington retractor
- Gelpi retractor

As the retractors are fixed to the bar on operation theater (OT) table, the assistant need not hold the retractor.

Retractors are available in various shape and sizes for special surgeries, e.g., and renal cell carcinoma (RCC) with inferior vena cava (IVC) thrombus, large renal tumor, and retroperitoneal lymph node (RPLND).

Disadvantage: Bars might be a cause of obstacle for assistant to stand and see the surgery.

Denis Brown Abdominal Retractor (Fig. 2)

Denis Brown abdominal retractor with:
- 2 blade 40 mm × 30 mm
- 2 blade 40 mm × 40 mm
- 1 frame 190 mm × 160 mm
- Used in any abdominal surgery for retraction and pediatric surgery.

Millin's Self-retaining Bladder Retractor with a Provision for Attachment of Third Blade (Fig. 3)

Two blades are fitted on horizontal bars which can slide and may be fixed by screws. In between these two blades, there is another screw which may attach the third blade when required. When finger bows are separated, the blades are lying closer. When finger bows are approximated, the blades are separated.

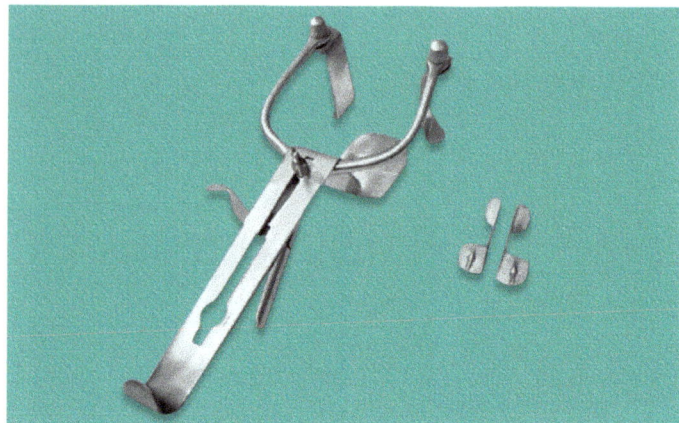

Figure 3: Millin's self-retaining bladder retractor.

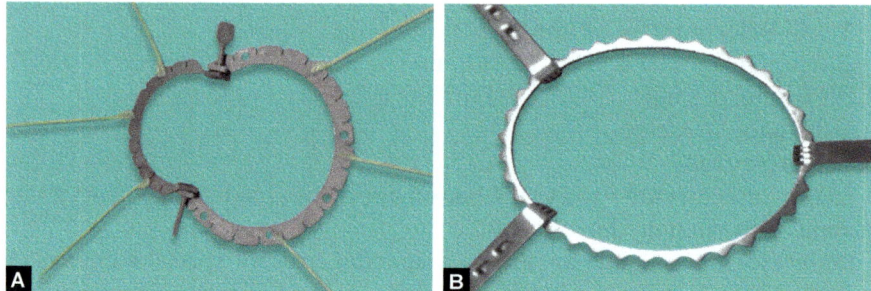

Figures 4A and B: Ring retractor.

This retractor is used during transvesical prostatectomy. The third blade retracts the fundus of the bladder. This keeps the bladder wide open and allows proper inspection of the prostate cavity and hemostasis under vision.

Ring Retractor (Figs. 4A and B)
- Turner Warwick retractor set, consisting of one circular ring 23 cm, four blades angled with lip 114 mm × 60 mm, and four blades curved 51 mm × 38 mm
- Used during urethroplasty for adequate exposure of the perineum.

Gil Vernet Hilar Retractor (Fig. 5A)
- Used for retraction of vein, renal hilum
- Available in various sizes; 20 cm (8 mm, 15 mm, 20 mm, and 23 mm)
- After creating plane of Gil Vernet, it can be used for retraction of tissues at renal hilum.

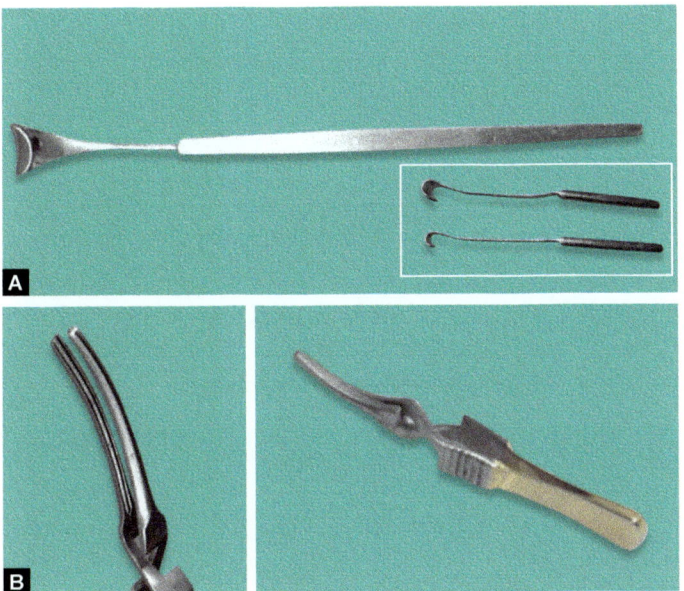

Figures 5A and B: (A) Gil Vernet hilar retractor; and (B) Bulldog clamp.

VASCULAR INSTRUMENTS

Bulldog Clamp (Fig. 5B)

It is used to grip blood vessels. DeBakey bulldog clamps, cross-action, 1 × 2 vascular teeth.
- *Shape*: Straight and curved
- *Material used*: Stainless steel.
- *Various sizes*: 1.5″, 2″, 2.5″, and 3″

Straight
- *Jaw length*: 20 mm, 30 mm, 45 mm, and 65 mm
- *Total length*: 79 mm, 89 mm, 105 mm, and 127 mm

Curved
- *Jaw length*: 20 mm, 30 mm, 45 mm, and 65 mm
- *Total length*: 76 mm, 86 mm, 105 mm, and 121 mm

Satinsky Vascular Clamp (Fig. 6)
- Satinsky classic vena cava clamps
- 1 × 2 vascular teeth Satinsky vascular clamp used to primarily clamp blood vessels
- *Material used*: Stainless steel

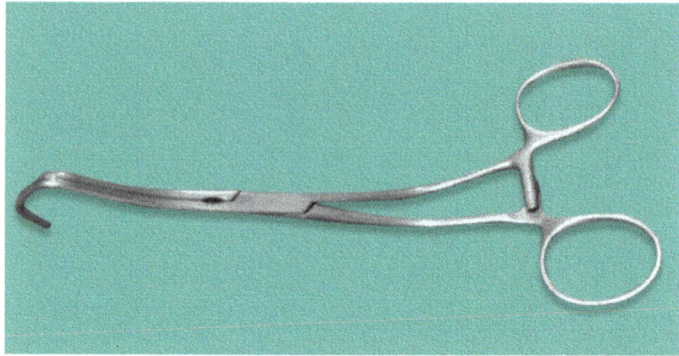

Figure 6: Satinsky vascular clamp.

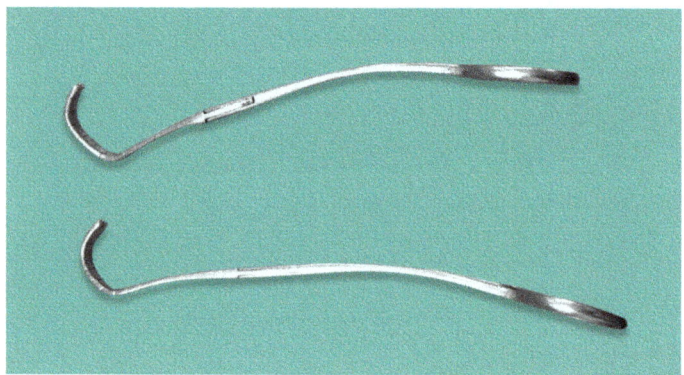

Figure 7: Cooley vascular clamp.

- Dimensions (inch) L × W × H: 11.1 × 3.8 × 2.0
- *Various sizes*: 8″, 9″, and 10″
- *Jaw length*:　68 mm　　　63 mm　　　57 mm
- *Jaw depth*:　12 mm　　　9 mm　　　6 mm
- *Total length*: 241 mm　　241 mm　　241 mm

Cooley Vascular Clamp (Fig. 7)

- Cooley classic anastomosis clamps
- Blades calibrated at 5 mm intervals, 2 × 2 vascular teeth
- Dimensions (inch) L × W × H: 7.0 × 3.0 × 0.25
- *Jaw length*: 73 mm
- *Jaw depth*: 17 mm
- *Total length*: 254 mm

DeBakey Vascular Clamps (Fig. 8)

- DeBakey classic multipurpose clamps
- 60° angle, 1 × 2 vascular teeth
- Dimensions (inch) L × W × H: 7.0 × 3.0 × 0.25

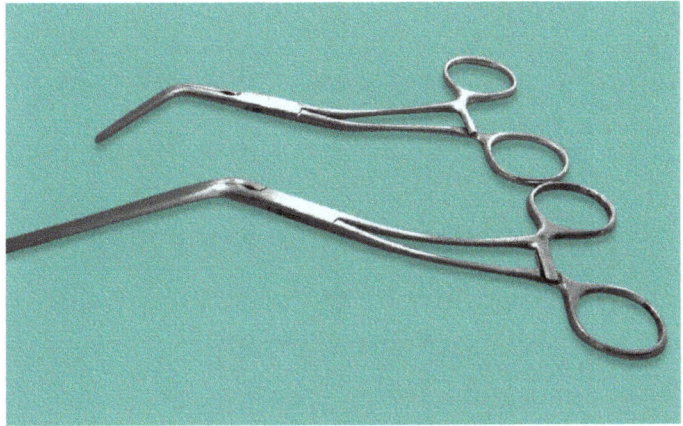

Figure 8: DeBakey vascular clamps.

- *Jaw length*: 40 mm, 50 mm, 70 mm, and 100 mm
- *Total length*: 244 mm, 203 mm, 241 mm, and 305 mm

DeBakey Vascular Forceps (Fig. 9)

DeBakey forceps is used to hold vascular vessels and tissues.

Lambert-Kay Vascular Inferior Vena Cava Clamp (Fig. 10)

- 1 × 2 vascular teeth
- *Jaw length*: 51 mm
- *Jaw depth*: 20 mm
- *Total length*: 191 mm

USES OF VASCULAR INSTRUMENTS

- *Used for temporary clamping of large vascular structures*: Iliac vessels, IVC, aorta, and renal artery
- Also used (bulldog clamp) during creation of arteriovenous (AV) fistula

STONE HOLDING FORCEPS

- *Desjardins forceps* (**Figs. 11A and B**): This is a long and slender instrument. There are finger bows but no catch. The shafts are curved, in some, it is gentle curve and in other varieties, there are different degrees of curvature. The blades are flat and fenestrated centrally. There are no fenestrations in the blade.

  It is used during removal of kidney, ureteric, or bladder stones.
- *Thompson Walker suprapubic cystolithotomy forceps* (**Fig. 12**): This forceps consists of finger bows—one finger bow for the thumb is ring-like, the other finger bow meant for other fingers is hook-like, a pair of shaft,

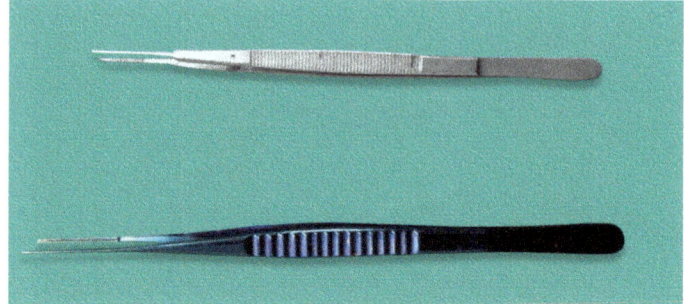

Figure 9: DeBakey vascular forceps.

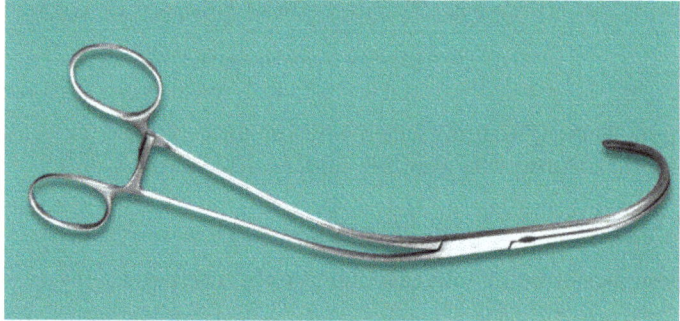

Figure 10: Lambert-Kay vascular inferior vena cava (IVC) clamp.

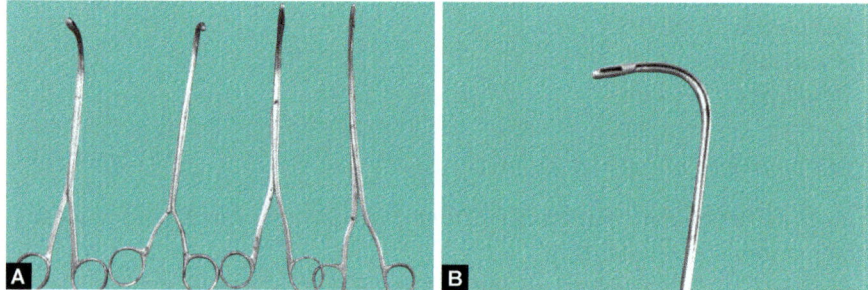

Figures 11A and B: Desjardins forceps.

and a pair of blades. The blades are longer and the inner surfaces of the blades are provided with fine knobs which help in better gripping of stones. There are no ratchets in this instrument.

USE

It is used for suprapubic cystolithotomy. After the bladder is opened by a suprapubic cystotomy, the instrument is inserted into the bladder and the stone is removed.

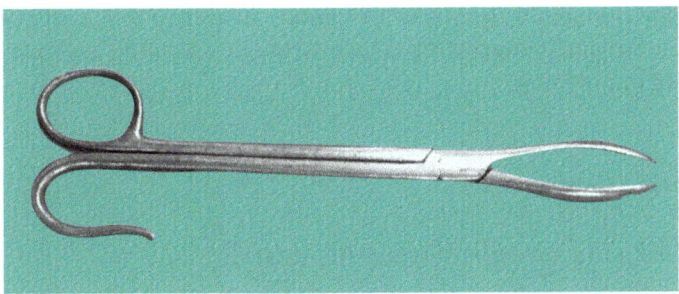

Figure 12: Thompson Walker suprapubic cystolithotomy forceps.

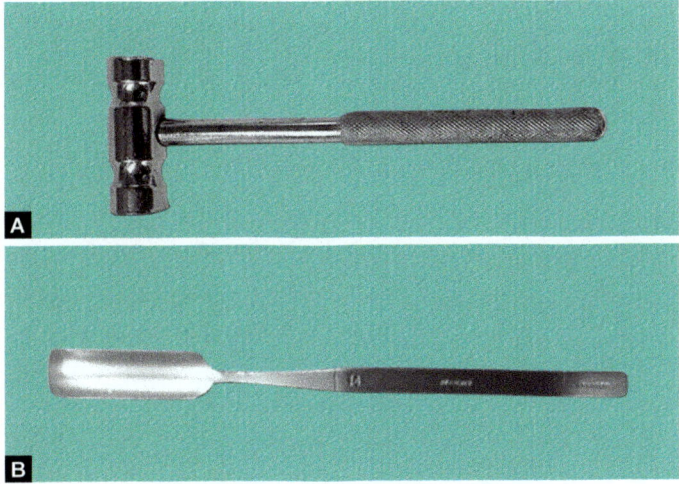

Figures 13A and B: Hammer and gouge.

INSTRUMENTS USED IN URETHRAL SURGERY

Chisel and Gouge (Fig. 13B)

It is used in progressive perineal urethroplasty during the step of inferior pubectomy.

Gouges (Fig. 13B)
- Length 8″ (203 mm)
- 1¼″ (32 mm)

Hammer (Fig. 13A)
- Diameter 1½″ (38 mm)
- Length 7″ (178 mm)
- Weight 15 oz (420 g)

Uses: Inferior pubectomy/excision of callous in transpubic urethroplasty. Gauge has a curved U-shaped tip which helps in removing the chip of the bone, during pubectomy.

Dilators

Metallic bougie: Characteristics

Clutton Metallic Bougie (Figs. 14A and B)

Clutton metallic bougie is a solid cylindrical metallic instrument. The handle is violin-shaped with a long shaft and the terminal end has a smooth curve

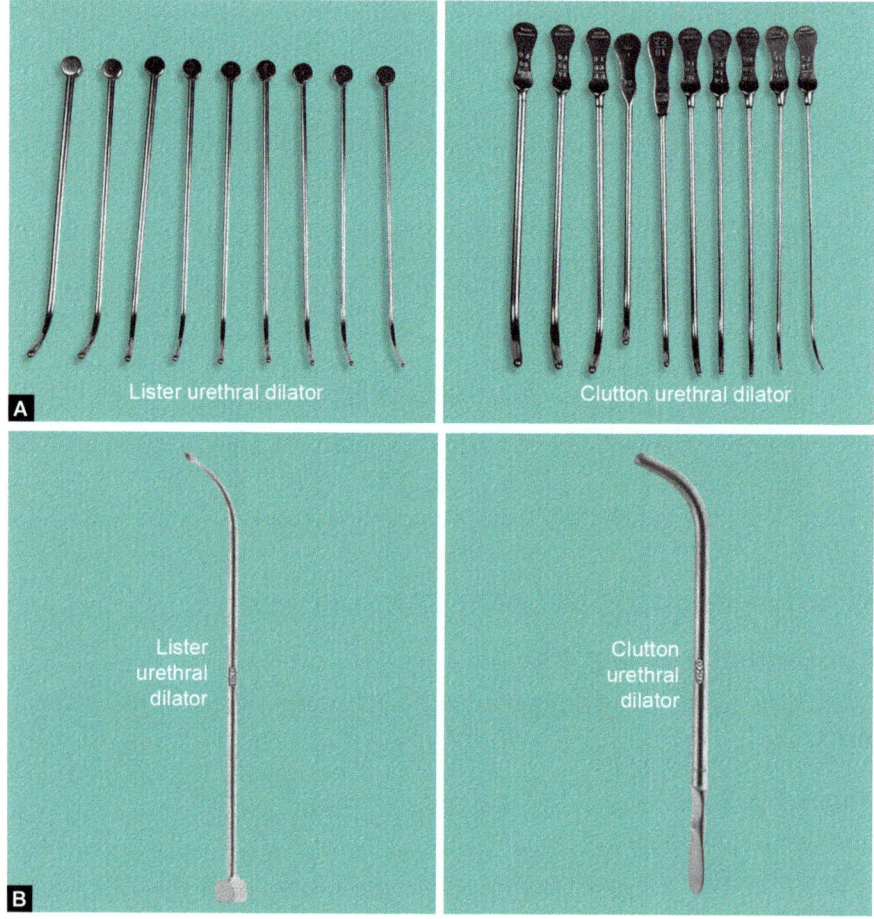

Figures 14A and B: Lister's and Clutton dilators. Lister's olive end with coin-shaped upper end with size marked. The upper figure is for tip and lower the broad part, Clutton round ended with violin-shaped upper end 3/6 size marked in millimeters upper for tip 4/8 for broad part. Both are used for dilating male urethra.

with a blunt tip. The denominator number denotes the circumference in millimeters. At the base and the numerator denotes the circumference in millimeters at tip. This is available in a set of 12 and the different numbers are 6/10, 8/12, 10/14, 12/16....28/32.

Lister's Metallic Bougie (Figs. 14A and B)

This is identical to a Clutton metallic bougie. The differences are—the handle is rounded and the tip is olive-pointed. The number written has a difference of three and has the same implication as in Clutton metallic bougie. This is also available in a set.

Uses of Metallic Bougie
- Used for dilatation of urethra in urethral stricture
- Used for dilatation of urethra prior to introduction of cystoscope
- Used during repair of rupture urethra by rail road technique
- Used for progressive perineal urethroplasty for identification of urethra

Haygrove Sound (Figs. 15A and B)

Haygrove sound is introduced into the suprapubic sinus and through the bladder neck to the distal limits of the posterior urethra.
Disadvantage: May go into false passage.

Kilian Septum Speculum (Fig. 16)
- *Total length*: 5¼" (133 mm)
- *With variable*:
  - *Blade length*: 2" (51 mm)
  - *Blade length*: 2½" (63 mm)
  - *Blade length*: 3" (76 mm)

Used during perineal urethrostomy, ventral onlay for buccal mucosal graft suturing at proximal urethra.

Thudicum (Fig. 17)
- The speculum is available in a wide range of other sizes, from size 0 to size 7.
- Size 70 mm
- Used during perineal urethrostomy—used for proper exposure of proximal urethra

Gorget

It is used for taking sutures from proximal urethra (**Fig. 18**).

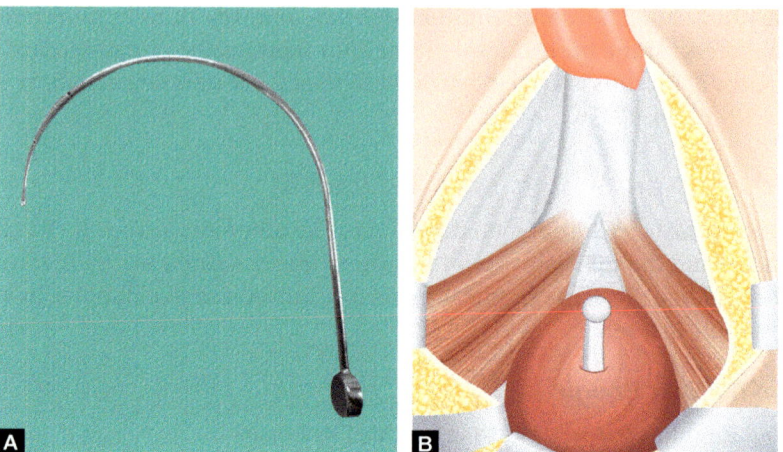

Figures 15A and B: Haygrove sound.

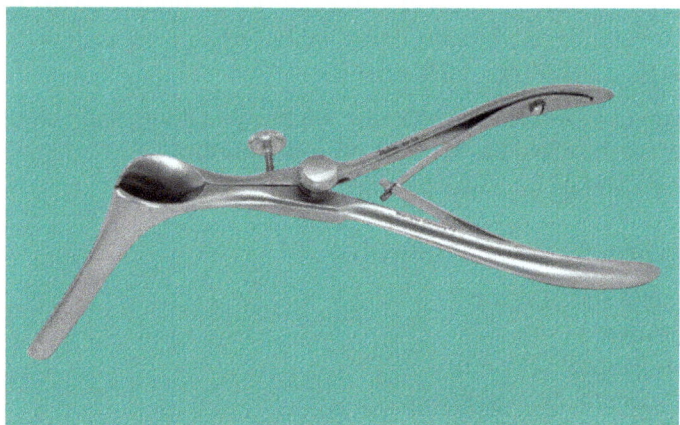

Figure 16: Kilian septum speculum.

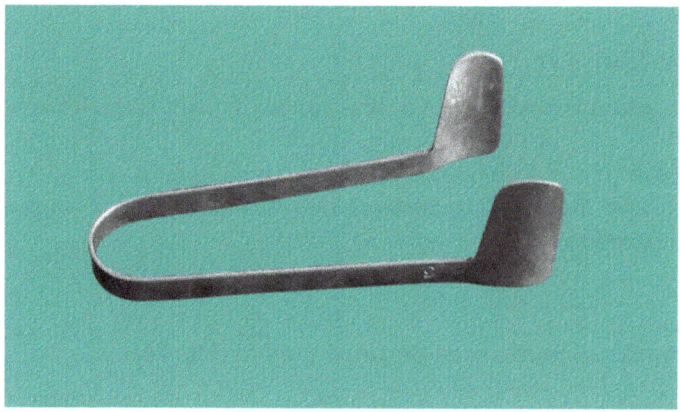

Figure 17: Thudicum.

CHAPTER 13: Open Urology Instruments | 185

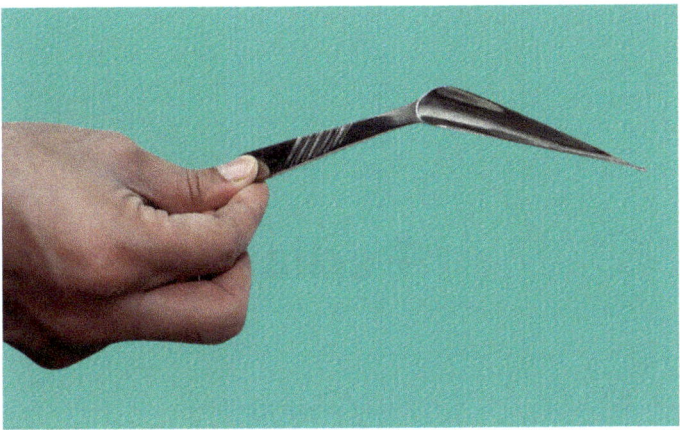

Figure 18: Gorget.

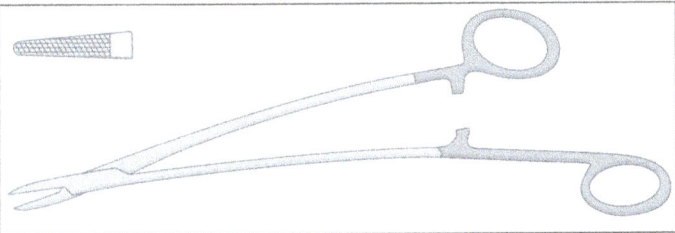

Figure 19: Turner Warwick.

Turner Warwick Needle Holder

Turner Warwick needle holder is an articulated needle holder. Thumb grip is at an angle to finger grip. Tip of the needle holder holding the needle is always visible. While taking suture from posterior urethra surgeon can always see direction of the needle (**Fig. 19**).

CHAPTER 14

Pediatric Urology

PEDIATRIC ENDOUROLOGY INSTRUMENTS

Various pediatric cystoscopes available are as follows:
- Rigid neonatal cystourethroscope
- Rigid pediatric cystourethroscope
- Compact cystourethroscope

For Neonates

Wolf Miniature Compact Fiber Cystourethroscope (Fig. 1)
- 4.5 Fr/6.5 Fr
- Angled eyepiece
- *Working length*: 120 mm
- *Viewing direction*: 5°
- *Working channel*: 3 Fr
- Oval irrigation
- Two lateral ports
- Autoclavable

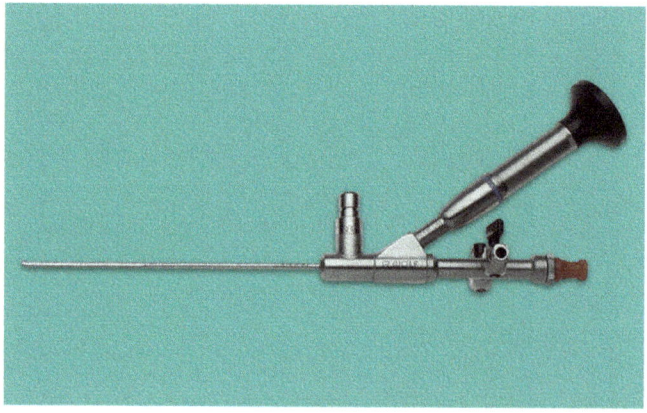

Figure 1: Compact fiber cystourethroscope (neonatal).

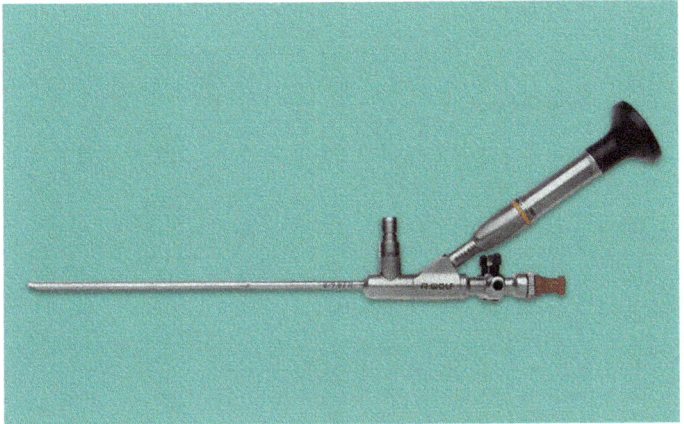

Figure 2: Fiber cystourethroscope (infant).

For Infants

Wolf pediatric cystourethroscope (**Fig. 2**)
- 8 Fr/9.8 Fr
- Angled eyepiece
- Atraumatic distal tip
- *Working length*: 150 mm
- 12-degree viewing angle
- Straight working channel of 5 Fr for rigid and flexible instruments
- Optimal for reflux therapy

Storz Pediatric Cystourethroscope (Fig. 3)
- *Tip*: 7 Fr, 1 step, 7–11 Fr
- With angled eyepiece
- 6-degree viewing angle
- *Length*: 13cm
- Autoclavable
- Fiberoptic light transmission
- Two lateral irrigation ports
- One working channel of 5 Fr for operating instruments of 4 Fr

For Adolescents

Wolf cystourethroscope (**Fig. 4**)
- Cystourethroscopes (12.5 Fr and 14 Fr) with working channel of 5 Fr and 7 Fr, respectively

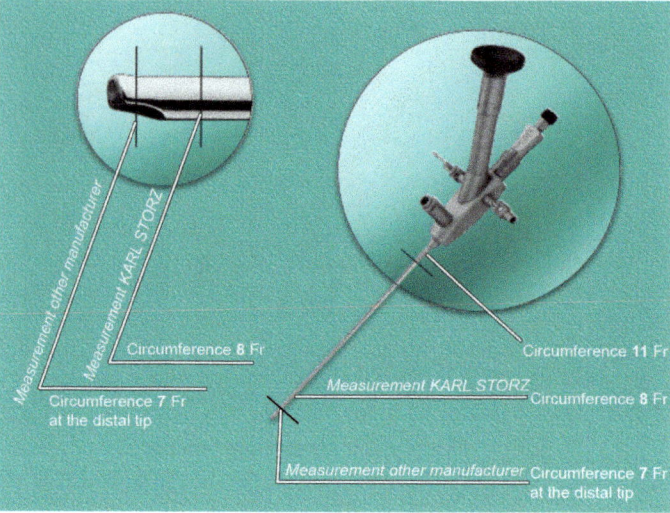

Figure 3: Pediatric cystourethroscope.

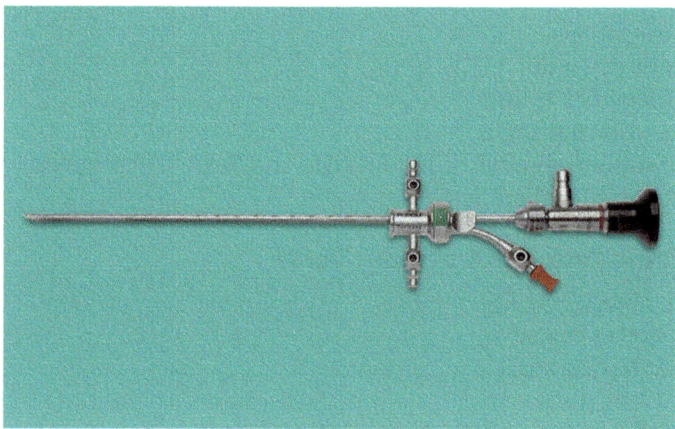

Figure 4: Adolescent cystourethroscope.

- Atraumatic distal tip
- Adaptor (bridge) with one/two ports available
- PANOVIEW telescope 2.7 mm diameter
- Viewing direction 30°
- Compatible with all common injection needles for endoscopic antireflux therapy

Cystoscope for Use with Deflux Needles
Cystoscope-urethroscope Sheath (Fig. 5)
- 8 Fr with 4 Fr working channel for Deflux needles
- With obturator and two Luer lock connectors
- With the proximally extended working channel in the Deflux sheath, the rigid needles can be gently inserted into the working channel, without becoming blunt.

Instruments for Use with Pediatric Operating Cystourethroscope
- Hook electrode—unipolar, 3 Fr (**Fig. 6**)
- Grasping forceps (**Fig. 7**)

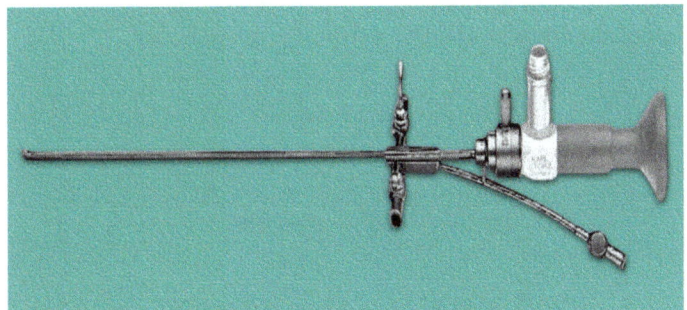

Figure 5: Cystoscope-urethroscope sheath.

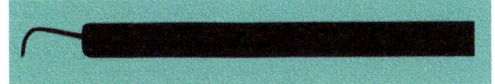

Figure 6: Hook electrode—unipolar, 3 Fr.

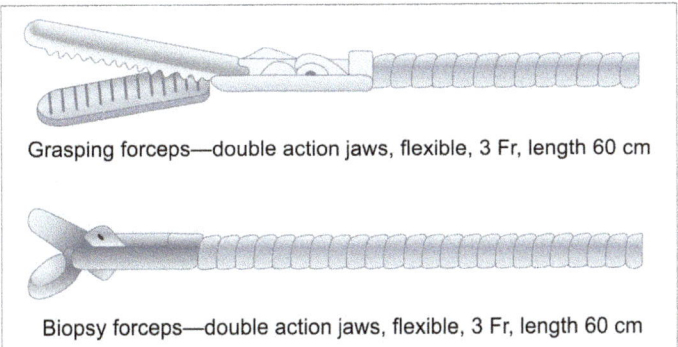

Grasping forceps—double action jaws, flexible, 3 Fr, length 60 cm

Biopsy forceps—double action jaws, flexible, 3 Fr, length 60 cm

Figure 7: Accessories used with pediatric cystoscope-urethro-fiberscope.

Monopolar coagulating bugbee electrode (**Fig. 8**)
- Bugbee electrode
  - *Diameter*: 3 Fr
  - *Working length*: 53 cm

Wolf Pediatric Optical Urethrotome (Fig. 9)
- 8.5 Fr
- 1.9 mm telescope
- 3-mm working channel
- 0-degree viewing angle

Pediatric Optical Urethrotome (Storz) (Fig. 10)
Features
- 8 Fr for use with miniature straightforward telescope
- Distal end of sheath is shaped in an atraumatic manner.

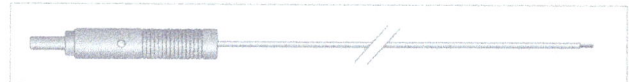

Figure 8: Bugbee electrode.

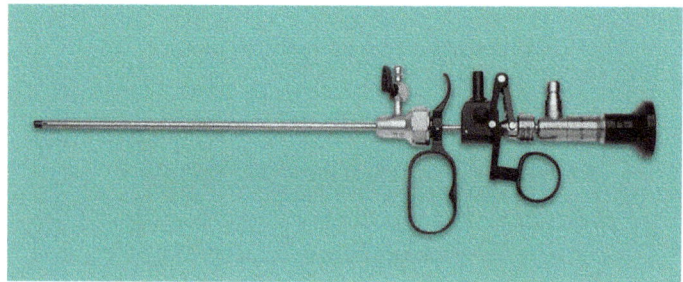

Figure 9: Pediatric cystoscope-urethro-fiberscope.

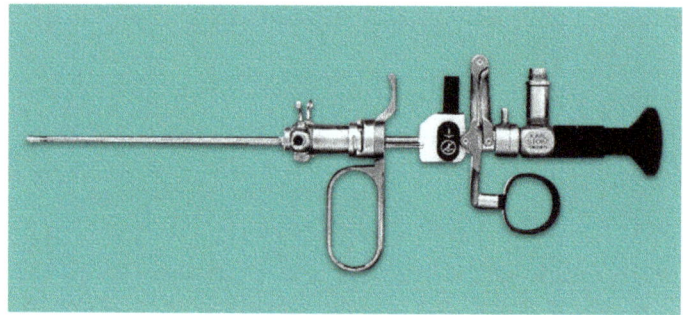

Figure 10: Pediatric optical urethrotome.

- Minimal sheath diameter
- Cutting by means of spring, in rest position, the electrode tip is inside the sheath
- *Working length*: 11 cm
- Various urethrotome knives are available for use (**Fig. 11**)

Resectoscope (Figs. 12 to 14)

(Richard Wolf)
- 9 Fr, 11.5 Fr, and 14.5 Fr
- *Telescope*: 1.9 mm, 2.7 mm, and 2.7 mm diameter, respectively
- Viewing direction: 0°

Pediatric Resectoscope (Storz)
- 9 Fr for use with miniature straightforward telescope (**Figs. 15A and B**)

Special Features
- Distal end of sheath is atraumatically shaped
- Minimal sheath diameter

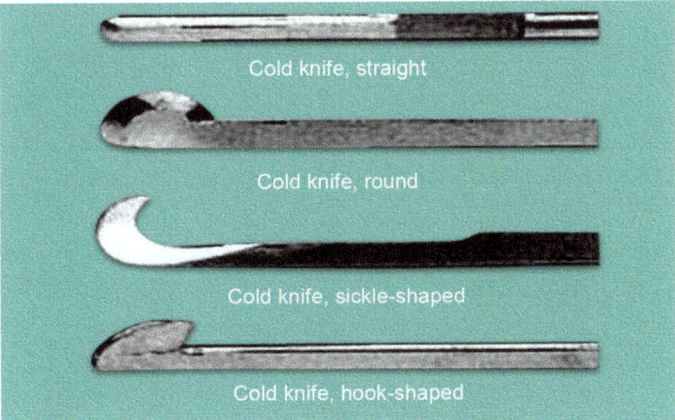

Figure 11: Urethrotome knifes.

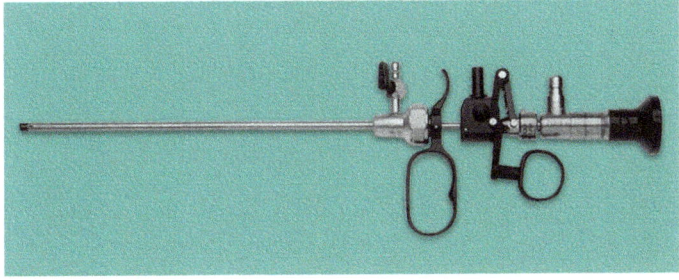

Figure 12: Pediatric resectoscope.

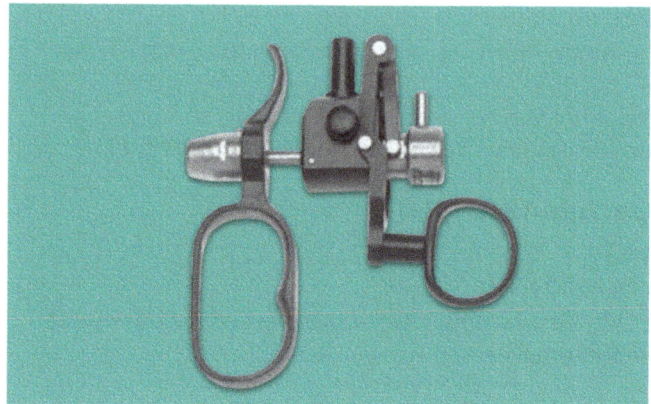

Figure 13: Passive working element.

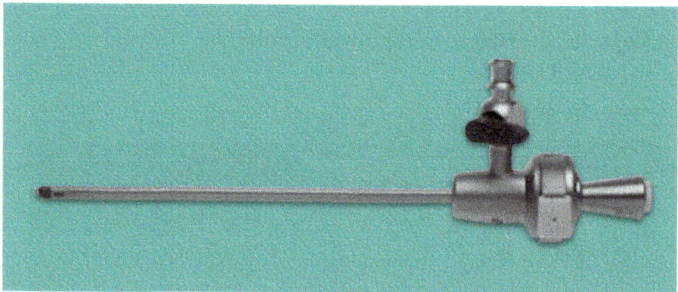

Figure 14: Sheath with fixed irrigation tap and obturator.

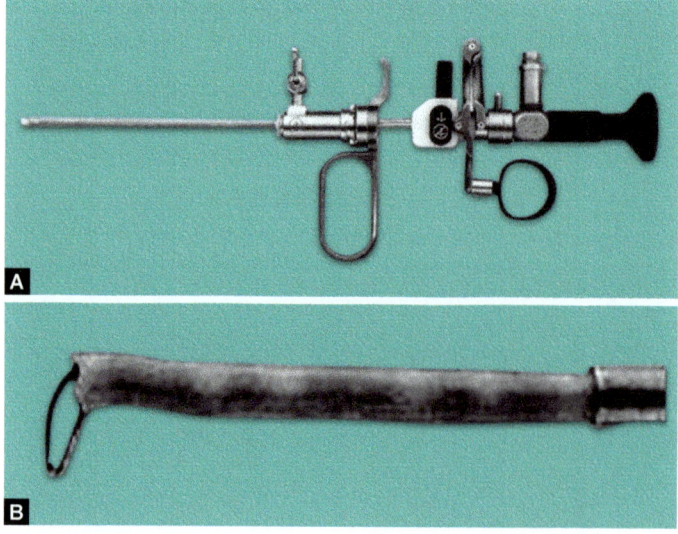

Figures 15A and B: (A) Pediatric resectoscope; and (B) Cutting loop—angled.

- Cutting by means of spring, in rest position, the electrode tip is inside sheath
- *Working length*: 12 cm
- Resectoscope sheath is 9 Fr with Luer lock stopcock, including connecting tube for inflow

Electrodes (Fig. 16)

Pediatric Ureterorenoscope (Storz) (Fig. 17)

Special Features
- *Distal tip*: 7.3 Fr
- Two lateral, right-angled irrigation ports
- *Instrument sheath*: 7.3 Fr, conical, 1step, 7.3–8 Fr
- *Working channel*: 3.6 Fr for use with instruments up to 3 Fr
- *Telescope*: Fiberoptic system, direction of view 6°
- Working length 25 cm

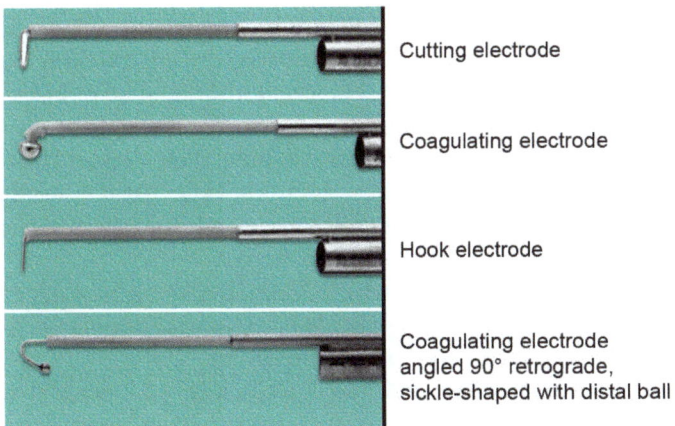

Figure 16: Resectoscope electrodes.

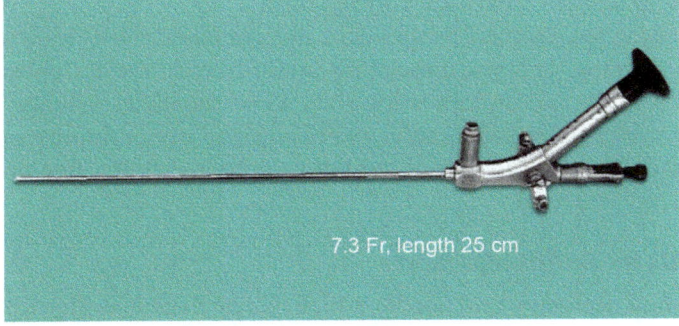

Figure 17: Pediatric ureterorenoscope.

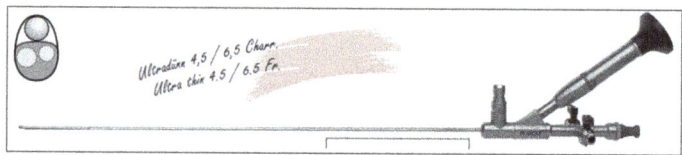

Figure 18: Wolf ureterorenoscope.

Wolf Pediatric Ureterorenoscope (4.5 Fr/6.5 Fr) (Fig. 18)
Lateral Eyepiece
- *Distal tip*: 4.5 Fr
- 5-degree viewing angle
- *Working channel*: 3 Fr admits lithoclast probe of 0.8 mm
- *Working length*: 430 mm
- *Total length*: 570 mm

Instruments for PUV Fulguration

In infants fulguration is done by inserting pediatric neonatal scope and through which bugbee electrode of 3 Fr can be passed and fulguration can be done using cautery pure current. Fulguration can also be done by using MIP XS nephroscope which is only 7.5 Fr size. Either bugbee or laser can be used for fulguration. In elder children, bigger cystoscope or 12 Fr miniperc can also be used. If these instruments are not available, then slender URS can be used with long length bugbee. Bugbee electrode (**Fig. 19**) it is available in different sizes 3 F or 5 F, Different length to be used through cystoscope or ureteroscope, Different tip design round tip, hook.

Bugbee is a wire with insulation which is attached to monopolar cautery. Generates current where it touches like PUV. Being monopolar it requires patient plate and foot paddle to complete the circuit.

In PUV fulguration is done at 5 and 7 o'clock or 12 o'clock if valve is prominent at roof. If you are using hook, then valves are engaged in hook and transient current is applied. Valves in children are flimsy and usually in one or two bursts fulguration is done. It is better to under do rather than over do. With round tip bugbee valves are only touched

Previously when neonatal scopes were not available valves were excised by Whitaker's hook. This was procedure under fluro control. Contrast was injected in bladder and urethra with valves were visualized. Whitaker hook was passed under fluoroscope valves were engaged under fluoroscopy and then mechanically excised by pulling hook which as sharp edge on inner side. No energy was used.

Instruments for Deflux Injection

Deflux can be injected by thin needle which can be flexible or rigid. Flexible needle can be introduced via cystoscope- and appropriate quantity can be

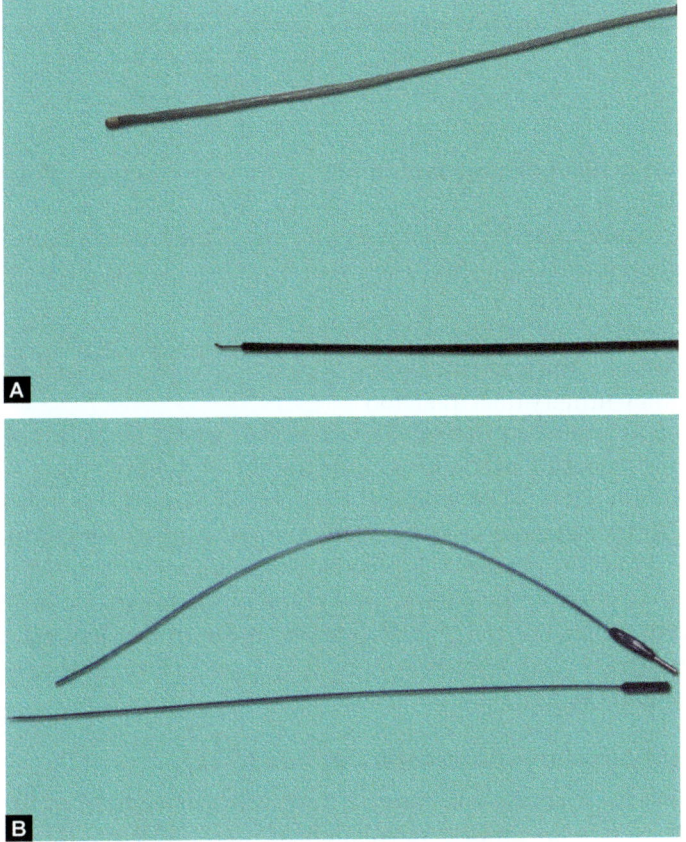

Figures 19A and B: Hook and round tip

injected submucosally at 6 o'clock position in ureteric orifice. Now days preferred instrument is MIPXS or MIP M nephroscope depending upon size of urethra. Advantage is long rigid needle can be use which has better control and precise injection can be done. 8F minimicroperc can also be used & through central channel needle can be passed.

Same needle and same instruments can used for injection of Botox in cases of neurogenic bladder, over active bladder or sometimes in sphincter in cases of spastic sphincter.

DEFLUX

Deflux is a sterile, highly viscous gel of dextranomer microspheres (50 mg/mL) in a carrier gel of nonanimal stabilized hyaluronic acid (15 mg/mL), constituting a biocompatible and biodegradable implant. The dextranomer microspheres range in size between 80 and 250 microns with an average size of about 130 microns. Deflux is supplied prefilled in a 1 mL syringe with a Luer lock fitting, and is intended for single use only. The syringe is equipped with a tip cap, plunger, and plunger rod. The syringe is terminally sterilized.

Indications

Deflux is indicated for treatment of children with vesicoureteral reflux (VUR) grades II–IV.
- Deflux is contraindicated in patients with any of the following conditions:
    o Nonfunctional kidney(s)
    o Hutch diverticulum
    o Ureterocele
    o Active voiding dysfunction
    o Ongoing urinary tract infection

It is recommended to use the Deflux metal needle (3.7 F × 23G tip × 350 mm) for safe and accurate administration of Deflux. The needle is introduced through a 4 Fr working channel. The needle is introduced under the bladder mucosa 2–3 mm below the refluxing ureteral orifice at a 6 o'clock position. The needle tip is positioned just under the urothelium and is advanced 4–5 mm in the submucosal plane of the ureter. Deflux is then injected until a prominent bulge appears, and the orifice has assumed a crescent-like shape. Only a small volume (0.5–1.0 mL) is needed to create a sufficient bolus (**Fig. 19**).

Pediatric Uretero-reno-fiberscope (Figs. 20 to 22)

With positive (or logical) deflection, a downward movement of the lever mechanism causes an upward movement of the endoscope tip and vice versa. Reverse this orientation by choosing the contrapositive mechanism; a downward movement of lever mechanism now causes a downward movement of the endoscope tip (**Table 1**).

A larger angle upward from 270° and downward from 270° allows for the intuitive orientation and visualization of the entire renal tract, including the intrarenal collecting system. The new angulation mechanism makes

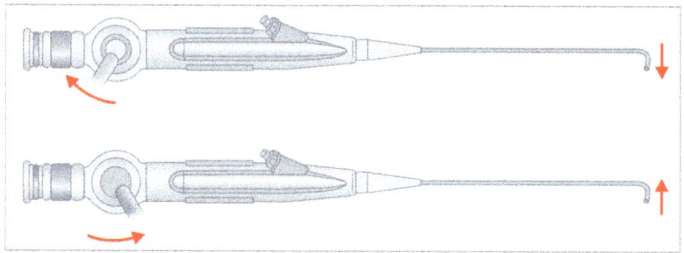

Figure 20: Pediatric cystoscope-urethro-fiberscope: Positive deflection mechanism.

it possible to use 200 μ laser fibers without compromising the angulation properties. Even large 365 μ laser fibers only result in a 10% loss of the angulation properties.

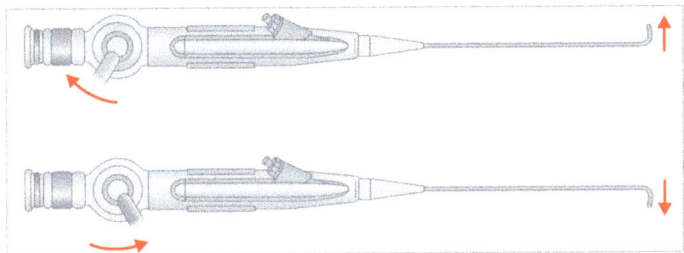

Figure 21: Pediatric cystoscope-urethro-fiberscope: Contrapositive deflection mechanism.

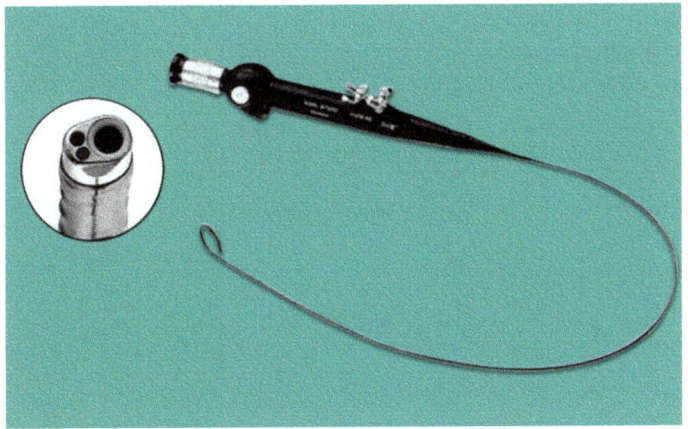

Figure 22: Pediatric uretero-reno-fiberscope.

TABLE 1: Pediatric ureterorenoscopes.						
Deflection of distal tip		Direction of view	Angle of view	Working length	Working channel inner diameter	Sheath size
Positive deflection		0°	88°	45 cm	3.6 Fr	7.5 Fr
With contrapositive deflection		0°	88°	45 cm	3.6 Fr	7.5 Fr

DIAGNOSTIC AND THERAPEUTIC INDICATIONS

- Lithotripsy and stone extraction in ureteral and renal tract
- Maximum angle of 270° permits access to the entire renal tract, including lower renal calyces
- Allows detection of pathology in anatomical areas difficult to access

DIAGNOSIS

- Identifying causes of hematuria
- Differential diagnosis of filling defects
- Diagnosis of ureteral tumors

THERAPY

- Removing calculi or foreign bodies
- Treating ureteral tumors
- Coagulating hemorrhagic
- Disintegrating ureteral calculi

CHAPTER 15

Lasers in Urology

INTRODUCTION

The term laser is basically acronym for "light amplification by stimulated emission of radiation." The use of lasers in urology started about half a century back. Ruby laser was used in carcinoma penis by Parsons et al. in 1968.[1] First commercial laser lithotripter was used in 1980s. Holmium laser is the work horse of laser lithotripsy in many parts of the world. The advent of Thulium laser fiber may change the situation in the coming years. Field of urology has always been at the forefront in the use of lasers, in fact about half of the published literature on lasers is pertaining to lasers in urology. Also, when it comes to laser lithotripsy, about 85-90% of the articles published are on urological applications.[2]

CLASSIFICATIONS OF LASER AS PER ITS USE IN UROLOGY

Laser for stone management	Laser for BPH management	Laser for stone and BPH management
Holmium:YAG (low watt)	Thulium laser	Holmium:YAG (high watt)
	Green light laser	Thulium laser fiber
	Diode laser	
	KTP/Nd:YAG	

(BPH: benign prostatic hyperplasia; KTP/Nd:YAG: potassium titanyl phosphate/ neodymium:yttrium aluminum garnet; YAG: yttrium aluminum garnet)

Classification as per Pulsed or Continuous Laser

Continuous laser	Pulsed laser
Thulium laser	Holmium:YAG
Green light laser	Thulium laser fiber
Diode laser	
KTP/Nd:YAG	
Thulium fiber laser	

(KTP/Nd:YAG: potassium titanyl phosphate/neodymium:yttrium aluminum garnet)

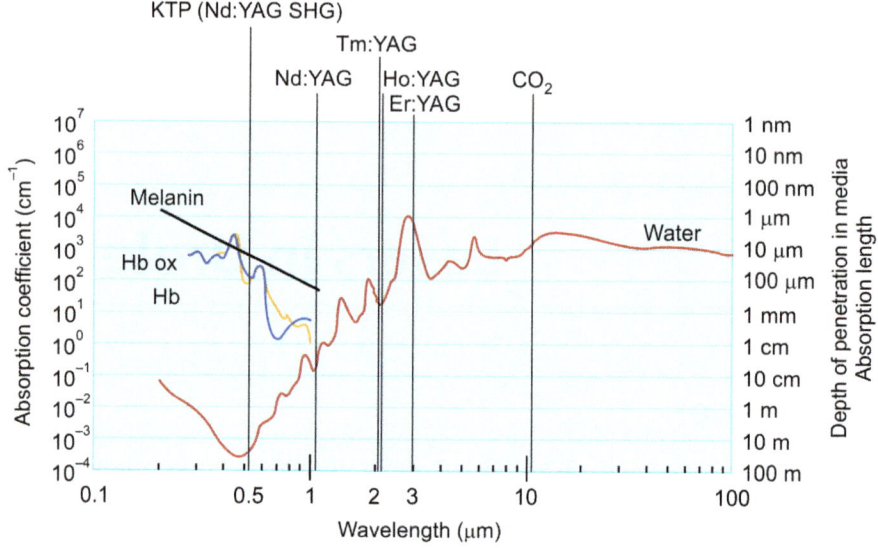

Figure 1: Depth of penetration of different lasers.

Solid State Lasers (Fig. 1)

- Holmium:yttrium aluminum garnet (YAG) laser
- Thulium:YAG laser
- Green light laser
- Diode laser
- Potassium titanyl phosphate/neodymium:yttrium aluminum (KTP/Nd:YAG)

Fiber-based Laser: Thulium Laser Fiber

Lasers properties and mechanism of action.

Holmium Laser

Holmium laser was developed years after the first reference to laser lithotripsy was made.

Properties of Holmium:YAG laser are as follows:
- Wavelength—2,100 nm
- Completely absorbed by water within 0.4 mm of fiber tip
- It is a contact laser.
- Can fragment all types of urinary calculi
- Can be transmitted by using fibers as small as 200 µm

The above properties make it safe, efficacious, and most commonly used tool for laser lithotripsy in urology.

MECHANISM OF LASER BEAM PRODUCTION IN HOLMIUM LASER

The Holmium:YAG is produced in an optical cavity. The YAG crystal is doped with holmium ions and this construction is referred to as a solid-state laser (**Fig. 2**). During each pulse, light is emitted from the flash lamp which contains xenon or a krypton. The emitted light interacts with holmium ions and results in emission of new photons with a wavelength of 2,120 nm. These photons in the optical cavity are reflected by mirror at the end of the cavity. This reflection results in further activation of the holmium ions and additional pump cycles are used to generate a particular energy pulse. A small cavity opening allows pulsed laser energy to exit the cavity when desired.

Most energy generated by flash lamp is broad spectrum and causes the cavity to heat. Only a part of the broad-spectrum energy emitted by flash lamp is absorbed by the holmium YAG system (**Fig. 3**).

This excess heating requires a cooling system. This water based cooling system adds to the bulk of the machine and makes it less portable. Maximum temperature range also determines the maximum energy and frequency a machine can reach; single cavity and generator systems can reach up to 30 W. High watt lasers >50 W require multiple cavities, a vapor compression refrigeration system is required as a cooling mechanism for the high power laser.

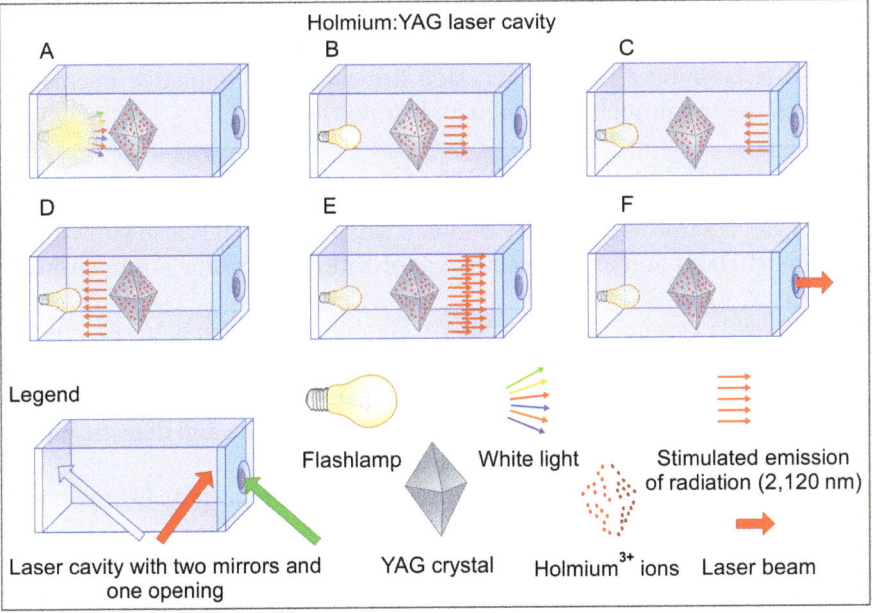

Figure 2: Holmium:yttrium aluminum garnet (YAG) laser cavity.

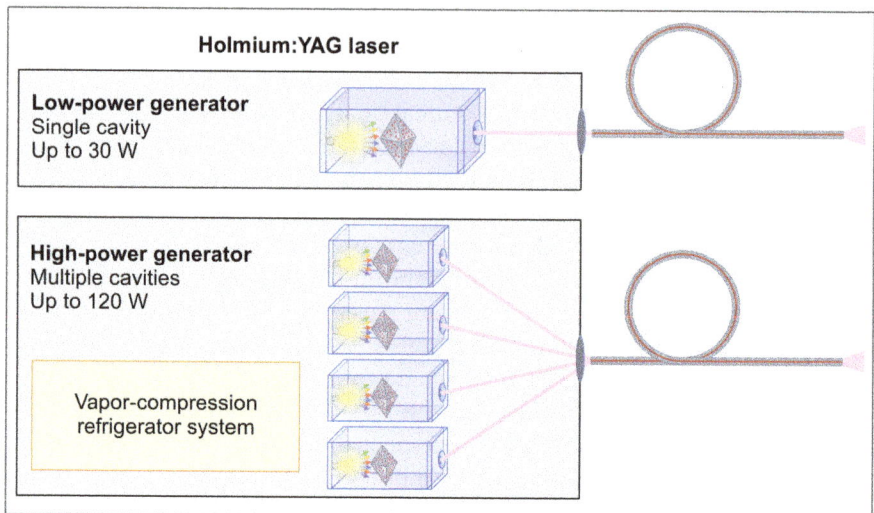

Figure 3: Holmium:yttrium aluminum garnet (YAG) laser.

NEODYMIUM:YTTRIUM ALUMINUM GARNET LASER

- It is a solid-state laser with a wavelength of 1,032 nm. It has a very low absorption coefficient and has a depth of penetration of 4–18 mm. It has a low-energy density in the tissue, therefore heat occurs below the boiling temperature. Coagulation and vaporization are possible but resection and enucleation are not possible.
- In this laser, energy is transmitted using a deflectable fiber tip. Prostatic tissue is laser by a noncontact, side firing laser. Coagulative necrosis occurs, tissue cannot be obtained for histology.

POTASSIUM TITANYL PHOSPHATE LASER

- KTP laser is same as frequency doubled Nd:YAG laser. It is also known as green light laser and photoselective vaporization of prostate is done using this laser.
- The invisible wavelength of the Nd:YAG is shifted to green light spectrum and frequency to 532 nm. This wavelength can be strongly absorbed by hemoglobin, but not by water. As the laser is absorbed by blood completely, it penetrates 1–3 mm in prostatic adenoma and delivers high energy causing photothermal vaporization.
- Tissue ablation rate of 0.3–0.5 g/min has been reported. Feasible in patients on anticoagulants.

HOLMIUM:YTTRIUM ALUMINUM GARNET LASER

It is a pulsed solid-state laser with a wavelength of 2,140 nm. Strongly absorbed by water. It is absorbed to a length of 0.4 mm in prostatic tissue. It causes heating of prostatic tissue to temperature of 100°C. This causes vaporization without deep coagulation. It is a sharp cutting tool along with coagulation of small- and medium-sized vessels up to depth of 2-3 mm. Enucleation, vaporization, resection, and vaporesection can be done.

THULIUM:YTTRIUM ALUMINUM GARNET LASER

- It is a continuous form laser with the wavelength of 2,013 nm. It is absorbed by water and depth of penetration is 0.25 mm. As well absorbed by water, it lowers depth of penetration and efficient absorption.
- It can be used for vaporization, enucleation resection, and vaporesection. It is a precise cutting and coagulating tools.

THULIUM FIBER LASER

Thulium fiber laser (TFL) consists of a very thin long silica fiber doped with thulium ions.[3] The core diameter of fiber is 10-20 μm and it is 10-30 meter long (**Fig. 4**). Diode lasers are used to excite the thulium ions. The wavelength of the emitted wave is 1,940 nm. It can be operated as both pulsed and continuous laser. A wide range of energy and frequency settings can be used with this laser. As it does not use a flash lamp, heat generation does not occur out of proportion and water-based cooling is not required. Cooling mechanism is composed of a forced fan ventilation.

Diode laser used for pumping thulium ions has energy spectrum that matches the thulium ions absorption line. This makes TFL more energy efficient and can operate at >50 W and frequency ranges of up to 2,000 Hz with forced fan cooling mechanism. As no mirrors are involved in construction of the TFL, it is more shock resistant as compared to the Holmium:YAG laser. The beam emitted from TFL has a more uniform distribution as it is emitted

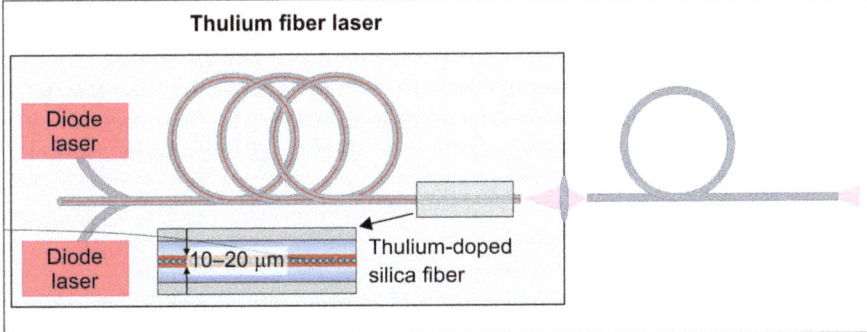

Figure 4: Schematic representation of a Thulium fiber laser. Laser pumping is achieved by electronically modulating diode lasers (pink boxes). A Thulium-doped, 10–20 μm core diameter, 10–30 m long silica fiber (red tube with green spots) is used as a gain medium for the generation of a laser beam. The uniform laser beam at the output connector allows for the use of laser fibers as small as 50 μm (blue).

from a small fiber rather than a large solid block of YAG. This allows focusing of the beam to very small spot and transmission through small diameter fibers (50-100 μm). The small diameter of surgical fiber is the conduit for laser energy and is different from the silica fiber which is doped with thulium ions and is present within the laser cavity of the TFL machine.

Thulium fiber laser is different from Thulium:YAG laser which is a solid-state laser and has a wavelength of 2,010 nm. It can be used as pulsed and continuous form. It can be used for enucleation. It has a wavelength of 1,940 nm.

	High watt Holmium laser	Thulium laser fiber
Wavelength	2,120 nm	1,940 nm
Pulse energy range	0.2–6 J	0.025–6.0 J
Pulse duration	0.05–1 ms	0.05–12 ms
Pulse frequency	120 Hz	2,000 Hz
Smallest fiber available	200 μm	150 μm
Cooling system	Water-based, vapor compression refrigeration for high watt lasers	Fan-based
Durability against shock	Low	High

Advantages of Thulium Fiber Laser

- Smaller size fiber can allow for better scope maneuverability in the pelvicalyceal system and the stones in the lower and inaccessible regions can be targeted better. Smaller fiber allows better irrigation and consequently vision. This can pave way for development of smaller size ureteroscopes.
- Use of pulse energy as low as 0.025 J will cause less heating and precise delivery of energy. TFL allows setting pulse duration as long as 12 ms, this pulse duration enables uniform distribution of energy in a flat top configuration.
- *Using high frequency*: As the fiber diameter decreases by half the energy has to be decreased by four times. To compensate for the same frequency can be increased up to 2,000 Hz in TFL. This would maintain the net ablation volume.

ANATOMY OF A LASER FIBER

Laser system transmits laser energy to the operative site through a flexible fiberoptic delivery system called the laser fiber or just the fiber.

Fiber Hub

The proximal end of the fiber is known as the hub; it has a threaded coupler to establish a secure connection with the machine. A stainless-steel ferrule aligns the fiberoptic part of the laser fiber with the optical output of laser system. The SMA 905 connector is a type of connector which provides cross-connectivity between different machines. Some fibers provide protective quartz insert in the hub. This insert absorbs the errant laser blast and protects the optical deck and the blast shield. Another feature that protects the laser fiber damage is the "Air well termination" in the connector.

Energy Transmission

The laser energy is transmitted via fiber core made of silica. Pulsed energy from the optical deck of the laser machine is transmitted to or focused through the fiber core. The fiber core is surrounded by a thin silica cladding; this cladding has a slightly lower index of refraction. The laser energy travels through the fiber core using the principle of total internal reflection, this implies that the all the energy travels via the dense silica core and reflects of the less dense silica cladding (**Fig. 5**).

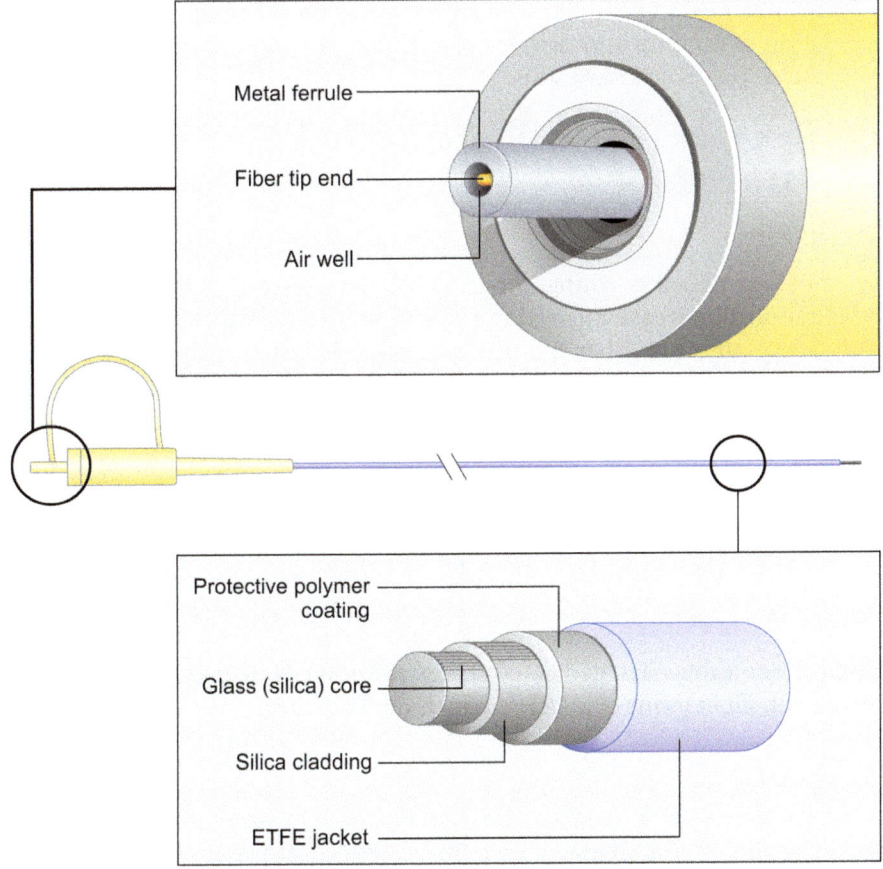

Figure 5: Anatomy of a laser fiber.

The thin silica cladding is further enforced by a polymer coating that protects the fiber damage during bending. Finally, the whole assembly is covered by ethylene tetrafluoroethylene (ETFE) jacket, this covering protects the fiber from the friction caused between fiber and the scope channel. Thus, the scope channel and the fiber are both protected.

FIBER SIZE

Various fiber sizes are available from 150 to 1,000 μm.

Fibers can be single use or multiple use depending on the make. Fiber size is inclusive of the fiber core and the cladding. The smaller the fiber, the more flexible it is and the lesser energy it will transmit. Larger fiber diameter creates wider ablation fissures, whereas smaller diameter fibers create a deeper ablation fissure. Larger fibers become less ablative if low energies (0.2 J) are used, in this situation the surface area of the fiber tip may be too high for the low energy delivered leading to decreased ablation. Larger fibers cause more retropulsion as compared to smaller fibers. As the fiber size increases, the flexibility of the scope decreases.

Back burn effect is the damage sustained at the fiber tip and causing degradation of fiber tip and damage to the fiber. It is caused by use of high energy, short pulse, and hard stone.

ROLE OF SHAPE TIP AND CONFIGURATION OF THE LASER FIBER

Ball Tip Fiber

It is proposed that this configuration will have higher ablation rate. This configuration allows easier insertion of the laser tip fiber into the scope. With the degradation of the fiber tip, this advantage is lost quickly. Also, these fibers are single use.

Leaving Fibers Coated

During lithotripsy leaving the fiber coated may allow for an easier insertion, it may potentially increase the stone ablation rate. It is safe than stripping the fiber and stripping may cause inadvertent damage.

Stripping the Fiber

Stripping is controversial, dedicated strippers are available to do the same. It may not benefit in terms of ablation rate or performance.

Tip Cleaving

Simple stainless steel scissors can be used to cleave the laser fiber tip it is as effective as the ceramic scissors. Benefits of cleaving are uncertain as it may not increase the ablation volume.

NEWER TECHNOLOGIES THAT ENHANCE THE PERFORMANCE OF A HIGH WATT HOLMIUM LASER

Moses Technology

Lumines™ technologies have introduced the Moses effect. Moses effect is based on the modulation of laser pulse which results in better laser and target interaction. Moses effect causes the current pulse to get divided into two adjacent peaks. The first peak separates water and the second one travels through a bubble created by the first peak. When delivered to the stone, less amount of energy is lost. Due to precise energy delivery, there is faster fragmentation and decreased retropulsion.

Burst Laser Therapy

It is a novel laser lithotripsy mode developed by certain manufacturers. In this each burst consists of three individual pulses, first one being more energy intense with the last one having the least energy. Each of the pulses has successively increasing pulse length and is emitted in rapid succession. Burst mode is significantly more ablative and can achieve about 60% more ablation volumes.

Laser Lithotripsy Settings

When we discuss about the laser lithotripsy settings, we are necessarily talking about three variables, namely pulse energy, pulse frequency, and consequently, the total power.

Total power (watt) = Pulse energy (J) × Pulse frequency (Hz)

By adjusting the above variables, the urologist decides how much energy is to be delivered at the level of fiber tip.

Pulse Energy

The higher the pulse energy, the higher the stone ablation rate. Keeping the total power constant when the energy is increased and frequency is decreased, the stone ablation volume increases. If the frequency is increased and the energy is decreased keeping the total power same, less stone ablation will occur as compared to a state when the energy is higher.

Pulse Frequency in Holmium Laser Lithotripsy

High frequency with low energy can produce smaller fragments and help the surgeon achieve fine dust. Keeping the frequency high and the energy low decreases the retropulsion of stones. Increased frequency and decreased energy for the same power decreases the total ablation volume (**Fig. 6**).

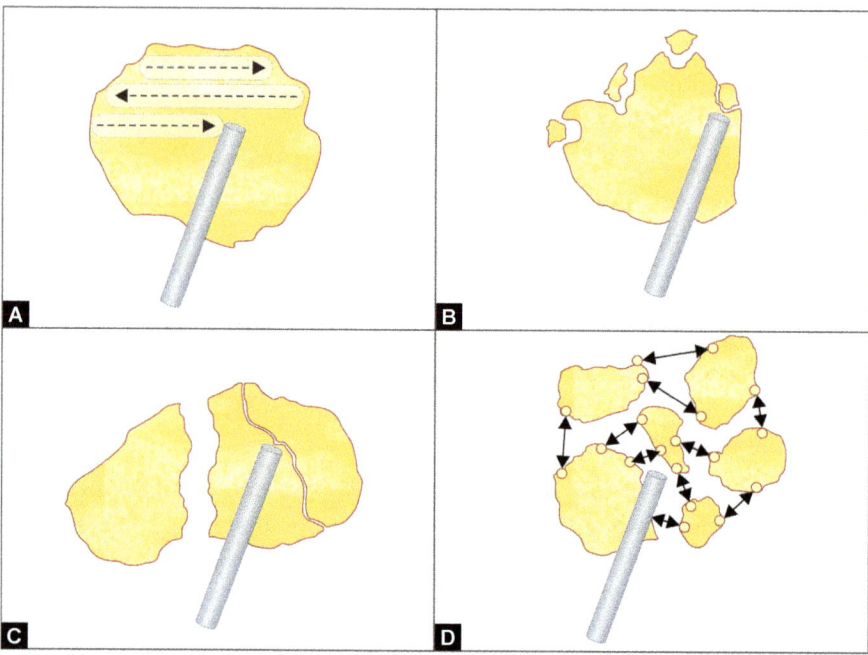

Figures 6A to D: Four techniques for intrarenal holmium laser lithotripsy. (A) The dancing technique is used for soft stones. The laser fiber is maintained in constant motion as it passes back and forth across the stone surface, ablating it layer by layer; (B) Chipping is the most commonly used technique. The laser is aimed at the stone periphery and fired continuously until a small fragment chips off. The laser is repositioned and the technique is repeated until the stone is whittled down to a small core fragment; (C) The fragmenting technique is used for hard stones that are resistant to chipping. The laser is aimed centrally and fired continuously until the stone fragments along natural cleavage planes. The technique is repeated on the resulting stone fragments; (D) The popcorn technique is best for collections of stones in dependent calyces. The fiber is positioned near the stones taking care to stay 1 mm away from the urothelium. The laser is pulsed or fired continuously; the laser effect and resulting stone motion produces rapid fragmentation.

Pulse Variation in Holmium Laser Lithotripsy

Pulse variation ranges from 0 to 1,500 µs for holmium laser lithotripsy. This effectively means that each pulse of a definite energy is delivered in a certain duration of microseconds. Generally, speaking duration of >700 µs is considered long pulse (180-330 µs—short pulse, 650-1,215 µs—long pulse). Short pulse mode is more ablative as large amount of energy is delivered in short duration as opposed to a long pulse where the same amount of energy is delivered in longer time. In an evaluation done by Kronenberg et al., short pulse ablated 25% more than long pulse in low frequency and high energy settings and 9.9% more ablation was achieved with short pulse as compared to long pulse when high frequency and low energy were used. In the same study when using the long pulse low frequency and high energy ablated larger volume.

Different effects of laser on stones are mentioned here.

Dusting Effect

Producing very small fragments which are smaller than 2 µm in size, resulting in fine dust. Low energy and high frequency help attain dusting effect.

For a low watt laser (30 W or less), this can be achieved by starting with a setting of 0.2 J, 20 Hz, and long pulse mode. The surgeon has to assess the stone fragmentation and if the stone fragmentation is not satisfactory, the frequency can go up to 40 Hz (depending on the machine) and energy to 0.4 J and then to 0.6 J.

In a high-power machine, higher frequency of 40 Hz can be used at the outset and can be increased to 60 Hz. The energy can be started from 0.4 J and can be increased.

Though high power lasers may allow energy up to 6 J, but as the energy increases, the fragment size will also increase.

Popcorn Effect

This technique is usually used for a conglomerate of larger stone fragments at the end of the procedure. Better suited for the high-power machines but can be replicated with low power machines also.

Principally all the fragments are gathered in a calyx, laser beam is defocused with distance of about 1–2 mm from the stones. The initial laser settings are 1 J and 20 Hz for low-power machines. For the high-power machines, the frequency can go up to 40 Hz and the energy can be increased to 2 J. This high wattage settings cause simultaneous fragmentation, ablation, and vaporization effect, decreasing the stone burden by up to 63% in 2 minutes. As there is retropulsion during the procedure, it should be done only in a calyx will relatively smaller mouth. All stone that get retropulsed eventually hit the wall of the calyx and are again directed toward the fiber tip.

Pop-dusting Effect

It is a relatively new terminology and is used by the surgeon in the second stage of the procedure.

The surgeons start the procedure by dusting, after a point and time no further dusting can be achieved as the stone is broken down into small fragments. At this stage, the energy is increased to 0.5–0.6 J and the frequency is kept between 20 Hz and 40 Hz, laser is kept in a noncontact mode and at a distance of 2 mm from the stone. Complete pulverization of stone is achieved using this technique.

DIFFERENT TECHNIQUES OF LASER LITHOTRIPSY

Painting

In painting technique, laser fiber tip is moved continuously on the surface of the stone in a mediolateral or lateromedial direction without direct contact with the stone. The settings are low energy (0.2–0.4 J) and high frequency (20–40 Hz).

Dancing

It is a technique similar to the painting technique where the aim is to produce fine dust. Similar settings to painting is used and the laser fiber is moved back and forth across the stones. The stone is dusted layer by layer, uniformly so that no large fragments are generated. The fiber has to be in constant motion and the speed of the movement depends on the hardness of the stones. The technique is more efficient in the softer stones. Harder stones tend to fragment more.

Chipping

Fine dusting is difficult to achieve in harder stones. So the aim in this situation is to achieve fragments <1 mm size which can be later popcorned to achieve fine dust.

In this technique, laser fiber is directed at the edge of the stone and held steadily till a small fragment of about 1 mm chips of the main stone. The process is repeated over and over till the whole stone bulk is fragmented into stones of 1 mm. Using the popcorn effect, the stone is eventually fragmented to dust.

Fragmentation/Drilling

In very hard stones even chipping is sometimes not possible as these hard stones tend to turn around if the surgeon tries to hit the edge of the stone. In these situations, the surgeon should directly target the middle of the stone and with high energy 1–2 J and frequency of 20 Hz try to drill the stone. The stone gets fractured along the natural cleavage lines and multiple large fragments are created. These individual fragments are again targeted with laser focused in center and held constantly till the fragment again breaks along the lines of cleavage. This process is repeated over and over to achieve a fragment size of 1–2 mm. After this, popcorn effect can be used to dust and ablate the stone.

Lasers Used for Management of Benign Prostatic Hyperplasia (BPH)

The lasers which can be used in management of BPH are as follows:
- Holmium laser:
    - Enucleation
    - Resection

- Thulium laser:
  - Enucleation
  - Resection
  - Vaporization
  - Vaporesection
- Thulium fiber laser
- Green light laser:
  - Vaporization
  - Vapoenucleation
- Diode laser:
  - Vaporization
- KTP/Nd:YAG:
  - Vaporization

TECHNIQUES OF ENUCLEATION

Three-incision Technique

Medial Lobe Resection

Incision marked at 5 o'clock and 7 o'clock. Deepened to capsular fibers by sweeping movements, the capsular fiber appears horizontally placed. The lobe is enucleated from the verumontanum toward the bladder neck and disconnected from the bladder neck by placing a horizontal incision at the level of bladder neck.

Lateral Lobe Excision

The lateral lobes are undermined on both the sides. This is done by undermining the initial incisions made at 5 o'clock and 7 o'clock. The undermining is done laterally and circumferentially toward 2 o'clock and 10 o'clock. Now incision is taken at 12 o'clock deepened up to the capsule. The incision is undermined laterally toward 2 o'clock and 10 o'clock. By doing this, the surgeon has to meet the precreated plane at 2 o'clock and 10 o'clock. The entire prostate is enucleated in three parts and pushed into the bladder and finally morcellated.

1. **What is the difference in using lasers, when used in ureter and kidney?**

   Ans. When used in ureter the total power should be less, as there can be thermal injury to ureteric wall. High energy and low frequency can result in migration of the stone. In an impacted ureteric stone, flow of irrigation is impeded so the dust created by lasing is not washed off quicky, the surgeon should be patient and allow all the snow storm to settle. The kidney stone is usually placed into the calyx and then dusted, towards the end of the procedure the laser beam can be defocused and total energy increased to create a popcorn effect.

2. **What is the ideal anesthesia for retrograde intrarenal surgery when you are going to do laser lithotripsy?**

   Ans. Ideally general anesthesia should be used so that respiratory movements of the patients can be controlled and subsequently laser can be properly directed to the stone.

3. **What are the problems that one can face while working with laser in upper calyx?**

   Ans. The movement of the kidney in the upper part of kidney is most pronounced as it is in contact with the diaphragm, hence the upper calyx moves maximum with respiration. The movements of the surgeon should be synchronized with respiration or in difficult situations respiratory gating technique with the help of anesthetist should be achieved. This means that the anesthetist should give apnea during which the lasing should be done and then when he ventilates, lasing is stopped.

4. **What is the difference between Thulium YAG laser and Thulium fiber laser?**

   Ans. Thulium:YAG laser is a solid-state laser and has a wavelength of 2,010 nm. It is a continuous form laser therefore cannot be used for stone management and is used for Prostate enucleation, vaporisation or vaporesection. Thulium Laser fiber can be used in pulsed and continuous form. It can be used for stone fragmentation as well as prostatic enucleation, vaporisation and vapo-resection. It has a wavelength of 1,940 nm.

5. **Do you actually need special type of scissors to freshen the tip of a laser fiber?**

   Ans. No, you don't need a special ceramic scissor to cleave the end of a laser fiber, it can be done with a stainless steel scissors.

6. **What is a difference between high watt and low watt laser?**

   Ans. Low watt laser are generally <30 W and require only a single cavity and generator. High watt lasers >50 W require multiple cavities, a vapor compression refrigeration system is required as a cooling mechanism for the high power laser.

REFERENCES

1. Parsons RL, Campbell JL, Thomley MW. Carcinoma of the penis treated by the ruby laser. J Urol. 1968;100(1):38-9.
2. US Corporate news. Laser medicine and surgery news and advances. News from Candela Corporation. 1988;6(5):24-5.
3. Traxer O, Keller EX. Thulium fiber laser: the new player for kidney stone treatment? A comparison with Holmium: YAG laser. World journal of urology. 2019 Feb 6:1-2.

SECTION 2

Uroradiology

CHAPTER 16

Stricture Disease

PAN ANTERIOR URETHRAL STRICTURE

Description of the Image (Fig. 1)
This is a retrograde urethrogram (RGU) which shows the whole of penile and bulbar urethra irregular and nondistensible. However, the contrast is seen filling in the posterior urethra and bladder. So, this is a pan anterior urethral stricture.

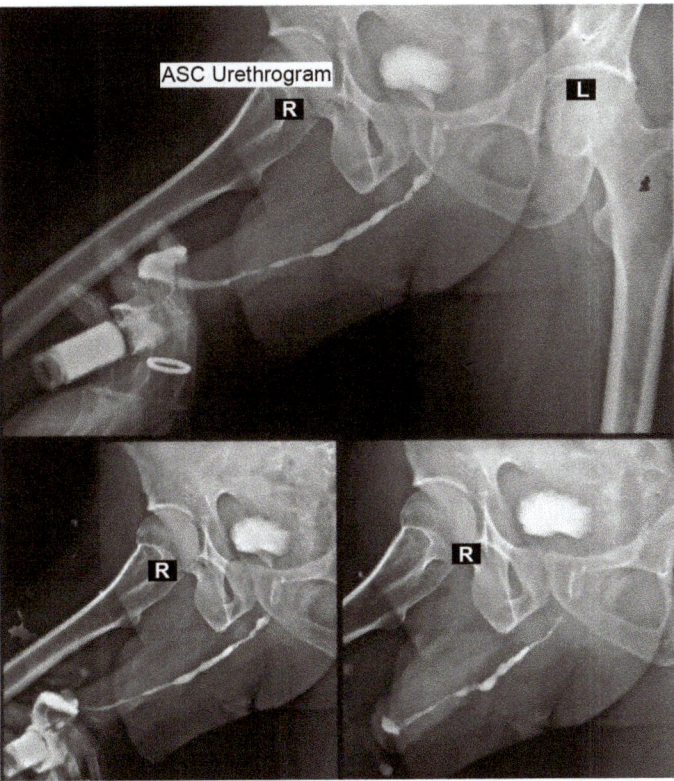

Figure 1: Retrograde urethrogram.

1. **Why do you say anterior urethral stricture?**

   Ans. Most of the times, in such types of strictures, posterior urethra is normal. In this X-ray also, very, prostatic urethra appears normal. However, to delineate that, we will require a micturating cystourethrogram (MCU).

2. **What do you think can be etiology of such stricture?**

   Ans. It could be iatrogenic—may be because of prolonged catheter, or instrumentation. It can also be associated with balanitis xerotica obliterans (BXO).

3. **Is it a properly done X-ray?**

   Ans. Position is satisfactory—as full length of urethra is visualized without any overlapping shadows.
   - Plain X-ray is always a prerequisite.
   - Exposure of hand of procedure performing surgeon should have been avoided.
   - External urethral meatus and submeatal portions are not properly visualized—but it may be because of very narrow meatus.

4. **Suppose this is a young adult, 45 years, family complete, what will you do?**

   Ans. I would like to do MCU—to delineate posterior urethra and then proceed with full length one-stage dorsal onlay buccal urethroplasty.

5. **Why do you need MCU?**

   Ans. Before any definitive surgery, it is better to delineate proximal limit, which can be done only by MCU.

6. **Can you do endoscopic management?**

   Ans. Results of any endoscopic management in such stricture are poor. Hence I will not do it.

7. **What are the ways to ensure occlusion of urethra to perform RGU?**

   Ans. By using Foley adapter, small size Foley's catheter, using clamps (Brodney and Knudson clamps).

8. **How will you identify different parts of urethra on MCU and RGU?**

   Ans. The penile urethra is identified by the soft tissue shadows of penis and scrotum. The membranous urethra is at the level of lower border of obturator foramen and just distal to the impression of verumontanum. The urethra between these two is the bulbar urethra.

CHAPTER 16: Stricture Disease | 217

9. **Describe the position in which RGU and MCU are done? What is it called?**

   Ans. Retrograde urethrogram: The operator stands to the right of the patient. The patient lies on the table supine on the fluoroscopy table and then rolled up slightly onto one hip (approximately to a 45° angle), with the dependent thigh flexed so that an oblique view of the lengthened urethra can be obtained and overlap can be avoided. The glans penis is cleansed with a sterile technique, and a contrast administration device is inserted into the meatus, either by Foley adapter, small size Foley's catheter or clamps. Sterile iodinated contrast is then injected into the urethra with the use of gentle pressure.
   - MCU: Done in standing position. For children, it is done in supine position.
   - Formulas for bladder capacity:
     - For age >1 year, Koff's formula is used

       Bladder capacity (mL) = [Age (years) + 2] × 30
     - For infants, Holmdahl formula

       Bladder capacity (mL) = [age (in months) × 2.5] + 38

       Other formula used is Fairhurst formula

       Bladder capacity (in mL) = 7 × body weight (kg)

DISTAL BULBAR STRICTURE

Description of the Image (Fig. 2)

This is a RGU, which shows well distensible distal penile urethra. Proximal penile urethra appears slightly nondistensible. There is narrowing at distal

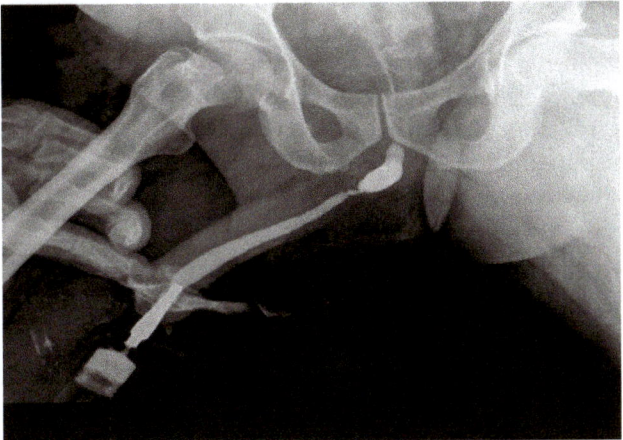

Figure 2: Retrograde urethrogram.

bulbar level. Length appears to be small about <1 cm. However, the position of the patient is not proper. Obliquity is not maintained during RGU and hence bulbar urethra is not completely opened. Mid and proximal bulb appears to be overlapped.

1. **What is the likely cause of such stricture?**

    Ans. The cause can be anything—iatrogenic, infective [postexposure to sexually transmitted disease (STD)], traumatic, or previous failed urethroplasty.

2. **How will you manage this case?**

    Ans. Both options can be discussed—visual internal urethrotomy (VIU) and urethroplasty.

3. **How do you decide which option is better?**

    Ans. Various points to be considered while taking such decision are as follows:
    - He is unmarried and a young boy
    - What is exact length of stricture—I will evaluate proximal penile urethra (which is nondistensible by looking at it by small cystoscope or ureteroscope—to see how is mucosa—whether it is pink and healthy or it is white, unhealthy, and irregular. If proximal mucosa is pink, then it is short length stricture.
    - What is the cause of stricture?
    - What is his choice?

4. **If urethroplasty is to be done—what is your choice of surgery?**

    Ans. Dorsal onlay buccal mucosa graft (BMG)

5. **Why not ventral onlay?**

    Ans. Usually, ventral onlay is done for mid and proximal bulbar urethra where there is good support of bulbospongiosus muscle and spongiosum is well developed and thicker. In this case, stricture appears to be distal bulbar and extending to proximal urethra.

POST TRAUMATIC POSTERIOR URETHRAL INJURIES

Description of the Image

This is MCU and RGU (**Fig. 3**). This X-ray is not taken in proper position and hence urethra is not properly opened up. RGU shows normal penile urethra. Distal bulb cannot be commented as probably it is overlapping. MCU—again is not in proper position, hence proximal and mid bulbar urethra appears to be overlapping. However, there appears to be complete cut off in distal or mid bulbar urethra.

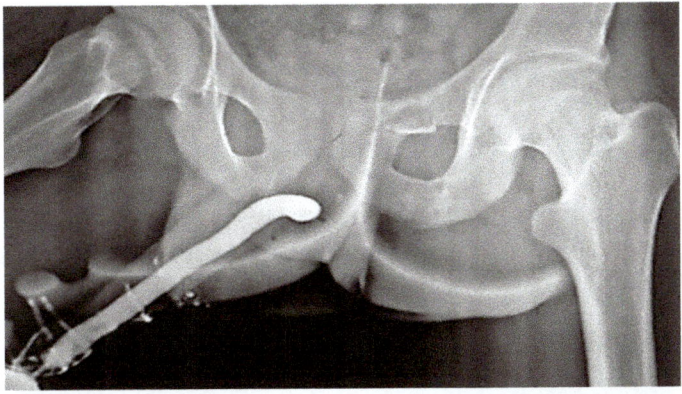
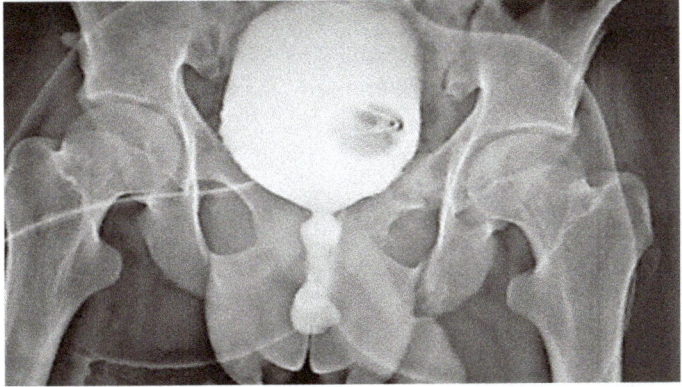

Figure 3: Retrograde urethrogram and micturating cystourethrogram.

1. **What can be the cause of this condition?**

   Ans. Most likely it is traumatic stricture as rest of urethra is well distensible and no irregularity.

2. **How will do RGU/MCU in PFUDD?**

   Ans.
   - Plain X-ray anteroposterior (AP) view with both hips
   - Cystogram phase (full plate—to look for reflux)
   - MCU is to be done in AP view. If it is high urethra, then it is appreciated well on AP view. Then it is done in oblique view.
   - Oblique position can be given if RGU has to be performed.

3. **How will you treat?**

   Ans. This requires end-to-end urethroplasty.

4. **Can you do core-through urethrotomy?**

   Ans. Results are poor and hence not recommended.

5. **Why results are poor?**

   Ans. In core-through urethrotomy, there is no urethra tunnel created in fibrous, scar tissue, and it is hoped that this tunnel gets epithelized. But this does not happen in majority of cases and hence not recommended.

6. **Would you do suprapubic scopy before surgery?**

   Ans. I would also like to see plain X-ray and cystogram plate to see for any stones and to assess competency of bladder neck. Suprapubic scopy can be done but reason is not to delineate the stricture length but to see if there are stones, especially if suprapubic catheter (SPC) is for long time.

Description of the Image

This is the X-ray where contrast is instilled in distal urethra and flexiscope is put in proximal urethra (**Fig. 4**). Other names for similar investigations are— to bugiogram, up-down gram, and gapogram.

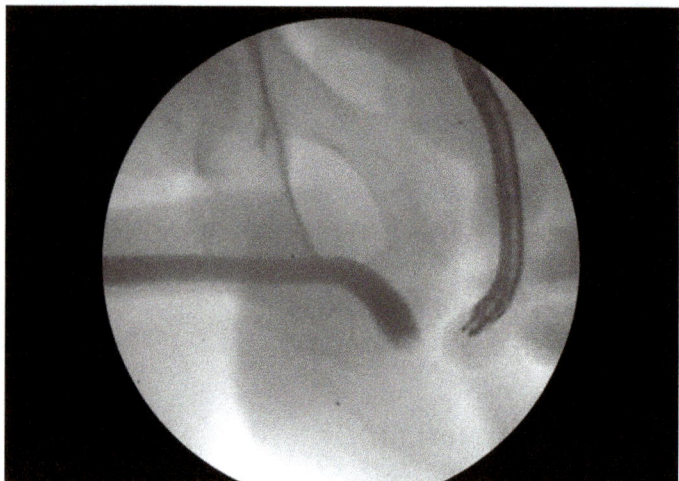

Figure 4: Retrograde urethrogram with flexible scope in posterior urethra.

1. **Why this investigation is done?**

   Ans. This is to delineate proximal and distal limit of stricture and to assess the gap between the two ends.

2. **What is expression cystogram?**

   Ans. It is MCU under general anesthesia (GA). Then, compression is given at suprapubic region with a wooden scale horizontally. So that the contrast delineates the posterior urethra.

Often, if deep anesthesia is given, the bladder neck opens up and contrast fills up the posterior urethra without any pressure.

3. **What is gapometry index?**
   Ans. Length of the defect/length of bulbar urethra. If it is <0.5, then the surgery will be relatively easier. If >0.5, then various maneuvers may be required to approach proximal urethra.

4. **What are the disadvantages of bugiogram?**
   Ans. It can cause false passage and may perforate the proximal blind end of urethra. It can excessively push the urethra and hence can give misleading picture—suggesting that stricture is low and gap is less.

5. **How will you overcome such problem?**
   Ans. The MCU can be done after giving alpha-blocker agent for few days. This causes relaxation of bladder neck and opens up the urethra and patient tends to void.

   Micturating cystourethrogram can done under GA in which bladder neck will open up and contrast will flow into the urethra in natural way and thus will give correct idea of gap if simultaneously RGU is done. To open bladder neck under GA, prerequisite is to take anesthesia at deep level. Bladder neck does not open with muscle relaxant. It opens up only by deep anesthesia.

Description of the Image (Fig. 5)

Plain X-ray pelvis AP view—showing bilateral fracture superior and inferior pubic rami. Not much displacement of bone and no free bony fragments seen. Next is cystogram picture with simultaneous RGU (**Fig. 6**). Again this is not done with proper positing, hence bulb has overlapped.

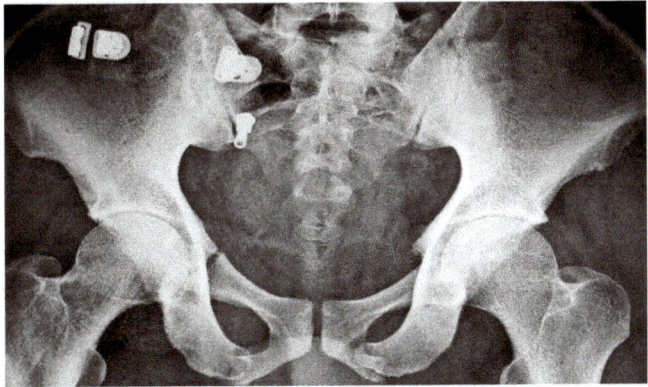

Figure 5: X-ray pelvis anteroposterior (AP).

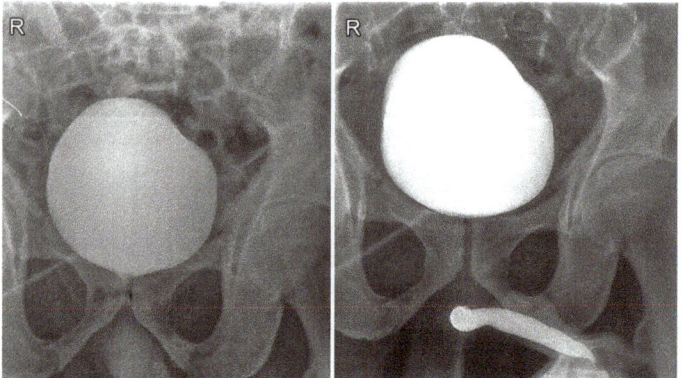

Figure 6: Retrograde urethrogram and micturating cystourethrogram.

1. **What is the fallacy in the RGU?**
   Ans. The length of the bulbar urethra cannot be delineated.

2. **If the first plate is micturating plate, then what is your opinion?**
   Ans. If it is micturating, then his bladder neck is not opening. This can happen due to many reasons which are as follows:
   - Because of unusual circumstances, patient is not able to pass urine, not properly straining or not understood command of urination as he is on catheter for a long time.
   - Sphincter has gone in spasm and hence posterior urethra is not visualized.
   - Bladder neck is closed due to stenosis—may be due to bladder neck injury: This is bit unlikely as usually bladder neck injury happens due to displaced bone fragment—which is not seen in this case.

3. **What will you do to visualize posterior urethra?**
   Ans.
   - Alpha blocker can be given few hours before MCU which can relieve spasm
   - Bugiogram
   - Suprapubic scopy
   - MCU under GA

4. **What is the ideal time to do surgery in such cases?**
   Ans. Usually, 3 months' gap between trauma and final surgery is better. However, this depends on various factors—if the bladder is not descended down (gap between inferior border of bladder and upper border of pubic bone is too large—which means still significant hematoma is present and it is better to wait). If active urinary tract infection (UTI) or epididymoorchitis, it is better to wait.

5. **If posterior urethra is properly visualized, will you still do suprapubic scopy?**

   Ans. Yes, it is a good idea to do suprapubic scopy as sometimes there are bladder stones which are not visualized in X-ray, sometimes there are stones in prostatic urethra and other benefit is that, if you keep scope, you can palpate the tip from perineum and get rough assessment whether proximal urethra is too high or low.

PROXIMAL PENILE URETHRAL STRICTURE

Description of the Image

Micturating cystourethrogram and RGU X-ray (**Fig. 7**) appears to be of a small child. MCU shows smooth bladder and dilated urethra with a smooth bulging at the level of proximal penile urethra. Rest of urethra is not properly visualized.

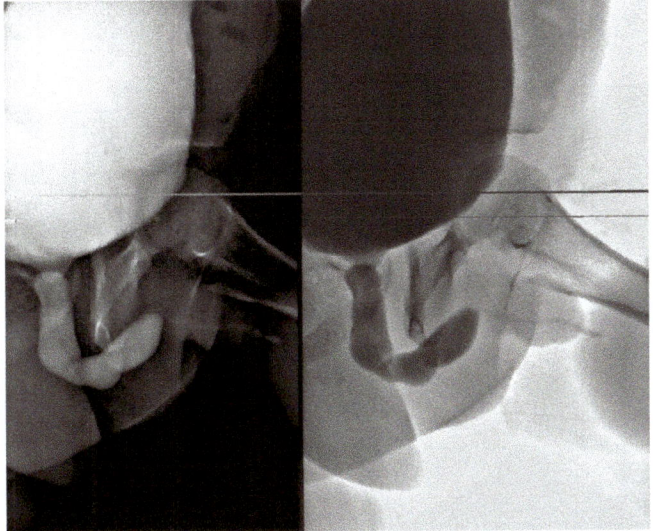

Figure 7: Micturating cystourethrogram and retrograde urethrogram.

1. **What do you think is the diagnosis?**

   Ans. It could be stricture in proximal penile urethra.

   Anterior urethral valve: An anterior urethral valve is a posteriorly directed semilunar fold arising from the floor of the anterior urethra and causing obstruction during micturition.
   - *Location*: 40% in the bulbar urethra
   - *30%*: Penoscrotal junction
   - 30% in the penile urethra

   Causes: Imbalance of tissue growth during urethral development, incomplete hypospadias, or an abortive process during urethral

duplication and a faulty union between glandular and urethral tissue during embryonal development.

Anterior urethral valve is a rare condition. Treatment is transurethral valve ablation by either cold cut, electrocautery, or laser.

2. **Do you think it is full length of penile urethral stricture?**

   Ans. That cannot be commented on this X-ray. As to comment on anterior urethra—RGU is required.

3. **What can be the cause of such stricture in children?**

   Ans. Iatrogenic—if any instrumentation is done, if catheter was kept for long time, trauma, impacted stone at that site in the past. These are some of the causes of stricture.

1. **This is an X-ray of the same patient—what is your comment on that?**

   Ans. It shows anterior urethra is well distensible and if we correlate MCU with RGU, then it appears short length stricture in proximal penile urethra. It may be at penobulbar junction (**Fig. 8**).

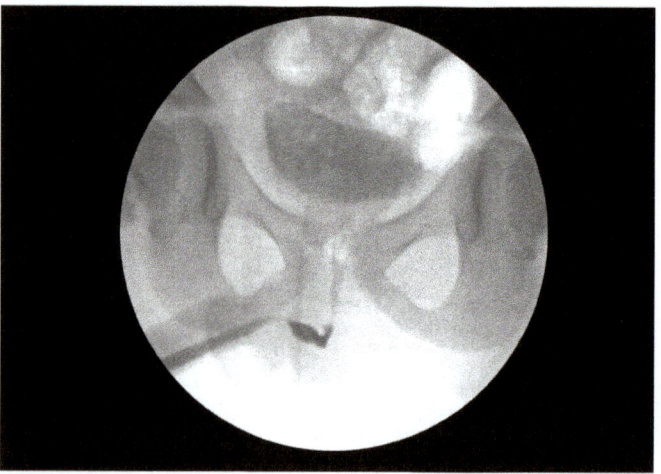

Figure 8: Micturating cystourethrogram (MCU) and retrograde urethrogram (RGU).

2. **Why stricture site in MCU and RGU appears to be different?**

   Ans. This is because of improper position. In MCU, position is proper—oblique position. While RGU is done more or less in AP view as evident by pelvis X-ray.

3. **What will you do if this child is of 6 years of age?**

   Ans. Options are: Endoscopic treatment—if the stricture is flimsy, then it can be dilated. However, if it recurs or if the stricture is very tight and rigid, then it is likely to fail, in that case, it is better to do urethroplasty. It could be one stage BMG—dorsal onlay or two-stage procedure.

CHAPTER 17

Benign Bladder Diseases

BLADDER DIVERTICULUM

Description of the Image

This is micturating cystourethrogram (MCUG) showing large bladder diverticulum. Bladder appears smooth walled, diverticulum is very big—almost size of the bladder or bigger and has narrow neck with significant postvoid residue in diverticulum. Bladder neck is wide open. Posterior urethra is visualized and is slightly dilated. Anterior urethra appears to be narrow; however, definitive comment cannot be made on MCUG. No reflux seen on any side and plain X-ray is lacking (**Figs. 1A to D**).

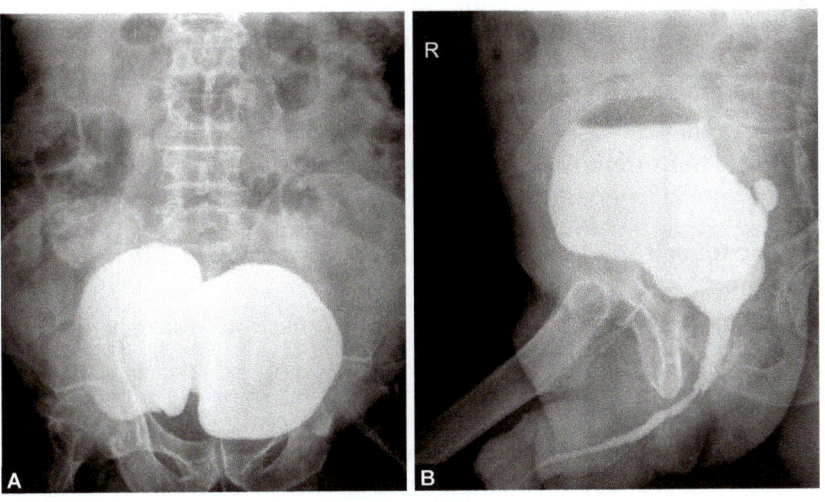

Figures 1A to D: *Contd...*

Contd...

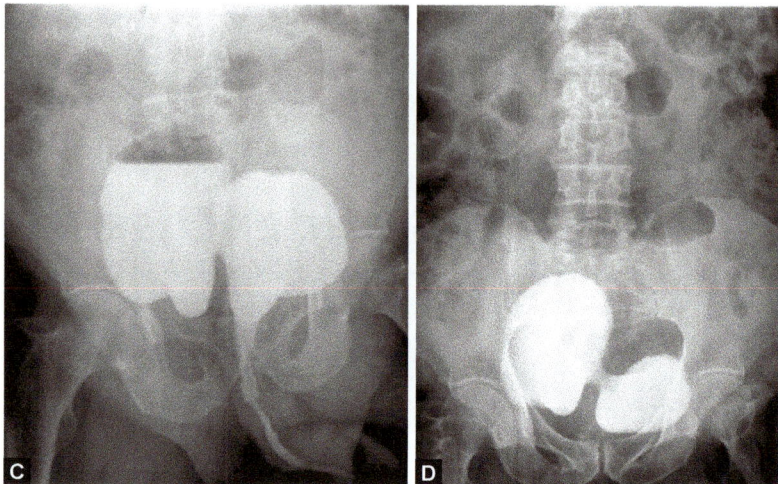

Figures 1A to D: (A) Cystogram; (B) MCUG right oblique; (C) MCUG left oblique; (D) Postvoid.

1. **What you think is the cause of diverticulum?**

   Ans. It appears to be unilateral big diverticulum. It could be congenital or acquired. When there is high pressure in bladder due to outlet obstruction, small diverticulum can become big. In pediatric age group, such diverticulum is usually congenital.

2. **Why you think it is acquired?**

   Ans. X-ray appears to be of an adult. B/N appears to be dilated which may be due to transurethral resection of prostate (TURP) and there is likely to be stricture in anterior urethra, which lead to big diverticulum.

3. **Do you think if stricture is taken care off, diverticulum also needs treatment?**

   Ans. Since it is big diverticulum and mouth is narrow, as seen in postvoid plate, diverticulum needs treatment.

4. **Which will you treat first?**

   Ans. Outlet needs to be treated first and then diverticulectomy. However, if there is sepsis due to residual urine in diverticulum, then it can be treated first and then the patient should be maintained on suprapubic catheter (SPC) postoperation till stricture is taken care off.

5. **Why oblique plate is necessary in such cases?**

    Ans. Oblique X-ray will give an exact idea to differentiate bladder from diverticulum.

6. **If it is associated with enlarged prostate, what will you treat first?**

    Ans. Diverticulectomy should be done first as the diverticulum has a narrow mouth and not emptying on postvoid plate. Often, diverticulum itself presses on the bladder neck and results in lower urinary tract symptoms (LUTS). In that case, patient may not need TURP or may be managed by medical therapy for prostate. Doing TURP first can have many problems like the chips may go into the diverticulum, postoperative persistent residue into the diverticulum may result into sepsis, if suprapubic catheter is required, then the fossa will remain dry which may cause stricture in the prostatic urethra. In case of large prostate with diverticulum, both can be done in the same sitting with open surgery.

7. **How will you diagnose outlet obstruction?**

    Ans. Generally, urodynamic study will have lot of fallacies, hence the obstruction is diagnosed by presence of trabeculations/sacculations in the bladder.

8. **How will you differentiate congenital and acquired diverticulum?**

    Ans. Congenital diverticulum is generally single, rest of the bladder is usually normal (smooth lined). It is usually in the pediatric age group and paraureteric in location.

NEUROGENIC BLADDER

Description of the Image

This is MCUG (**Fig. 2**) in adult female patient—which shows bladder which is relatively of small capacity, severely trabeculated, with multiple saccules and diverticula. Right reflux is present however full pelvicalyceal (PC) system is not visualized. Right lower ureter is visualized which shows slight tortuosity and significant dilatation. Postvoid shows insignificant residue. Spina bifida is evident in sacral vertebrae. Impression is neurogenic bladder.

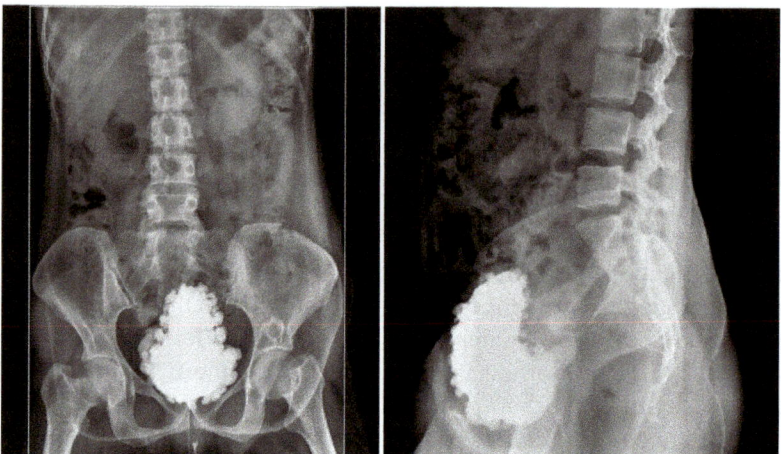

Figure 2: Micturating cystourethrogram anteroposterior (AP) plate and lateral plate.

1. **What do you think is type of neurogenic bladder it is?**

   Ans. This appears to be high pressure bladder. So likely to be upper motor neuron type of bladder.

2. **How this patient would have presented with?**

   Ans. Frequency, urgency, urgency incontinence, features of renal failure, repeated episodes of urinary tract infection (UTI), and constipation.

3. **What this appearance is described as?**

   Ans. This is fir tree or Christmas tree or pine tree appearance, which is typical of high pressure neurogenic bladder.

4. **Why do you say it is neurogenic bladder?**

   Ans. Since spina bifida is evident, it is more likely to be a neurogenic bladder. However, in the absence of such signs, the d/d can be non-neurogenic neurogenic bladder.

5. **What other relevant investigations will you do which are diagnostic?**

   Ans. Complete blood count (CBC), ultrasonography (USG), serum creatinine, magnetic resonance imaging (MRI) of the spine.

6. **What are the likely finding in the urodynamic study?**

   Ans.
   - Poor compliance
   - Detrusor instability
   - Low cystometric capacity
   - High voiding pressures
   - Poor or maintained urinary flow
   - On electromyography (EMG), it could be nonrelaxing sphincter or detrusor sphincter dyssynergia

CHAPTER 18

Pediatric Urology

BILATERAL PRIMARY OBSTRUCTIVE MEGAURETER

Description of the Image

This is computed tomography (CT) intravenous pyelogram (IVP) (**Figs. 1A to C**) which shows bilateral gross hydronephrosis and hydroureter. Ureters are grossly dilated up to ureteropelvic junction (UPJ) and tortuous as compared to pelvicalyceal (PC) system. PC system is well-dilated; however, cortical thickness on the left side is good, while on the right side, parenchyma is of variable thickness. Bilateral function appears good. Bladder is not visualized by contrast filling; however, the bladder appears partially full and normal. Diagnosis is likely to be bilateral primary obstructive megaureter.

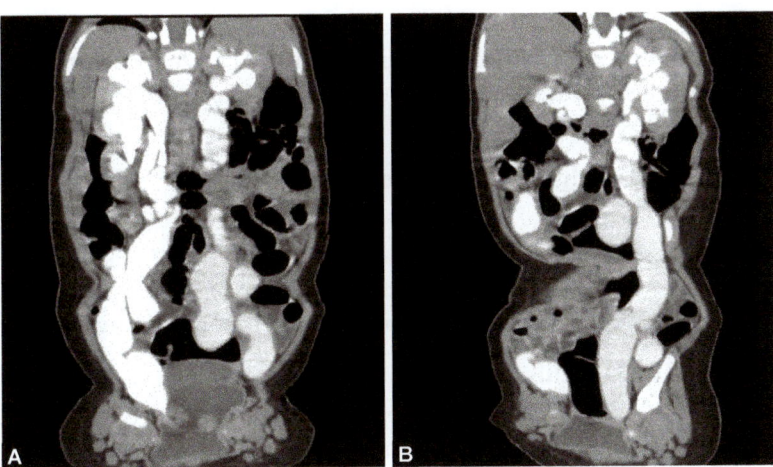

Figures 1A to C: *Contd...*

Contd...

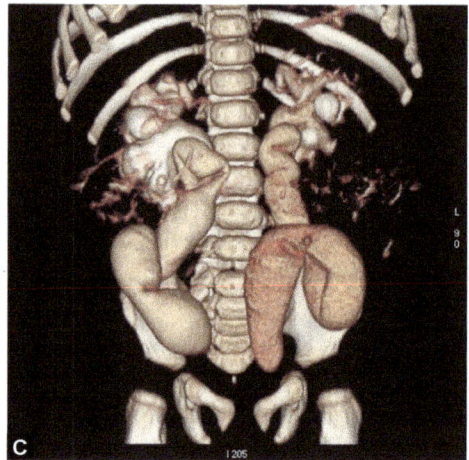

Figures 1A to C: CT IVU images.

1. **Can you rule out reflux disease?**
   Ans. Micturating cystourethrogram (MCU) is required; however, if it was grade V reflux then bladder should have been visualized in CT IVP.

2. **What are the diagnostic features of primary obstructive megaureter (POMU) on CT scan or plain IVP?**
   Ans. The features are as follows:
   - Lower ureter is twice the diameter of upper ureter.
   - The ureteric dilatation is disproportionate to calyceal dilatation.
   - There is a smooth tapering of the lower end like a bird beak.
   - Sometimes, the atretic segment may be seen.

3. **How this child might have presented with?**
   Ans.
   - Vague pain in abdomen
   - Recurrent urinary tract infection (UTI)
   - Failure to thrive—not taking proper feeds and not gaining weight

4. **Will you do MCU in this case?**
   Ans. Yes, MCU is necessary as reflux is necessary to be ruled out. Sometimes, it could be refluxing and obstructive megaureter. Also, the bladder and urethra need to be visualized.

5. **How do you classify megaureters based on radiology imaging?**
   Ans. The megaureters can be classified as obstructing, refluxing, obstructing and refluxing, nonobstructing, and nonrefluxing. All can be primary or secondary.

- Anything >7 mm is a megaureter.
- If the bladder is normal on intravenous urography (IVU) and MCU, then it is primary megaureter.
- If it is abnormal, then it is secondary megaureter.
- If the contrast is draining in delayed films, then it is nonobstructive, otherwise it is obstructive.

6. **How will you treat this child?**

   Ans. The child needs bilateral ureteric reimplantation. However before surgery, his bladder capacity needs to assessed, in 2 years child I expect capacity to be low, which may not allow me to do tapering and reimplant on both sides. In that case, I will do bilateral Sober cutaneous ureterostomies. Allow the child to grow further and also allow the ureter to regress in size. This will help in reimplant.

7. **Why you want to do Sober ureterostomy?**

   Ans. If loop ureterostomy is done, bladder will not get any urine—which will become dysfunctional. This will create additional problem. Hence, with Sober ureterostomy, some amount of urine will go down and bladder cycling will continue to some extent.

8. **What is the role of DTPA renogram?**

   Ans. If it is borderline obstructing, then DTPA renogram will show the clearance. However, during the DTPA renogram, the focus should be on vesicoureteric junction (VUJ). Also, the patient should be catheterized during DTPA renogram.

9. **What is the etiology of megaureter?**

   Ans. It is because of the adynamic segment of the lower ureter.

POSTERIOR URETHRAL VALVES WITH REFLUX

Description of the Image

This is MCU of a child (**Fig. 2**). Bladder is of adequate capacity with irregular walls. Posterior urethra is dilated with abrupt narrowing at bulbomembranous junction. Bilateral grade V reflux is present. Bladder neck appears to be hypertrophied. Some pooling of contrast appears to be present under the preputial skin, suggestive of phimosis. My diagnosis is posterior urethral valves with bilateral grade V reflux with likely phimosis and secondary bladder neck hypertrophy.

232 | **SECTION 2:** Uroradiology

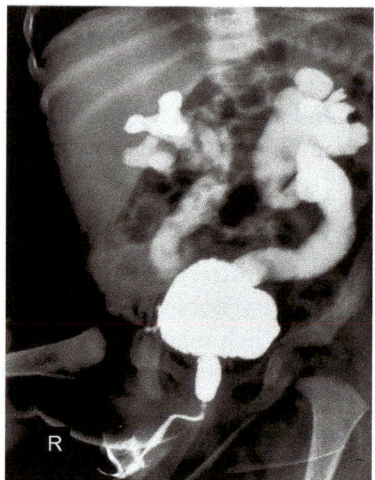

Figure 2: Micturating cystourethrogram.

1. **Are you happy with the X-ray?**

   Ans. Plain X-ray is required as part of study. Oblique plate is needed to see of any diverticula in bladder and postvoid plate is necessary to see if both ureters are draining and how much is residual urine in bladder.

2. **What is keyhole sign?**

   Ans. The trabeculated bladder with bladder neck hypertrophy and dilated posterior urethra gives an appearance of a keyhole and hence the term keyhole sign. It is typically seen in posterior urethral valves. Antenatally, in ultrasonography (USG), dilated posterior urethra is noted.

3. **How this child would have presented with?**

   Ans. Poor stream since birth, recurrent episodes of UTI, failure to thrive, not gaining weight, crying while passing urine, or features of renal failure.

4. **What other investigations are required?**

   Ans. Complete blood count (CBC), urine, and creatinine.

5. **How will you treat this child?**

   Ans. Treatment depends on age, amount of infection, and what is creatinine level.

6. **If the child is 3 years of age, no infection at present, and creatinine is 0.3, what will you do?**

   Ans. I will like to do fulguration of valve, small cystoscopes are available –7.5 Fr or 9 Fr. I will do cystoscopy, confirm presence of valve, see the bladder for any diverticula, amount of trabeculations, ureteric openings, etc. Valves are fulgurated with bugbee electrode passed through cystoscope, and fulguration is done at 5 o'clock and 7 o'clock.

7. **Any other methods to fulgurate?**
   Ans. Other methods to fulgurate valve are as follows:
   - Laser
   - Hook electrode

8. **What problems do you anticipate after fulguration?**
   Ans. Postoperative and follow-up is required to prevent valve bladder syndrome. Child will need alpha blockers, anticholinergic, and constant monitoring of flow, nocturnal incontinence, upper tract dilatation, and renal function tests.

9. **If on presentation, creatinine is high, and child is in sepsis, what will you do?**
   Ans. I will place a urethral catheter, drain the bladder, start intravenous (IV) antibiotics, and assess the response. If child improves remarkably, creatinine becomes normal, then I will consider primary fulguration. If not, then vesicostomy is preferable.

10. **What is the earliest age at which MCU can be done?**
    Ans. It can be done any time after birth.

11. **What are the types of valves?**
    Ans.
    - *Type I*: Valves representing folds extending inferiorly from the verumontanum to the membranous urethra [~95% of posterior urethral valves (PUVs)]
    - *Type II*: Bicuspid valves as leaflets radiating from the verumontanum proximally to the bladder neck—rare (misnomer)
    - *Type III*: Valves as concentric diaphragms either above or below the verumontanum with a small perforation near the center (~5% of PUVs)

12. **What is windsock sign?**
    Ans. Type 3 PUV is called windsock valve due to its characteristic appearance as the membrane looks elongated like a windsock reaching the bulbar urethra.

BILATERAL POSTERIOR URETHRAL VALVES

Description of the Image

This is MCU in a female child showing full and overdistended bladder, which shows smooth margins (**Fig. 3**). Bilateral grade III–IV reflux is present. Bladder

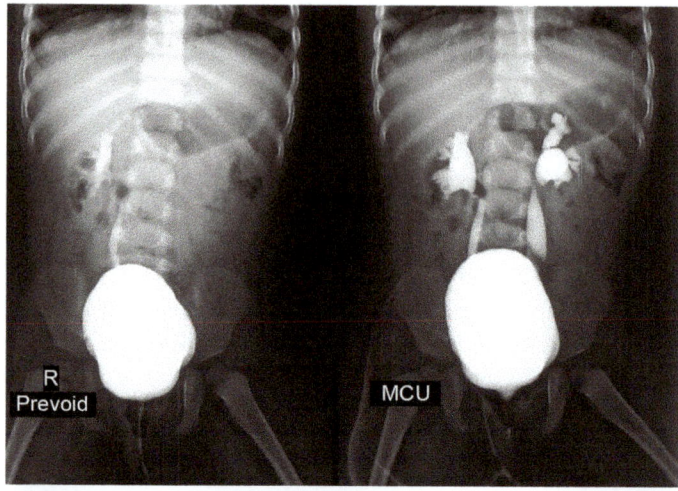
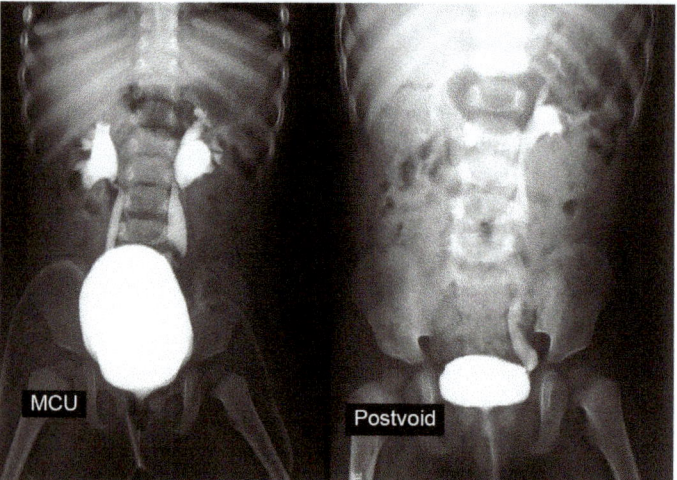

Figure 3: Micturating cystourethrogram.

neck is opening well and urethra is normal. Postvoid plate shows mild residual urine and complete emptying of right system, while left is partially drained. Oblique plate would have been advisable to see of any diverticula present.

Suppose this is a 1½-year-old girl.

1. **How this girl would have presented with?**
   Ans. Recurrent UTI, crying while passing urine, not taking feeds, failure to thrive, and antenatal presentation may be there.

2. **Is it primary reflux or secondary?**
   Ans. Appears primary reflux because the bladder wall is smooth and urethra is normal.

3. **What is your comment on the bladder capacity?**
   Ans. While doing MCU, bladder should be distended according to the estimated capacity according to age. If the bladder outline goes beyond bony pelvis, it is an overly distended bladder. It implies large capacity.

4. **How will you do MCU in a child?**
   Ans. It can be done by placing a small feeding tube and distending the bladder. Or if the bladder is full, then injecting the contrast by a suprapubic puncture. If the child is given command to void and X-ray is taken on an oblique plate. In infants, often, suprapubic pressure is given which stimulates voiding.

5. **What are the grades of reflux?**
   Ans.
   - *Grade I*: Lower ureter is visualized
   - *Grade II*: Whole PC system is visualized
   - *Grade III*: PC system is visualized with dilatation of calyces
   - *Grade IV*: Dilatation of PC system and ureter
   - *Grade V*: Associated with dilated tortuous ureters, dilated PC system with loss of papillary impressions

6. **What is low pressure and high pressure reflux?**
   Ans. Low pressure reflux is the one which appears in the cystogram phase. While in high pressure reflux, the reflux appears only in the voiding phase.

7. **What are the points to be noted in voiding phase?**
   Ans.
   - Opening of bladder neck
   - Delineation of the whole urethra
   - Vaginal pooling of contrast in females
   - Pooling of contrast under the prepuce in boys
   - Appearance or increase of reflux
   - Any prominence of diverticulum (oblique plate)

8. **How do you diagnose secondary pelviureteric junction obstruction (PUJO) in MCU?**
   Ans. Marked tortuosity of the ureter with delayed entry of contrast into the PC system followed by a delayed persistence of contrast in the PC system even after the dye is washed out from ureter in the postvoid phase.

9. **Why do you want oblique plate in this child?**
   Ans. Even though this is primary reflux, oblique plate can give idea if there are any paraureteric (Hutch) diverticula present or not. If it is present, it

has bearing on the management as in those cases, often reflux does not subside as age grows.

10. **How will you treat?**

    Ans. First I will get baseline dimercaptosuccinic acid (DMSA) scan—just to document split function and if any scars present. Then will start culture-specific antibiotics as chemoprophylaxis. Parents should be advised about proper cleaning after passing stools. Constipation should be avoided and toilet training should be properly done.

11. **If she continues to have breakthrough infection, what will you do?**

    Ans. Generally, children respond well. If breakthrough infection occurs, then underlying factors should be checked such as hygiene, compliance of medication, sensitivity of medication, over activity of the bladder, and constipation should be ruled out. If all is ok, then child needs bilateral ureteric reimplantation.

12. **Will you do deflux?**

    Ans. This is grade III–IV reflux—deflux can be tried. It has good result in grade III reflux. However, success rate is inferior to open surgery (surgical management).

CHAPTER 19

Urolithiasis

BILATERAL RENAL CALCULI

Description
This is a plain KUB X-ray showing right pelvic and lower calyceal stones and left pelvic ureteric junction (PUJ) stone (**Fig. 1**).

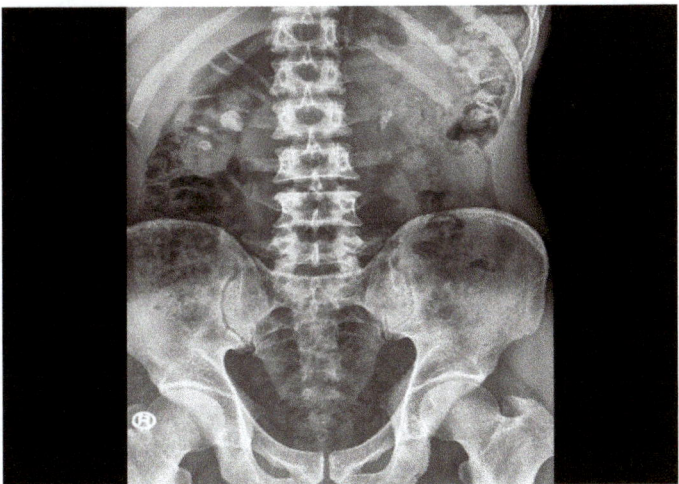

Figure 1: Plain KUB X-ray showing right pelvic and lower calyceal stones.

1. **What is the likely presentation?**
   Ans.
   - Bilateral flank pain
   - Renal failure
   - Recurrent episodes of urinary tract infection (UTI)
   - Acute pyelonephritis
   - Hematuria
   - Can be asymptomatic

2. **How will you investigate this patient?**

   Ans. Specific investigations would be serum creatinine, USG, and if creatinine is normal, then CT intravenous urogram (IVU). If the serum creatinine is high, then noncontrast CT KUB.

3. **How will you treat this patient?**

   Ans. It depends on various factors such as age, creatinine, infection, function, and pelvicalyceal anatomy.

4. **Will you do metabolic work-up in this case?**

   Ans. Since this is a case of bilateral stones, it is one of the indications of metabolic work-up. The other indications are:
   - Recurrent stone formers
   - Pediatric stones
   - Multiple stones
   - Radiolucent stones

5. **What metabolic work-up will you do and when?**

   Ans. Abbreviated work-up and extended work-up.

   Abbreviated work-up consists of blood investigations including sodium, potassium, chloride, carbon dioxide, blood urea nitrogen, creatinine, calcium, intact parathyroid hormone, uric acid, urine analysis, urine culture, and radiographic imaging.

   Extended work-up includes three 24-hour urine samples.

   First two 24-hour specimens—on random diet, reflective of their usual dietary intake.

   Third 24-hour sample—after 1 week, on a calcium-, sodium-, and oxalate-restricted diet.

   When all the stones are cleared and patient is on his normal diet and his routine activities, then a metabolic work-up should be done.

6. **What is stone clinic effect?**

   Ans. If patient knows that he is going to follow up on a stone clinic, then he may alter his diet and fluid intake, which may give fallacious metabolic evaluation of blood and urine.

STAGHORN STONE

Description

This is a plain X-ray KUB, which is well exposed, well prepared and properly centralized. Both psoas shadows are well visualized. It is showing complete staghorn stone on the left side with extension of stone in all the calyces. The lower calyceal stones appear to be a bunch of multiple secondary stones (**Fig. 2**). Renal outline is faintly seen in the lower pole suggesting

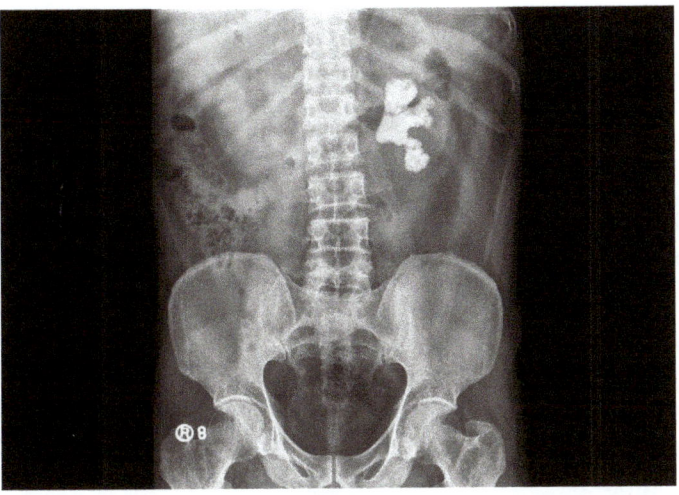

Figure 2: KUB X-ray showing complete staghorn stone on the left side.

thin parenchyma. No radiopacity is seen in opposite side or ureter or bladder area.

CT intravenous pyelogram (IVP) shows right side normal kidney. Left side kidney is about three vertebra size. Left side pelvicalyceal system is opacified with the contrast. The calyces are dilated, and the extension of staghorn stone is occupying all the calyces. There is variable thickness of parenchyma. Ureter is well opacified and normal. The upper calyx on the left side is above the level of 12th rib (**Figs. 3A to D**).

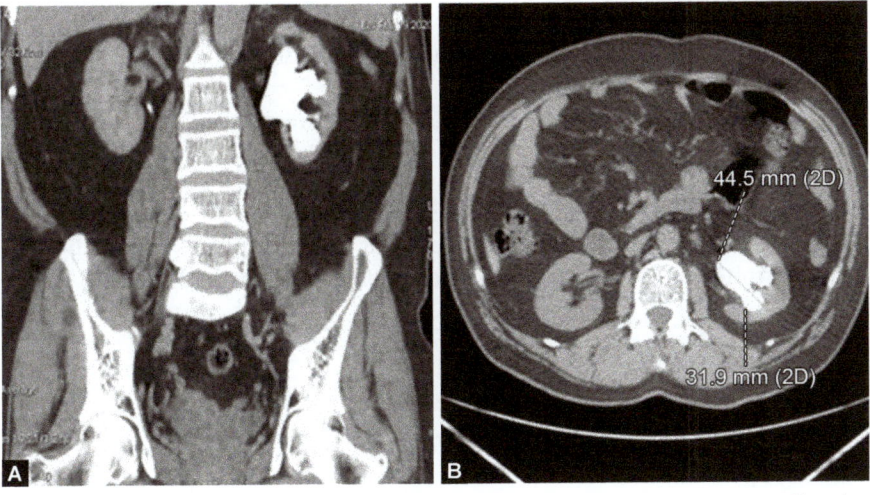

Figures 3A to D: *Contd...*

Contd...

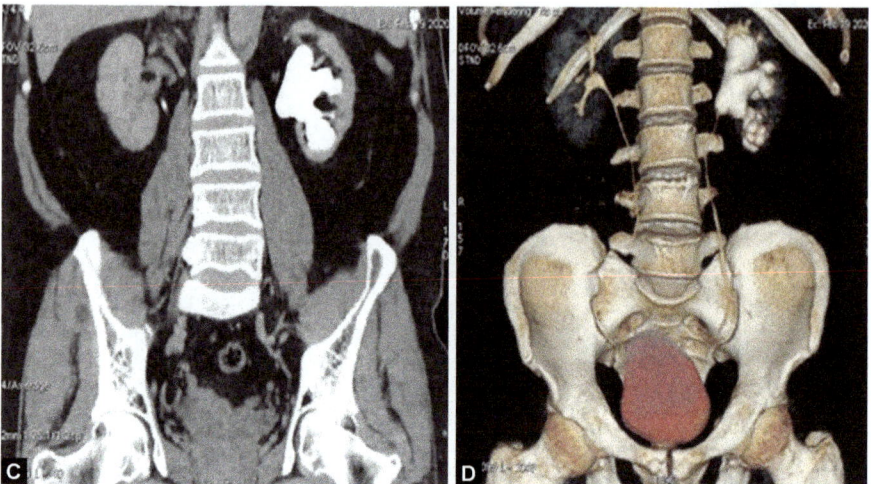

Figures 3A to D: CT intravenous pyelogram (IVP) shows pelvicalyceal system.

1. **How this patient would have presented?**

   Ans.
   - Left side flank pain off and on
   - Recurrent episodes of UTI
   - Acute pyelonephritis
   - Asymptomatic

2. **If the patient is asymptomatic, will you treat this stone?**

   Ans. Yes. This patient requires treatment even though he is asymptomatic because:
   - Kidney is still functioning. If untreated, kidney will become non-functioning.
   - There is hydronephrosis and thinning of parenchyma.
   - Stone is of a staghorn nature.

3. **How relevant is HU and how will you measure it?**

   Ans. Hounsfield unit (HU) is measured at different places especially at the periphery and the center and then average HU is calculated.

Measuring HU is very relevant to measure the hardness of the stone or to understand the density of the stone which can give indirect idea about the nature of the stone. For Example, HU around 1,300 suggests hard stones such as calcium oxalate monohydrate; HU around 1,100 suggests calcium oxalate dihydrate; HU around 100 suggests uric acid stone; and HU around 600 suggests infected stone in which you can expect slough-like material during surgery.

4. **What is the common composition of staghorn stones?**

    Ans. Triple phosphate stones (calcium-ammonium-magnesium phosphate) are common in patients with paraplegia or in patients who are nonambulatory with orthopedic illness.

    Struvite stones are infective stones because of urea splitting organisms. Calcium oxalate and uric acid are also a component in some cases.

5. **How will you treat this patient?**

    Ans. The treatment of choice is percutaneous nephrolithotomy (PCNL). However, it is likely to be multistage and multi-tract.

6. **How the stone burden is calculated in a staghorn stone?**

    Ans. The stone burden can be calculated by stone morphometry. The volume of the stone is important. Just measuring the size of the stone in AP view is not important. Various ways to calculate the stone volume are by:
    - 3D reconstruction during CT scan which will give exact volume
    - Stone volume can be calculated by ellipsoid formula (length × height × width × pie/6).
    - Also, the stone can be drawn on graph paper and volume can be calculated.

7. **What are the different types of stone scores?**

    Ans. Most commonly used stone scoring systems are Guy's stone score[1] (**Fig. 4**), S.T.O.N.E score (**Table 1**), and CROES nomogram (**Fig. 5**).

8. **What are the complications of PCNL for staghorn stone?**

    Ans. Bleeding (intraoperative, early postoperative, and delayed), perforation of pelvicalyceal system, extravasation, surrounding organ injury, sepsis, residual stones, scarring of kidney, and recurrent UTI.

Grade I

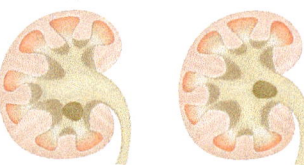

A solitary stone in the mid or lower pole with simple anatomy
or
A solitary stone in the pelvis with simple anatomy

Grade II

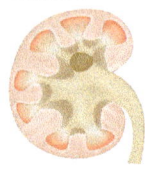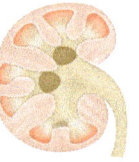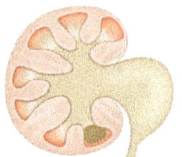

A solitary stone in the upper pole with simple anatomy
or
Multiple stones in a patient with simple anatomy
or
Any solitary stone in a patient with abnormal anatomy

Grade III

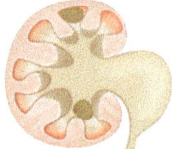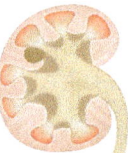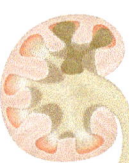

Multiple stones in a patient with abnormal anatomy
or
Stones in a calyceal diverticulum
or
Partial staghorn calculus

Grade IV

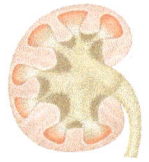

Staghorn calculus
Any stone in a patient with spina bifida or spinal injury

Figure 4: Guy's S.T.O.N.E score.

TABLE 1: S.T.O.N.E score.				
Variable	Score			
	1	2	3	4
Stone size (mm^2)	<400	400–799	800–1599	>1599
Tract length (mm)	≤100	>100	NA	NA
Obstruction	No or mild hydronephrosis	Moderate-to-severe hydronephrosis	NA	NA
Involved calyces (n)	1–2	3	Staghorn	NA
Stone essence (HU)	≤950	>950	NA	NA

Source: Okhunov Z, Friedlander JI, George AK, Duty BD, Moreira DM, Srinivasan AK, et al. S.T.O.N.E. nephrolithometry: novel surgical classification system for kidney calculi. Urology. 2013;81:1154.

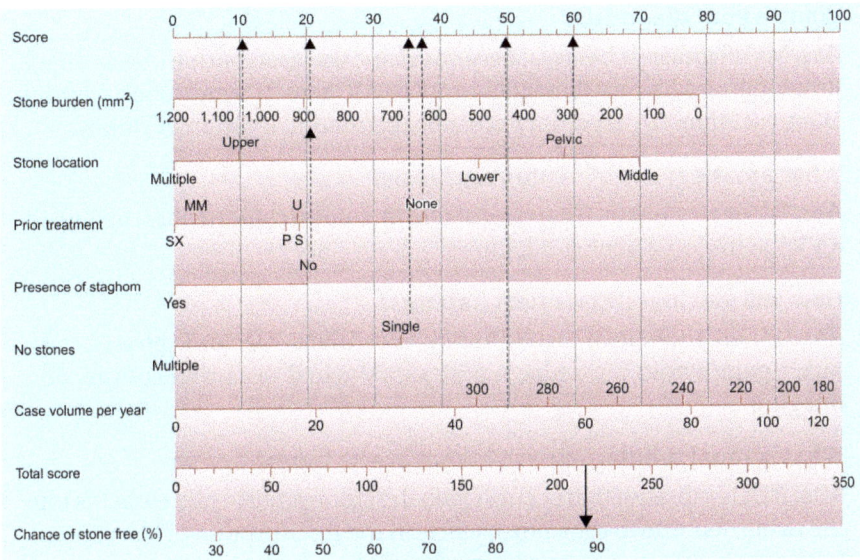

Figure 5: CROES nomogram.

Source: de la Rosette J, Assimos D, Desai M, Gutierrez J, Lingeman J, Scarpa R, et al. The clinical research office of the endourological society percutaneous nephrolithotomy global study: indications, complications, and outcomes in 5803 patients. J Endourol. 2011;25:11-7.

NEPHROCALCINOSIS

Description

This is a plain KUB X-ray showing multiple stones in the periphery of both kidneys (**Fig. 6**). No stone is seen either in the ureter or bladder.

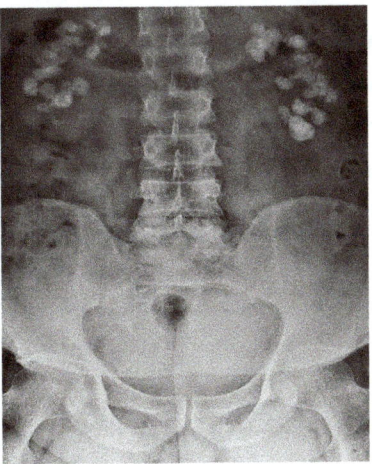

Figure 6: KUB X-ray showing multiple stones.

1. **What is your diagnosis?**

   Ans. My diagnosis is bilateral nephrocalcinosis. It can be due to hereditary tubulopathies [renal tubular acidosis (RTA)], genetic syndromes, vitamin D intoxication, hyperparathyroidism, and medullary sponge kidney.

2. **What are the types of nephrocalcinosis?**

   Ans. Types are chemical nephrocalcinosis, microscopic nephrocalcinosis, and macroscopic nephrocalcinosis.

3. **How will you investigate such patients?**

   Ans. Blood investigations including creatinine, calcium, phosphorus, intact parathyroid hormone, magnesium, urinalysis, urine culture, and imaging.

4. **What is renal tubular acidosis? What are its types?**

   Ans. RTA is a disease that occurs when the kidneys fail to excrete acids into the urine. It is due to transport defects in the reabsorption of bicarbonate (HCO_3^-), the excretion of hydrogen ion (H^+), or both.

   Clinically and pathophysiologically, RTA has been separated into three main categories—distal RTA or type 1; proximal RTA or type 2; and hyperkalemic RTA or type 4.

   Type 3 is rare and is a combination of type 1 and type 2 RTA.

5. **What are the types of hyperoxaluria?**

   Ans. Primary hyperoxaluria (PH1, PH2, and PH3), dietary hyperoxaluria, and enteric hyperoxaluria.

6. **Do you think these are calcifications or stones?**

   Ans. These are stones which are located in the collecting ducts.

7. **How will the patient present?**

   Ans. The patient can present with history of recurrent passage of stones, multiple attacks of colic or retention.

8. **How will you treat the patient?**

   Ans. We have to treat the patients as and when they become symptomatic for the stone. If the stones are all in the calyces, they can be treated by retrograde intrarenal surgery (RIRS). If the primary cause cannot be cured, then bilateral ileal replacement of ureter to prevent recurrent episodes of obstruction.

BILATERAL URETERIC STONE

Description

This is KUB X-ray which is showing right ureteric stone at the level of transverse process of L3 and left ureteric stone at the level of L5 which has got an oblique axis with longitudinal length three times more than the width

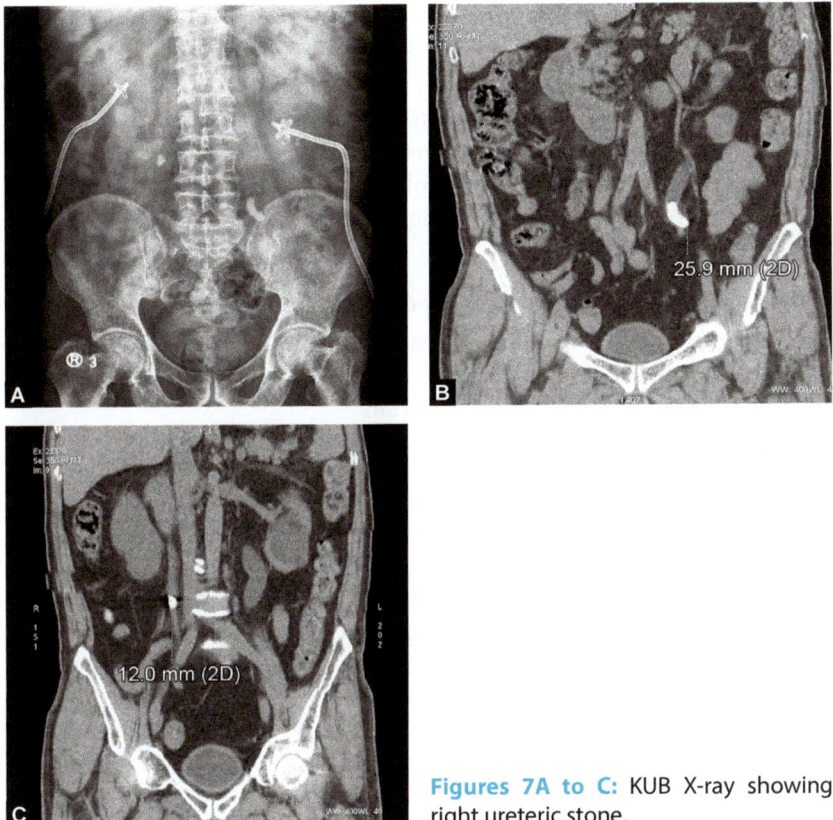

Figures 7A to C: KUB X-ray showing right ureteric stone.

(**Figs. 7A to C**). Bilateral malecot nephrostomies are seen. No radiopacity is seen in kidney or bladder region.

1. **How this patient would have presented with?**
   Ans.
   - Symptoms of acute renal failure
   - Infection/pyonephrosis on one or both sides
   - Anuria/oliguria
   - Bilateral flank pain
   - Recurrent UTI

2. **After placing nephrostomy, what things will you observe?**
   Ans.
   - Output from each side
   - Clearing the purulent urine if it was a pyonephrotic kidney
   - Resolution of hydronephrosis
   - Creatinine clearance on each side
   - Urinalysis with reference to pH, specific gravity, urinary sodium
   - Creatinine trend
   - Improvement of symptoms

3. **If this patient had come with anuria with bilateral hydronephrosis, would you have done bilateral DJ stent?**

   Ans. The left side stone appears to be oblique in axis and appears to be severely impacted. So, it appears that the DJ stenting may not be successful. Secondly, if it is pyonephrosis, nephrostomy drains the pus effectively and efficiently. Nephrostomy can be done under LA. DJ stenting may need some anesthesia. Hence, I would have preferred bilateral nephrostomy.

4. **Which kidney do you think is better?**

   Ans. Right kidney has better cortical thickness. Left kidney appears to have thin parenchyma and sac like.
   So, right kidney appears to function well.

5. **How will you treat the patient?**

   Ans. If both the kidneys are functioning well, then right ureteroscopy (URS)/RIRS/antegrade URS or push PCNL. Left side, the stone is angulated, hence URS may have difficulty. For antegrade, the stone is lower down. Hence, both the options may be tried. However, if both the options fail, then laparoscopic ureterolithotomy or open ureterolithotomy.

CALCULUS IN ECTOPIC KIDNEY

Description

This is a plain KUB X-ray which shows radio opacity in the region of the left lower portion of the SI joint (**Fig. 8**). The stent is in position. The lower end

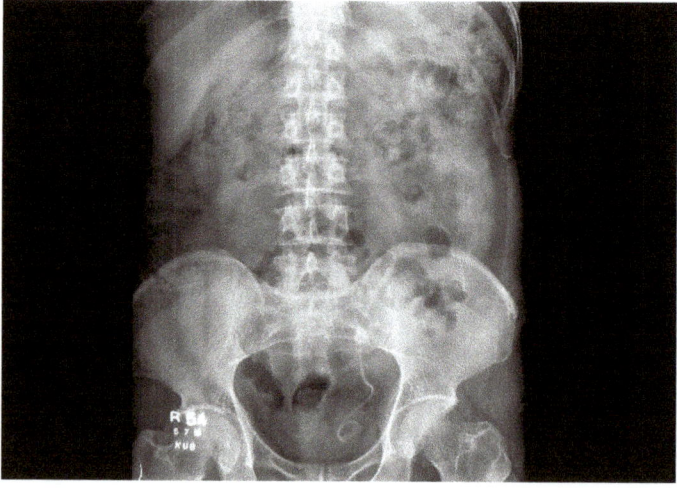

Figure 8: KUB X-ray shows radiopacity in the region of the left lower portion of the SI joint.

is properly coiled. However, the upper end is not properly visualized. There is no radio opacity in any other region. The likely possibility is left ectopic kidney with stone with stent in situ.

1. **Why is it not a forgotten in an orthotopic kidney with a mid ureteric stone stent?**

   Ans. If it was a forgotten stent, the upper portion of the stent is not seen even if the stent is broken, upper portion should be visualized as a migrated stent in the kidney.

2. **How do you confirm the diagnosis?**

   Ans. By doing USG and CT IVU.

3. **What is the differential diagnosis of radiopacity in that region?**

   Ans.
   - Ureteric calculus
   - Calcified lymph node
   - Calcification in the vessel
   - Stone in a transplant kidney
   - Fecolith/tablet

CT IVU of the same patient:

Description: This is the CT IVU which shows left pelvic ectopic kidney with pelvis facing anteriorly (**Figs. 9A to C**). Stone is in the renal pelvis with minimal hydronephrosis and normal ureter.

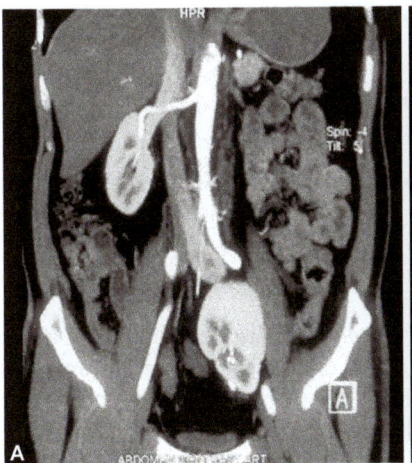
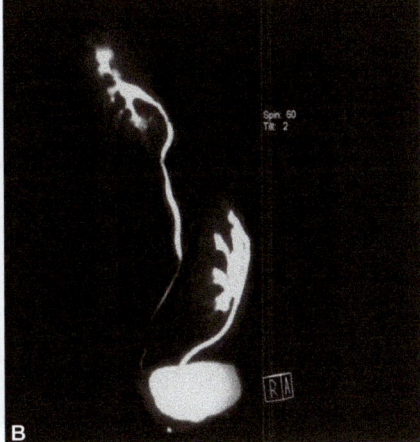

Figures 9A to C: *Contd...*

Contd...

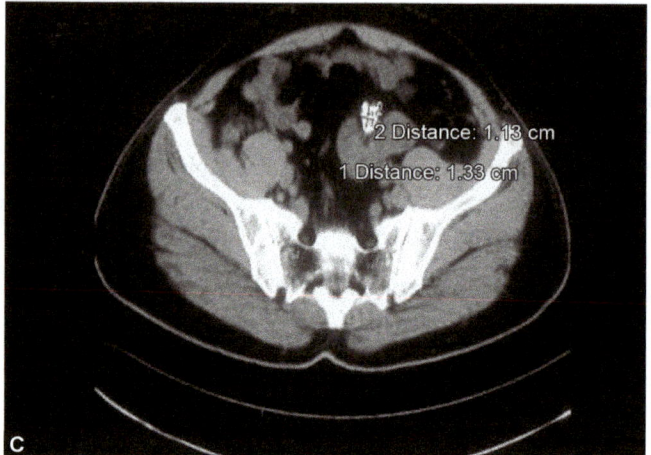

Figures 9A to C: CT IVU of the same patient.

1. **What anatomical facts would you note on USG or CT IVP?**
   Ans.
   - Lie of the kidney
   - Position of the kidney
   - Whether pelvis is anterior or posterior and position of calyces
   - Vascular supply of kidney
   - Concomitant PUJ obstruction
   - Any solid or hollow viscus or bone between the target calyx and abdominal wall

2. **What are the different treatment options?**
   Ans.
   - PCNL—USG/laparoscopy guided
   - Laparoscopic pyelolithotomy
   - RIRS

3. **Will you do ESWL in this case?**
   Ans. Extracorporeal shock wave lithotripsy (ESWL) is difficult because the kidney is situated in the bony pelvis and it would be difficult to localize the stone without intervening bony structures. Also, ESWL is to be done in prone position. Also, the drainage of such kidneys is impaired due to high insertion of ureter.

4. **What are the difficulties anticipated in RIRS?**
   Ans.
   - Ureter has multiple curves and may not get dilated. Hence may need preprocedure stenting.

- There could be acute kink at the PUJ, and hence difficulty in negotiating the scope in the pelvis, especially if it is a high riding ureter.
- While fragmenting, some fragments may go into inaccessible calyx, which may be difficult to remove with RIRS.
- RIRS is done without access sheath. If access sheath is used, it should be short and it is to be kept below the PUJ.

5. **How will you do laparoscopically guided PCNL?**
    Ans. The puncture of the pelvicalyceal system is done under the laparoscopic control to ensure there is no bowel injury, the puncture is from the cortex, and not directly on the pelvis. Once the puncture is done, subsequent steps are done under fluoroscopy without any pneumoperitoneum. Generally, peritoneal drain is kept along with nephrostomy drainage and a DJ stent.

6. **What are the salient steps of laparoscopic pyelolithotomy?**
    Ans.
    - It is to be done only when the pelvis is facing anteriorly
    - Patient is in steep Trendelenburg position
    - Sigmoid mesentery is mobilized
    - Pelvis is exposed
    - Incision kept on pelvis
    - If required, flexible nephroscope with the port
    - DJ stent to be placed
    - Closure of pelvis
    - Peritoneal drain to be kept

    Generally, the vessels come from the posterior side and it is unlikely that the vessels will be injured in the procedure.

REFERENCE

1. Thomas K, Smith NC, Hegarty N, Glass JM. The Guy's stone scored grading the complexity of percutaneous nephrolithotomy procedures. Urology. 2011;78:277.

CHAPTER 20

Renal Imaging

PELVIC URETERIC JUNCTION OBSTRUCTION

Description

This is the CT intravenous urogram (IVU) of a child which shows delayed excretion and good concentration of the contrast in a hugely dilated extrarenal pelvis, with thin parenchyma (**Figs. 1A to F**). Calyces are also dilated and abrupt narrowing of pelvic ureteric junction (PUJ) with visualization of ureter. The likely diagnosis is primary PUJ obstruction.

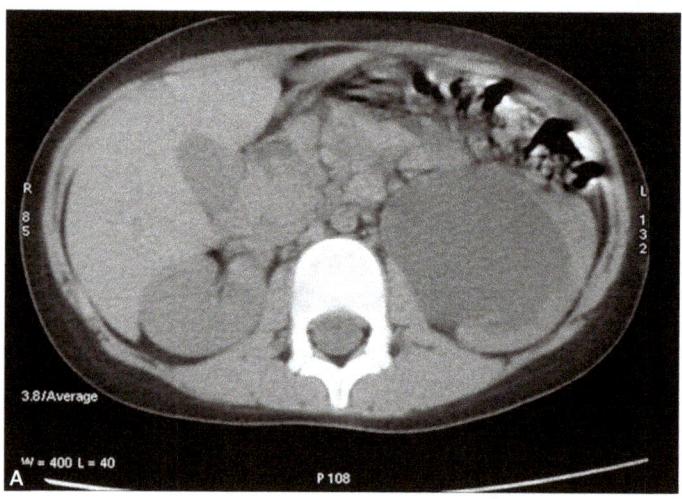

Figures 1A to F: *Contd...*

Contd...

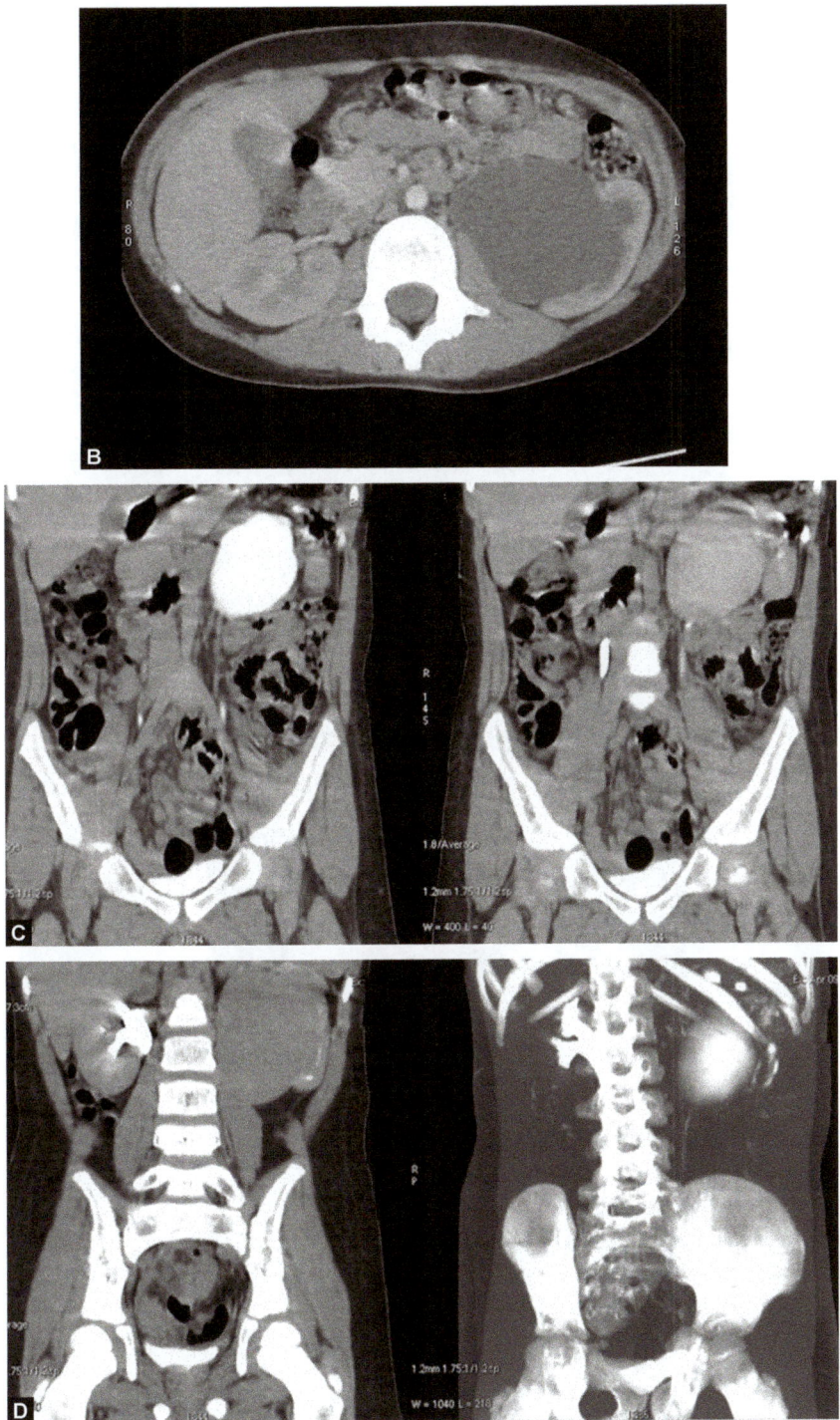

Figures 1A to F: *Contd...*

Contd...

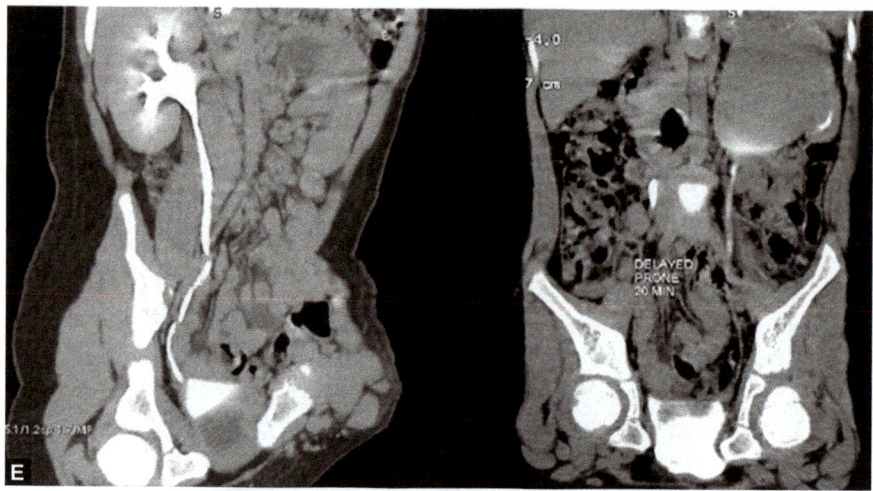

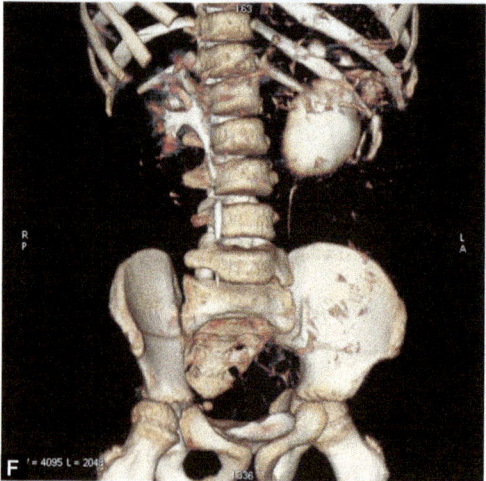

Figures 1A to F: CT intravenous urogram (IVU) of a child which shows delayed excretion on left side.

1. **What are the likely ways of presentation in this child?**
   Ans.
   - Vague left side flank pain
   - Recurrent episodes of urinary tract infection (UTI)
   - Asymptomatic (USG done for some other reason)
   - Antenatally detected PUJO

2. **What are the ways to classify hydronephrosis?**
   Ans. It can be classified by SFU (Society of Fetal Urology) classification:
   - Grade 0: No dilatation; calyceal walls are opposed to each other
   - Grade 1: Dilatation of the renal pelvis without dilatation of the calyces

CHAPTER 20: Renal Imaging | 253

- Grade 2: Dilatation of the renal pelvis (mild) and calyces (pelvicalyceal pattern is retained); no parenchymal atrophy
- Grade 3: Moderate dilatation of the renal pelvis and calyces; blunting of fornices and flattening of papillae; mild cortical thinning may be seen
- Grade 4: Gross dilatation of the renal pelvis and calyces; loss of borders between the renal pelvis and calyces; renal atrophy seen as cortical thinning

3. **Will you do isotope renogram in this case?**
   Ans. In this case, the isotope renogram is not required for the diagnosis of obstruction or functioning of the kidney. However, it is required from the follow up point-of-view. It has to be kept in mind that in an obstructed kidney, isotope renogram may give over estimation of function.

4. **In a suspected PUJO on USG, what are the indications of CT IVU in a child?**
   Ans.
   - Failed previous pyeloplasty
   - Suspected secondary PUJO obstruction
   - Secondary stones—noncontrast CT can be done to identify the exact number of stones. CT IVU will give you the calyceal anatomical details and will suggest which calyces contain stones.
   - Anomalous kidney (horseshoe kidney, ectopic kidney, malrotated kidney)
   - On USG, there is a suspected PUJ stone leading to hydronephrosis.

5. **What are the hazards of CT IVU in children?**
   Ans.
   - The radiation dose is very high (8–10 mSv which is equivalent to 400 chest X-rays).
   - CT IVU cannot be utilized as a follow-up tool.

6. **Do you want to know about crossing vessel preoperatively?**
   Ans. It is not necessary to know the crossing vessels by any investigation. Crossing vessel can be identified intraoperatively and can be tackled accordingly.

7. **How do you know the length of the stenosed segment?**
   Ans. It is not necessary to know the exact length of the stenosed segment. Whatever is the length can be tackled intraoperatively and hence RGP also is not required.

8. **Will you do MCU in this case?**
   Ans. Although the reported incidence of reflux is high (10–22%), micturating cystourethrography (MCU) is routinely not required when USG does not show any hydroureter. Even if the reflux is detected these

are low grade and of no consequences. If the USG shows any dilatation of the ureter, MCU is indicated. However in case of bilateral hydronephrosis even when USG does not show any hydroureter MCU may be indicated.

9. **How do you know the extrarenal pelvis?**

   Ans. Draw a line parallel to the lie of the kidney:
   - In axial section—from medial border of the anterior and posterior parenchyma
   - In sagittal section—from medial end of the upper and lower pole
   If the pelvis is seen medial to this line, then it is intrarenal pelvis.

10. **What are the investigations of choice in suspected case of primary PUJO in children and in adults?**

    Ans.
    - In children, only isotope renogram
    - In adults, CT IVU and isotope renogram

    In adults, the hydronephrosis can be because of various reasons such as impacted PUJ stone, genitourinary tuberculosis, and upper ureteric strictures. In adults, the radiation of one CT IVP is not as hazardous as in children.

ANGIOMYOLIPOMA

Description

There is a mass lesion seen in the lower pole of the kidney.

On USG, the mass appears hyperechoic, mainly endophytic in nature. On CT scan, the renal contour is maintained, and the mass does not have exophytic component and does not reach the hilum (**Figs. 2A and B**).

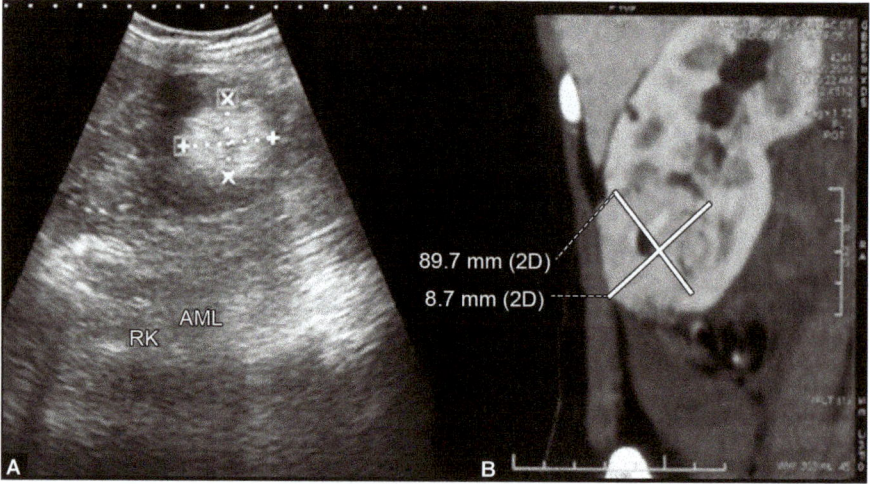

Figures 2A and B: (A) USG showing kidney mass appears hyperechoic; (B) CT scan, the mass does not have exophytic component.

1. **What is the diagnosis?**

    Ans. The diagnosis is likely to be angiomyolipoma (AML) of kidney as the mass is hyperechoic in USG. The hyperechogenicity on USG is due to fat content.

2. **What do you think are characteristic features of AML on CT scan?**

    Ans.
    - The negative HU in the mass suggests fat content which is highly suggestive of AML. Very rarely, the renal cell carcinoma (RCC) also can contain fat.
    - Significant enhancement of the lesion
    - Well circumscribed in nature

3. **What are the likely presentation?**

    Ans.
    - Asymptomatic and incidental detection on USG
    - Vague pain on the ipsilateral side
    - Hematuria

4. **What are the syndromic associations with AML?**

    Ans.
    - Clinical triad of TSC: K/s Vogt triad
    - Facial lesions (adenoma sebaceum) seizures
    - Mental retardation

5. **How will you treat the patient?**

    Ans. The AMLs which are asymptomatic, <4 cm, and in old ladies or male patients can be kept under observation.

    In young ladies, during pregnancy, the AML may increase and rupture, and hence require treatment.

    If excessively symptomatic, even a small AML may need treatment. Any lesion >4 cm requires treatment which can be either selective angioembolization of the feeding vessel if it is present or, nephron sparing surgery.

6. **What are the complications?**

    Ans.
    - The rupture of AML can cause severe sudden perirenal hematoma (Wunderlich syndrome)
    - Severe hematuria
    - Sudden intrarenal hemorrhage causing acute severe pain
    - Large size AMLs are more prone for bleeding even from trivial trauma.

7. **What are the indications for angioembolization?**
   Ans.
   - AML with active bleeding
   - Large mass with a definitive bleeding vessel
   - AML in a solitary kidney
   - Bilateral AML
   - Central tumors

8. **Is there any medical management for AML?**
   Ans. Yes, everolimus and sirolimus are used for medical management, especially in cases of TS, patients not been considered for angioembolization or NSS.

RENAL MASS

Description

There is a large heterogeneously enhancing mass occupying the upper and middle pole of right kidney abutting the liver cranially, maintaining the fat plane, laterally, abutting the psoas, fat plane is maintained. Neoangiogenesis is seen all around the mass.

There is a single renal artery with additional collaterals supplying the tumor.

There is a single renal vein which is free of thrombus.

There is no obvious lymph nodes enlargement seen.

Most likely diagnosis is RCC (**Figs. 3A to D**).

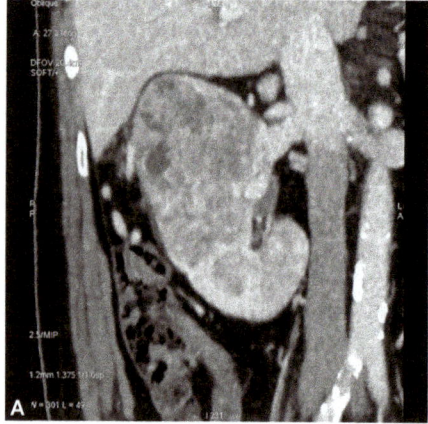 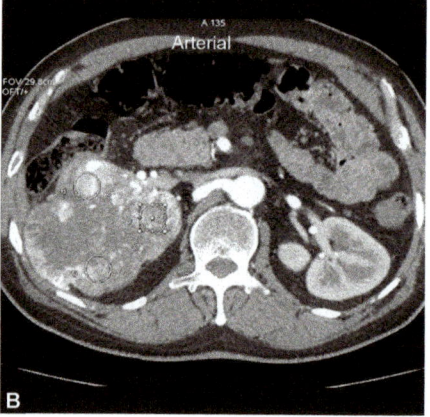

Figures 3A to D: *Contd...*

Contd...

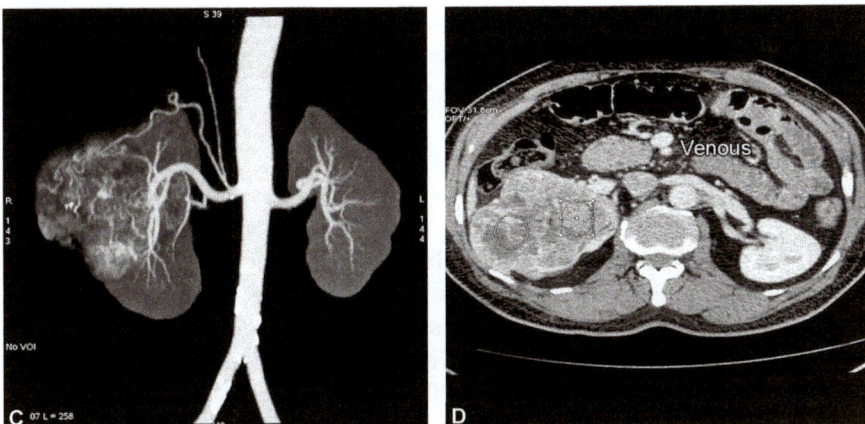

Figures 3A to D: CT scan images of a right renal mass.

1. **What do you think is the T stage of the tumor?**

   Ans. The tumor appears to be >7 cm, sinus fat is not seen separately, and there are no obvious lymph nodes seen.
   So, it could be cT3aN0.

2. **What this patient would have presented with?**

   Ans.
   - Flank pain
   - Hematuria
   - Lump in abdomen
   - Paraneoplastic syndrome
   - Fever, jaundice, hypertension
   - Constitutional symptoms

3. **What more work-up is required in this case?**

   Ans. Metastasis evaluation to be done by chest CT.

4. **Will you do FDG PET in this case?**

   Ans. Routine use of fluorodeoxyglucose (FDG)-positron emission tomography (PET) scan in case of RCC is discouraged.

5. **How do you risk stratify a metastatic disease?**

   Ans. If metastasis is positive, then further investigations are Hb, serum calcium, serum LDH, ANC, ESR, and LFT to risk stratify the patient according to IMDC (International Metastatic RCC Database Consortium) criteria or Motzer criteria.

6. **Will you remove adrenal in this case?**

   Ans. If the plane between the adrenal gland and the kidney is preserved, then there is no need to remove the adrenal gland even if it is an upper polar mass.

RENAL MASS WITH IVC THROMBUS

Description

Left kidney shows heterogeneously enhancing mass occupying the whole kidney mainly arising from the lower pole. There is no excretion of contrast in the pelvicalyceal system (PCS) on left side. Left renal vein shows thrombus which is going into the inferior vena cava (IVC) up to its retrohepatic course but not extending above the diaphragm. Thrombus is not occupying the whole IVC (**Figs. 4A to C**). The tumor does not appear to infiltrate the surrounding structures. No obvious grossly enlarged lymph nodes are seen. No metastasis is seen in the liver. The diagnosis is RCC with IVC thrombus.

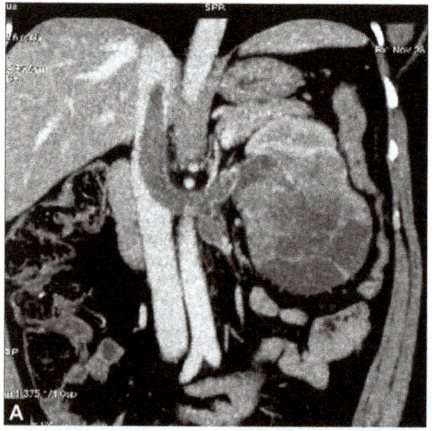
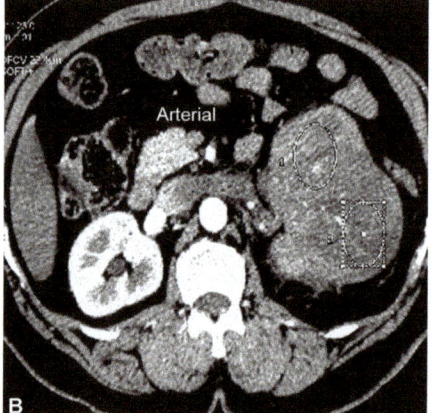
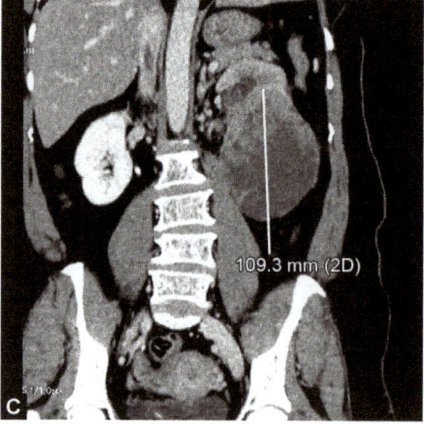

Figures 4A to C: CT scans show renal mass with thrombus.

1. **How this patient would present?**

   Ans. In addition, there could be varicocele and bilateral pedal edema. However, since the IVC is not completely obstructed and there is flow in the IVC, lower limb edema may not be significant or may be absent.

2. **What is role of MRI?**

   Ans. MRI gives accurate diagnosis about the level of thrombus and it will give the idea about the renal vein invasion. It is a preferred investigation in patients with raised creatinine.

3. **How do you classify the venous thrombus in RCC??**

   Ans. AJCC level:

T3a	Tumor grossly extends into the renal vein or its segmental (muscle-containing) branches, or tumor invades perirenal and/or renal sinus fat but not beyond the Gerota fascia
T3b	Tumor grossly extends into the vena cava below the diaphragm
T3c	Tumor grossly extends into the vena cava above the diaphragm or invades the wall of the vena cava

   Mayo classification:

Level	
0	Limited to renal vein or its tributaries
I	Extends into IVC but <2 cm above renal vein orifice
II	Extends into IVC, >2 cm above renal vein orifice but below hepatic veins
III	Extends above hepatic veins but below diaphragm
IV	Extends above diaphragm

4. **How do you differentiate bland thrombus from tumor thrombus? What are its implications?**

   Ans. The tumor thrombus will enhance in a post contrast phase. However, bland thrombus will not enhance. Tumor thrombus consists of tumor tissue which goes inside the vein; however, bland thrombus is formed due to hypercoagulable state and obstruction of IVC.

   Bland thrombus is usually distal to renal vein, and tumor thrombus is usually proximal to renal vein.

5. **During surgery with lower polar exophytic large mass, what precautions will you take?**

   Ans. Often, large lower polar mass infiltrates the transverse mesocolon, therefore, while doing nephrectomy, that portion of mesocolon needs to be excised. If large portion of mesocolon is infiltrated, then a part of colon also needs to be excised.

SMALL RENAL MASS

Description

This is a CT scan which shows 3.3 × 2.5 cm mainly exophytic enhancing mass arising from the lateral aspect of mid pole. Rest of the PCS and parenchyma is normal. Left kidney is normal (**Figs. 5A and B**). The mass is likely to be RCC.

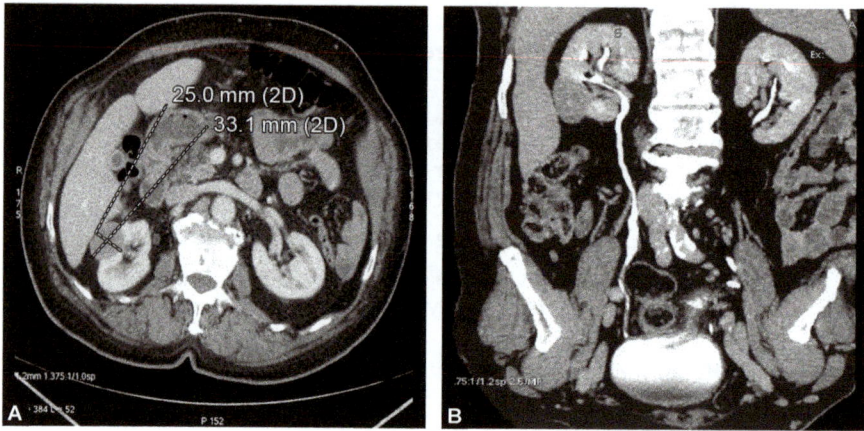

Figures 5A and B: CT scans show exophytic mass.

1. **What is the likely presentation of such patients?**
   Ans.
   - Asymptomatic
   - Flank pain
   - Hematuria

2. **Will you do biopsy in this case?**
   Ans. I will not do a biopsy in this case as it is clearly an enhancing mass. The indications of biopsy are:
   - Radiologically indeterminate lesions (enhancement is <20HU)
   - Patients planned for active surveillance
   - Patients planned for local therapy
   - In cases of metastatic disease, to plan for medical or surgical treatment
   - Mass is suspected to be metastasis in kidney, for example, lymphoma

3. **What is nephrometry score?**
   Ans. Different nephrometry scores are available. RENAL and PADUA are the most commonly used scores. These scores are used to measure

the complexity of the surgery. All these scores take into consideration exophytic nature, size of tumor, nearness of tumor to sinus fat, relation with polar lines, and location of tumor.

4. **Will you do renal angiography if you do partial nephrectomy in this case?**

    Ans. Renal angiography gives idea about the number of vessels, and if the tumor is near the hilum, it gives the relation of vessels to the tumor. However, in the peripheral exophytic small tumor, angiography may not be required.

5. **What are the concerns of doing partial nephrectomy in cT2 tumors?**

    Ans. T2 means tumor is >7 cm. In such big tumors, often the left-out kidney is small. Also, there is a high chance of margin positivity and multicentricity. Also, upstaging of tumor on final histology is likely.

6. **What is the definition of SRM?**

    Ans. A tumor <4 cm is known as small renal mass (SRM).

CHAPTER 21

Bladder and Ureteric Imaging

LOWER URETERIC MASS

Description

The CT scan shows a filling defect in the lower ureter (**Figs. 1A and B**). There is no stone on the plain CT.

So there is a possibility of a lower ureteric tumor.

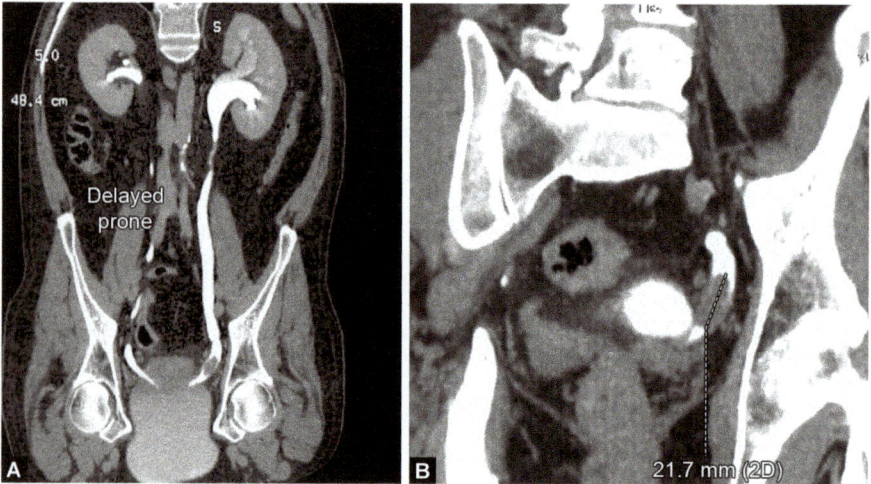

Figures 1A and B: CT scans show a filling defect in the lower ureter.

1. **What are the different types of tumors in the ureter? What is this filling defect likely to be?**

    Ans. The different types of filling defects in the ureter are tumor (benign or malignant), stone, clot, papillary necrosis, polyp, and fungal ball.

The plain CT does not show any stone, the kidney is well functioning, no perinephric stranding, and no back pressure changes are seen. It seems to be arising from the wall, so it seems to be ureteric tumor.

2. **How do you differentiate benign tumor from malignant?**
   Ans. Benign tumors are generally polyp or a small papilloma which are generally of a small size. Malignant tumors are larger in size, irregular surface, solid and broad based, enhancing in nature, and often show thickening of the wall and infiltration outside the ureter. Often, malignant tumors cause back pressure changes.

3. **What would you do next?**
   Ans. Diagnostic ureteroscopy and biopsy

4. **How will you take biopsy?**
   Ans. The biopsy can be taken by:
   - Forceps
   - Basket
   - If the mass is pedunculated, the whole specimen can be cut with the help of a laser and can be taken for a biopsy.

5. **Suppose this is a malignant tumor, what advise will you give?**
   Ans. The advice will depend on the biopsy report.
   If it is a low-grade tumor, pedunculated and small tumor, then complete endoscopic resection can be done. If complete resection cannot be done, then resection and ureteric reimplantation can be done.
   If it is a high-grade tumor, then nephroureterectomy has to be done.
   If it is a high-grade tumor in a solitary kidney and provided the tumor has not gone outside and no lymph node enlargement, then lower ureteric excision and reimplantation/Boari flap has to be done. Patient has to be on a strict follow-up after surgery.

TRANSITIONAL CELL CARCINOMA

Description

The CT images show a large ill-defined renal mass occupying almost the whole of kidney with evidence of filling defect in the proximal renal vein suggestive of a renal vein thrombus (**Figs. 2A to C**). The axial cut shows evidence of perinephric stranding suggesting extension of the disease. At places, the mass lesion appears to be involving the psoas. There is an evidence of a large conglomeration of lymph nodes in the hilar region. There is evidence of hydronephrosis with significant calyceal dilatation of the upper calyx. There is nonexcretion of contrast. The wall of the ureter shows significant

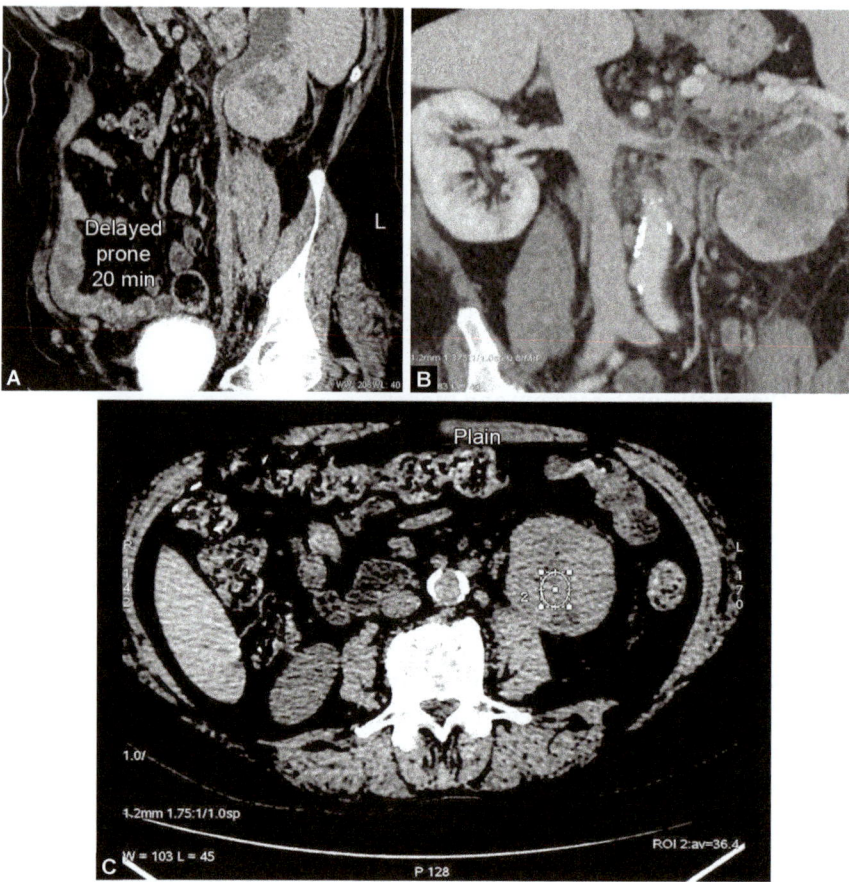

Figures 2A to C: CT images show a large ill-defined renal mass suggestive of a renal vein thrombus.

enhancement with extensive periureteric stranding along the whole course of the ureter. There is thickening of the wall of ureter.

1. **What would be the possible diagnosis?**

   Ans. The possible diagnosis is renal cell carcinoma (RCC) and transitional cell carcinoma (TCC).

   RCC can be diagnosed because the kidney is completely destroyed and there is renal vein thrombosis. TCC, because the ureteric wall is enhancing, thickened, and there is hydronephrosis.

2. **What will be the patient presentation in this case?**

   Ans. The patient may present with:
   - Hematuria
   - Flank pain
   - Weight loss
   - Fever

3. **How would you differentiate RCC and TCC on imaging and CT scan?**

   Ans.
   - The RCC is more of peripheral tumor and then comes in center while TCC is more of central tumor which expands from center to periphery.
   - RCC is well defined and well capsulated while TCC is ill defined.
   - The enhancement is more in RCC and less in TCC.
   - The calyces are destroyed in TCC while they are often stretched in RCC.
   - Hydronephrosis is often associated with TCC.

4. **If the tumor is TCC, what will be the clinical stage of the disease?**

   Ans. The stage of the disease is T4 because the surrounding structures are infiltrated.
   N2 because there are multiple big lymph node masses.

BLADDER MASS

Description

This is the USG film of bladder which shows a small mass arising from the bladder wall which appears to be papillary in nature (**Fig. 3**).

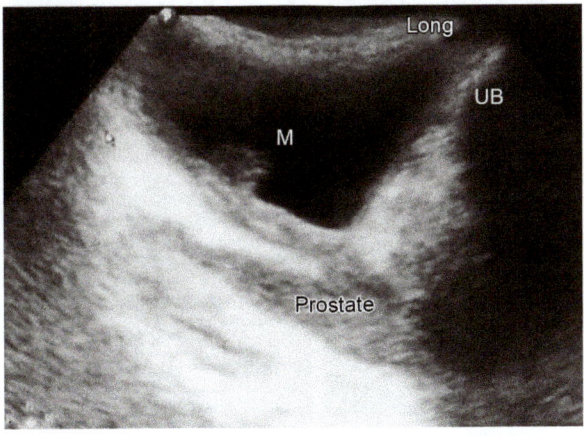

Figure 3: USG showing bladder mass.

1. **What is the likely diagnosis?**

   Ans. The likely diagnosis is nonmuscle invasive bladder tumor.

2. **How do you differentiate clot from the mass?**

   Ans. Mass is fixed to the bladder wall while clot can move. Hence, on changing the position of the patient, the clot will move. Mass is echogenic while the clot will be of mixed echogenicity with multiple areas of hypoechogenicity. The mass will show hypervascularity on color Doppler.

3. **How will you proceed?**

   Ans. If the mass is small, <2 cm, pedunculated, and there is no evidence of hydronephrosis in upper tracts, then further evaluation of upper tracts is not necessary. The next step will be cystoscopy and transurethral resection of bladder tumor.

   If the mass is large, broad based, multiple, sessile, with hydronephrosis, the next step is CT intravenous urogram.

BLADDER MASS WITH NONFUNCTIONING KIDNEY

Description

The CT IVU shows evidence of a large ill-defined broad-based mass occupying almost whole bladder and seem to arise at the UV junction (**Figs. 4A and B**). The lower ureter is thickened. The mass shows significant enhancment on the postcontrast images. Right kidney shows hydronephrosis, thinned out parenchyma, and no excretion of contrast. No obvious lymph node enlargement is seen.

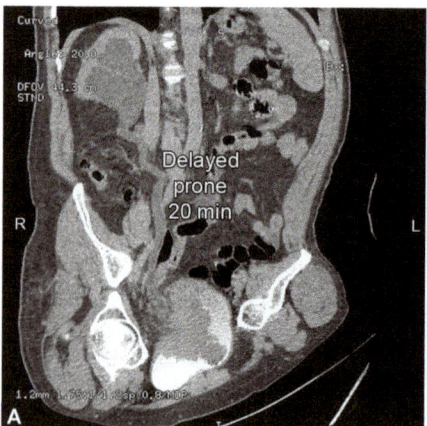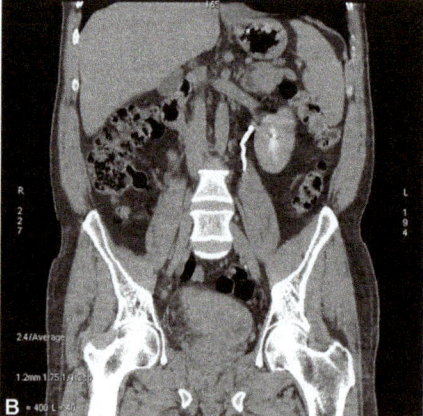

Figures 4A and B: CT IVU shows evidence of a large ill-defined broad-based mass.

1. **What would be the presentation of the patient?**

   Ans.
   - Hematuria
   - Frequency
   - Urgency
   - Urge incontinence

- Passage of clots, necrotic tissue
- Flank pain
- Anorexia
- Cachexia
- Fever

2. **What will you do next?**

    Ans. Metastatic work-up in the form of CT chest. And then, cystoscopy, bimanual examination under general anesthesia and transurethral resection biopsy of the mass.

3. **Will you remove the mass completely or take only biopsy?**

    Ans. Since on the CT scan, it appears to be invading the muscle, UVJ, broad based, and a large mass which suggests to be an invasive bladder cancer, hence, only biopsy with deep muscle inclusion is necessary to get the histological evidence of grade and stage.

4. **If biopsy shows high-grade muscle invasive disease, what will you do?**

    Ans. Since the local disease appears to have gone outside at the UV junction, i.e., T3 stage, it is preferable to give neoadjuvant chemotherapy and after that, right nephroureterectomy with radical cystectomy with ileal conduit.

CHAPTER 22

Adrenal Mass

ADRENAL MASS

Description

These are the plain and contrast CT scans of abdomen and pelvis (**Figs. 1A and B**). The plain scan shows a well-circumscribed lesion in suprarenal area on right side. In the contrast scan, the mass lesion is enhancing and shows some necrotic areas within. No fat density areas are seen within the lesion.

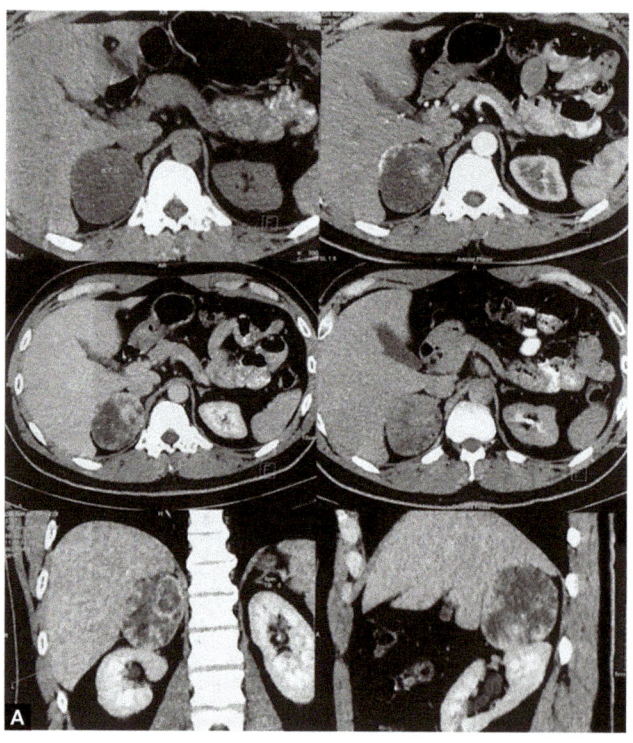

Figures 1A and B: *Contd…*

Contd...

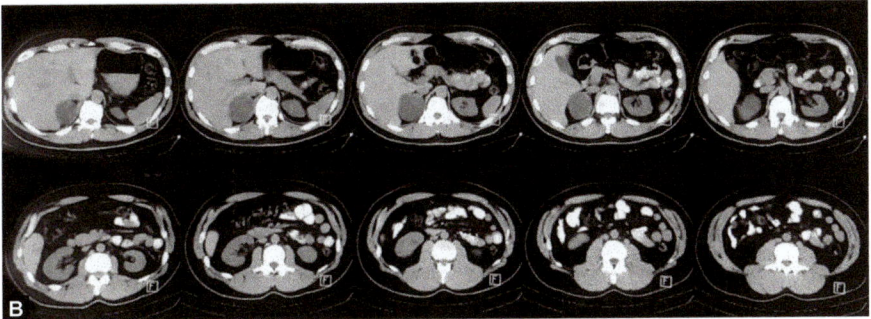

Figures 1A and B: Plain and contrast CT scans of abdomen and pelvis.

No lymph nodes are visible. The wash out study cannot be commented upon in these images. All the above findings suggest a diagnosis of right pheochromocytoma.

1. **What are the characteristic features to diagnose pheochromocytoma from adenomas?**

   Ans. Usually, the average size of pheochromocytomas is approximately 4–6 cm while that of adenomas is smaller.

   In plain CT scan, the attenuation value of pheochromocytoma is always >10 HU. This is due to absence of intracytoplasmic lipids within pheochromocytoma tumors. In adenoma, there are 10% or more negative pixels.

   After the administration of contrast medium, pheochromocytomas usually have enhancement >130 HU. In smaller solid lesions, the enhancement is relatively homogeneous, while in larger lesions the character of the enhancement is more or less heterogeneous. It is typical of pheochromocytomas with central necrosis and the enhancement of the peripheral rim is due to the viable tumor tissue.

   The adrenal CT protocol includes 1-minute contrast-enhanced scan and late-enhancement scans, i.e., 15 minutes, which allows the measurement of the absolute and relative decrease in post-contrast attenuation. It shows the rate of contrast medium washout. Adenomas have rapid washout compared to the slower washout of pheochromocytomas.

2. **What is early washout and late washout?**

   Ans. An absolute percent washout (APW) is comparing noncontrast values with 15-minute post-contrast density values.

   Relative percent washout (RPW) is comparing arterial phase density measurements with 15-minute post-contrast density values.

   An APW of >60% and RPW of >40% on delayed (washout) imaging are indicative of adenoma (**Flowchart 1**).

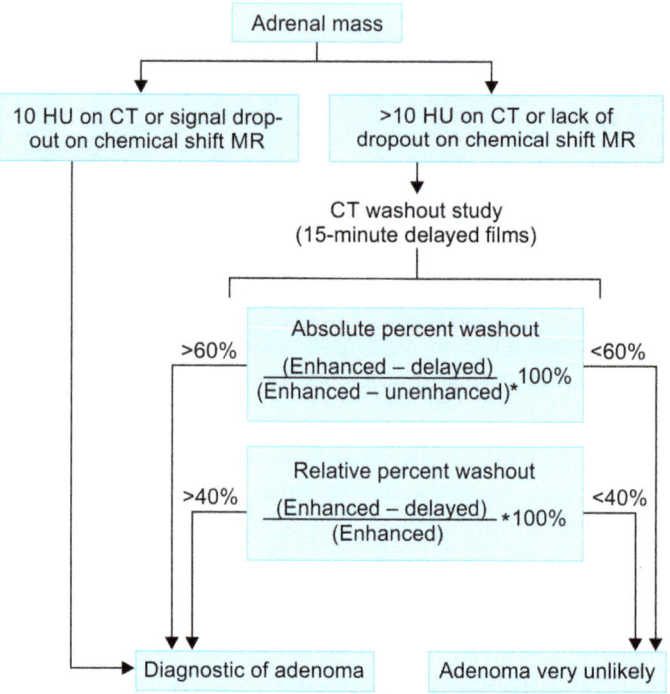

Flowchart 1: Absolute and relative percent washout.

3. How do you differentiate ACC from other tumors?

Ans. On imaging, adrenocortical carcinomas (ACCs) tend to be larger than benign adrenal tumors, with an average size of 10–12 cm on presentation. There are irregular borders, irregular enhancement, calcifications, and necrotic areas with cystic degeneration. Mean attenuation on noncontrast CT scan in ACC is significantly higher (39 HU) compared with adenomas (8 HU). Also, ACCs do not exhibit rapid contrast washout which is characteristic of adenomas. The presence of lymph nodes and local tumor invasion to inferior vena cava and other adjacent organs are other indicators of ACC.

4. What is incidentaloma?

Ans. Adrenal incidentalomas are unsuspected adrenal masses >1 cm in diameter which are identified on imaging performed for unrelated causes.

5. When will you intervene?

Ans. The surgical indications for intervention are:
- Functional adrenal mass
- Mass >4 cm with exception of myelolipoma

- Mass with imaging findings suggestive of malignancy (e.g., lipid poor, heterogeneous, irregular borders, infiltrates surrounding structures)
- Adrenal incidentaloma that grows >1 cm on follow-up imaging
- Extremely large and/or symptomatic myelolipoma
- Isolated adrenal metastasis
- Failed neurosurgical treatment of Cushing's disease which requires bilateral adrenalectomy

6. **What hormonal testing will you do for this patient?**
   Ans.
   1. Overnight dexamethasone (1 mg) suppression test
   2. Measurement of fractionated metanephrins or
   3. Metanephrins in a 24-hour urinary specimen

7. **When will you do a measurement of the plasma aldosterone concentration and plasma renin activity ?**
   Ans. In patients with adrenal mass having hypertension and hypokalemia plasma aldosterone concentration and plasma renin activity should be measured

8. **What is the indication of doing a MIBG scan?**
   Ans. MIBG is useful in diagnosis of
   1. Extra adrenal pheochromocytoma
   2. Recurrent pheochromocytoma
   3. Metastatic pheochromocytoma
   4. Tumor > 5 cm
   5. Mass lesion with positive serum and urinary normetanephrine and normal serum and urinary metanephrins

9. **What is role of DOTATATE-PET/CT in preoperative assessment of phaeochromocytoma and paragangliomas ?**
   Ans. Ga-68 DOTATATE is a somatostatin receptor imaging (SRI) agents used for diagnosis of phaeochromocytoma and paragangliomas. It is highly sensitive and specific for phaeochromocytoma and paragangliomas and is the first approved FDA agent for the same.

10. **What is the TNM staging adrenocortical carcinoma?**
    Ans.
    T1 < 5 cm in size
    T2 > 5 cm in size
    T3 infiltration of surrounding adipose tissue
    T4 invasion of adjacent organs
    N1 any node positive disease
    M1 and non contiguous spread to site outside adrenal
    Stage 1 : T1 N0 M0
    Stage 2 : T2 N0 M0

Stage 3 : T1-T2 N1 M0
   T3 N0 M0
Stage 4 : T1-4 N0-1M1
   T3 N1 M0
   T4 N0-1 M0

11. **What are the poor prognostic features of ACC?**

    Ans. 1. Advance stage
    2. Tumor > 12 cm
    3. Positive surgical margin
    4. High mitotic rate
    5. Cortisol production
    6. Tumour necrosis
    7. Atypical mitotic figures
    8. High Ki 67 staining

12. **What is the difference in paediatric and adult ACC?**

    Ans. More than 90% ACC's in children are functional. Virilisation is the most common presentation and occurs in 55-70% patients. They may be associated with Li-Fraumeni syndrome.

CHAPTER 23

Miscellaneous

TRAUMA

Case 1

Short History
- A 32-year-old male with history of road traffic accident (RTA)—fell from the motorcycle 10 days back; patient was managed conservatively at local hospital and was discharged.
- Patient followed up after 6 days with history of gross, continuous hematuria, and right flank pain. Pain was continuous, dull, and aching in nature.
- History of fever with chills for one day
- On examination, pulse—122 beats/min
- BP—104/70 mm Hg
- Multiple abrasions over abdomen with fullness in right lumbar region. There was tenderness, guarding, and rigidity in lumbar region and renal angle.
- Air entry was decreased on right lower chest region.
- **CT scan revealed shattered right kidney in mid portion with large hematoma. there is a evidence of contrast extravasation around the kidney (Figs. 1A to C).**

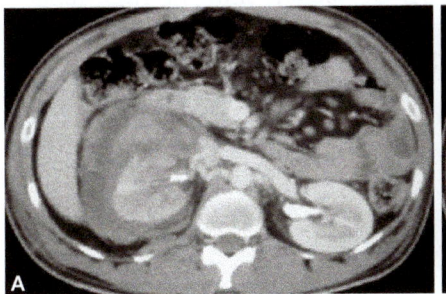
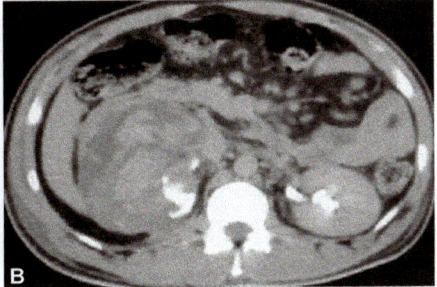

Figures 1A to C: Contd...

Contd...

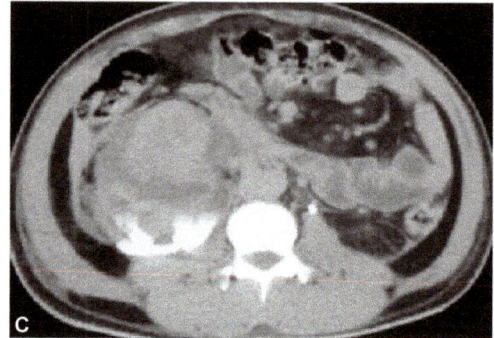

Figures 1A to C: Case1 Renal Trauma.

Case 2

- An 18-year-old male patient was brought by relatives with history of RTA.
- The patient complained of pain in abdomen.
- On examination:
    - Pulse—100 beats/min
    - Respiratory rate—30 breaths/min
    - Blood pressure—100/70 mm Hg
    - Tenderness in right lumbar region and renal angle. There was local guarding.
    - On catheterization, hematuria was noticed.
    - Hb: 10 g%
- Noncontrast axial CT section showing heterogeneous enlarged right kidney with hyperdense contusions, hyperdense fluid collections in right perinephric region suggestive of hematoma and intra-abdominal free fluid (**Figs. 2A and B**).
- Contrast-enhanced arterial phase axial CT section showing right renal lacerations, perinephric hematoma, and hemoperitoneum (**Figs. 2C to H**).
- Contrast-enhanced venous phase axial CT section showing right renal lacerations, devascularization of anterior parenchyma, perinephric hematoma, and hemoperitoneum (**Figs. 2I and J**).

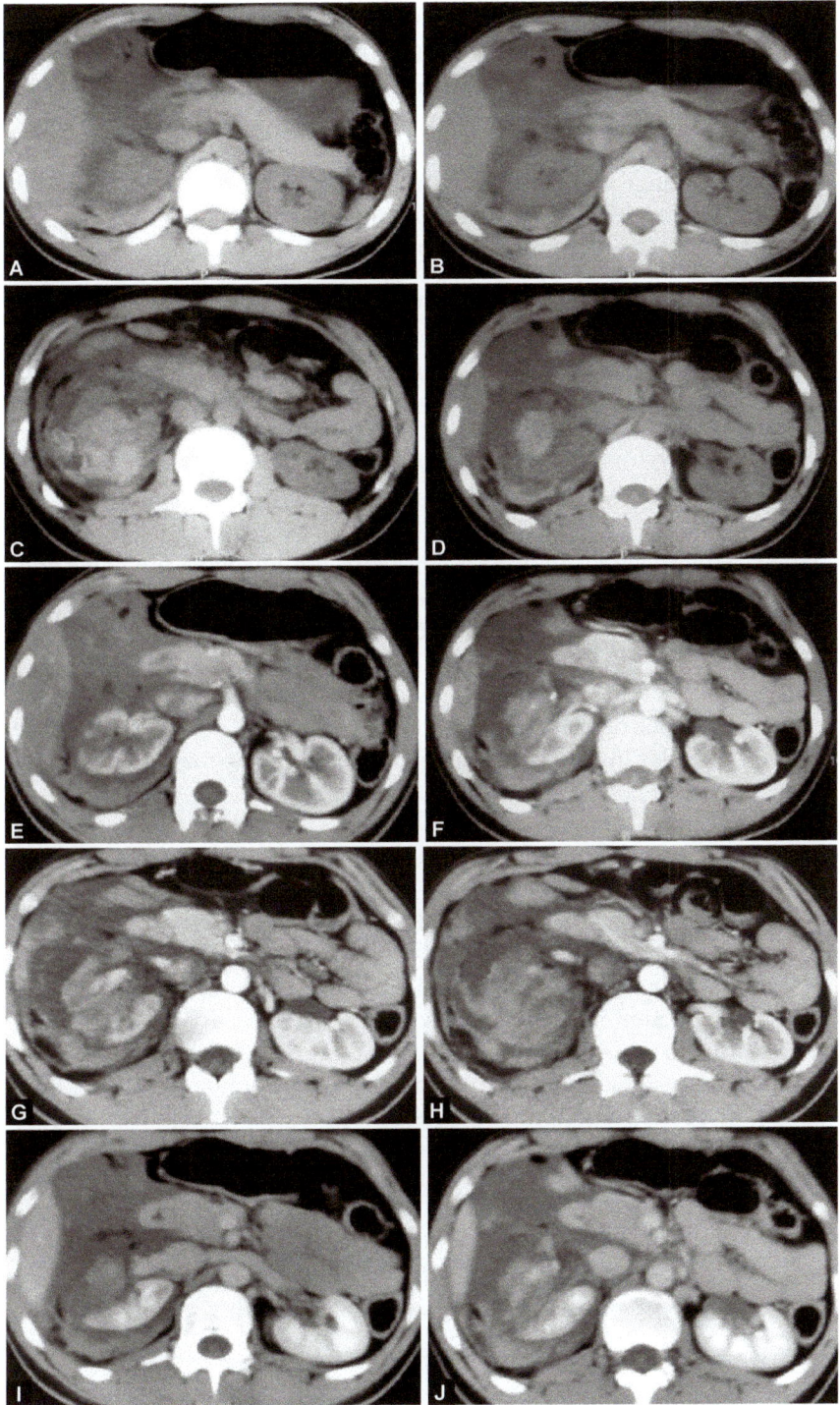

Figures 2A to J: Case 2 Renal Trauma.

1. **What are the determining factors for evaluating a renal injury?**

   Ans. The determining factors to evaluate a renal injury are:
   - Penetrating abdominal trauma with likelihood of renal injury
   - Rapid decelerating injury
   - Polytrauma
   - Blunt trauma with gross hematuria
   - Microscopic hematuria with shock/hypotension
   - All pediatric patients with microscopic hematuria

2. **What is classification of renal trauma?**

   Ans. Severity of renal trauma is assessed according to AAST classification (American Association for the Surgery in Trauma), which includes depth of parenchymal involvement, pelvicalyceal system (PCS), and renal vessels.
   - **Grade I:**
     - Subcapsular hematoma or contusion, without laceration
   - **Grade II:**
     - Superficial laceration ≤1 cm depth not involving the collecting system (no evidence of urine extravasation)
     - Perirenal hematoma confined within the perirenal fascia
   - **Grade III:**
     - Laceration >1 cm not involving the collecting system (no evidence of urine extravasation)
     - Vascular injury or active bleeding confined within the perirenal fascia
   - **Grade IV:**
     - Laceration involving the collecting system with urinary extravasation
     - Laceration of the renal pelvis and/or complete ureteropelvic disruption
     - Vascular injury to segmental renal artery or vein
     - Segmental infarctions without associated active bleeding (i.e., due to vessel thrombosis)
     - Active bleeding* extending beyond the perirenal fascia (i.e., into the retroperitoneum or peritoneum)
   - **Grade V:**
     *Advance one grade for multiple injuries up to grade III
     - Shattered kidney
     - Avulsion of renal hilum or laceration of main renal artery or vein:
       - Devascularization of kidney due to hilar injury
       - Devascularized kidney with active bleeding

3. **Which are the best radiological investigations for renal trauma?**

   Ans. The best radiological investigation for a renal trauma is contrast-enhanced CT scan of abdomen and pelvis with delayed views. In emergency and unstable patients, initially FAST (Focused Assessment with Sonography for Trauma) can be done or a single shot intravenous pyelogram (IVP) can be done.

4. **What would you do if called during a laparotomy for abdominal trauma for a retroperitoneal hematoma with no preoperative CT scan?**

   Ans. If called during an emergency surgery for a retroperitoneal hematoma without a preoperative CT scan, a single shot IVP on table or renal ultrasound with assessment of renal blood flow to verify contralateral renal function can be done. This makes sure that the contralateral kidney is functioning. After that, renal exploration can be proceeded.

   Renal salvage by renorrhaphy or partial nephrectomy requires complete exposure of the injured kidney, debridement of nonviable tissue, suture ligation of bleeding arterial vessels, and repair of the collecting system injury.

   Defects in the renal parenchyma can be closed primarily.

   If a major injury to PCS is present, placement of intraoperative DJ stent or a nephrostomy tube should be considered. Adequate drainage of the perinephric area following repair should also be done.

   If there is an expanding hematoma or shattered kidney, then nephrectomy is indicated.

5. **What is the role of angioembolization in renal trauma?**

   Ans. Angiographic embolization can be used to stop significant renal bleeding. Also, it can be used for persistent or delayed bleeding during nonoperative conservatively managed patients. Vascular traumatic injuries such as arteriovenous fistula and pseudoaneurysms can be managed by angioembolization.

6. **What are the indications for conservative management in renal trauma?**

   Ans. Grade 1, grade 2, isolated grade 3, and stable patients of grade 4 can be managed conservatively.

7. **Describe conservative management.**

   Ans. Conservative management consists of bed rest, close monitoring of vital signs and urine output, serial abdominal examination, serial hemoglobin/hematocrit measurement, antibiotics, and blood transfusion, if indicated. Patient is allowed to ambulate when gross hematuria has resolved. An imaging study like CT scan at 3 months can be repeated if the patient had a grade 3 injury which was treated conservatively.

8. **What are the indications for surgery in renal trauma?**

   Ans. Absolute indications for renal exploration following trauma are:
   - Hemodynamic instability resulting from renal bleeding

- An expanding or pulsatile retroperitoneal hematoma
- Inability to stop persistent or delayed hemorrhage by selective vascular embolization

Relative indications for renal exploration are:
- Finding a retroperitoneal hematoma at the time of surgical exploration for intra-abdominal injuries in a patient with inadequate preoperative radiographic staging.
- CT-documented presence of a grade 3 or higher renal injury coexisting with intra-abdominal injuries that require abdominal exploration.

9. **What are the principles for renal exploration in renal trauma?**
   Ans.
   - Surgical exploration by a transabdominal approach
   - Early vessel control to provide the immediate capability to occlude them if massive bleeding encountered ensue when the Gerota fascia is opened.
   - Complete renal exposure
   - Limited debridement of nonviable tissue
   - Watertight closure of the pelvi calyceal system if possible
   - Reapproximation of the parenchymal defect with fascio-adipose tissue
   - Liberal use of drains

10. **Describe the various surgical techniques for renal reconstructive surgery in renal trauma.**

    Ans. The surgical approach is usually transabdominal approach in supine position. The renal vessels should be isolated before exploration. The small bowel is eviscerated. An incision over the aorta in the retroperitoneum just superior to the inferior mesenteric artery extended superiorly to the ligament of Treitz, allows the exposure of the anterior surface of the aorta. This is followed superiorly to the left renal vein, which crosses the aorta anteriorly. A vessel loop can be placed on the right or left renal vein as necessary. The vein must be retracted cranially, and the left and right renal arteries will be found. The artery is secured with vessel loops. The right renal vein also can be secured through this incision.

    In large hematomas, the inferior mesenteric vein can be used as landmark. The retroperitoneal incision just medial to the inferior mesenteric vein, the anterior surface of the aorta can be identified and followed superiorly to the crossing left renal vein.

    The kidney is then exposed by incising the peritoneum lateral to the colon, followed by mobilization off the Gerota fascia. The Gerota fascia is then opened, and the kidney with injury is completely dissected from the surrounding hematoma.

11. **What are the renovascular injuries possible?**

    Ans. The renovascular injuries possible are arteriovenous fistula, pseudoaneurysms, lacerations of renal artery or vein, segmental infarct, and avulsion of renal hilum.

12. **What are the indications for nephrectomy in renal trauma?**

    Ans. Nephrectomy should be considered only in irreparable grade 4 or grade 5 renal injuries.

13. **Enumerate the postoperative complications of renal trauma.**

    The postoperative complications include:
    - Infection
    - Secondary hemorrhage
    - Trauma-induced renal vascular hypertension
    - Trauma-induced chronic flank pain

RETROCAVAL URETER

Description

These are IVP plates showing hydronephrosis with upper ureteric dilatation. Upper ureter shows acute curve. Lower ureter is not visualized. Kidneys and bladder appear normal (**Figs. 3A and B**).

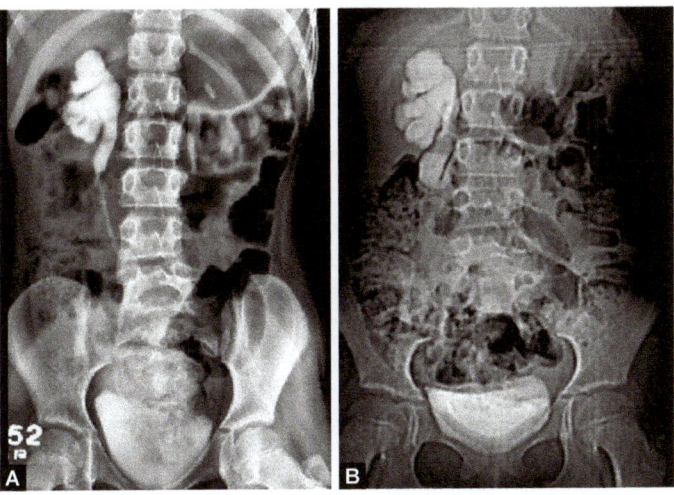

Figures 3A and B: Case 3: IVP showing Retrocaval Ureter.

1. **What is your diagnosis?**

   Ans. First diagnosis is retrocaval ureter. It could still be impacted ureteric stone.

2. **What will you do?**

   Ans. CT intravenous urogram is necessary, which will confirm the diagnosis, stone as well as retrocaval ureter.

3. **What is the treatment for retrocaval ureter?**

   Ans. Depends upon severity of symptoms—in any case, since it is showing significant hydronephrosis, even if patient is asymptomatic, treatment is required. Ureteroureterostomy is required, which can be done laparoscopically/robotic or open. Principle of surgery is to excise the segment of ureter which is behind the inferior vena cava (IVC) and to do wide oblique anastomosis of ureter which is anterior to IVC above and below. Sometimes stricturous segment below the IVC cannot be mobilized, in that case it can be left as it is. Ureter above and below is transected and anastomosis is done.

4. **What is developmental perspective for retrocaval ureter?**

   Ans. It results from anomalous development of the vena cava and not from anomalous development of the ureter. The aberrant embryology is the persistence of the right posterior cardinal vein instead of the right subcardinal vein as the renal segment of the IVC. As the right posterior cardinal vein lies ventral to the ureter, the ureter effectively comes to lie in a "retrocaval" or "circumcaval" position.

5. **What are the radiological signs known as?**

   Ans. The signs are known as fish-hook, shepherd crook, and reverse J sign.

6. **What are the types of retrocaval ureter?**

   Ans. In type I, the ureter crosses behind the IVC at the level of the third lumbar vertebra and it has an "S" or fish-hook type shape at the point of obstruction. Marked hydronephrosis is seen in 50% of patients. In the type II, the crossover occurs higher at the level of the renal pelvis. There is sickle-shaped appearance. Mild hydronephrosis is usually seen in the majority of these.

SECTION 3

Uropathology

CHAPTER 24

Renal Pathology

SPECIMEN 1: NEPHRECTOMY WITH UPPER URETERIC STONES

Description
- Cut Open nephrectomy specimen showing grossly dilated pelvicalyceal system (PCS) with thinned out cortex (**Fig. 1**).
- Yellowish brown stone present in the renal pelvis
- Petechial hemorrhage present in pelvic mucosa
- The diagnosis is impacted pelviureteric junction (PUJ) stone with hydronephrosis with thinned out parenchyma (nonfunctioning kidney).

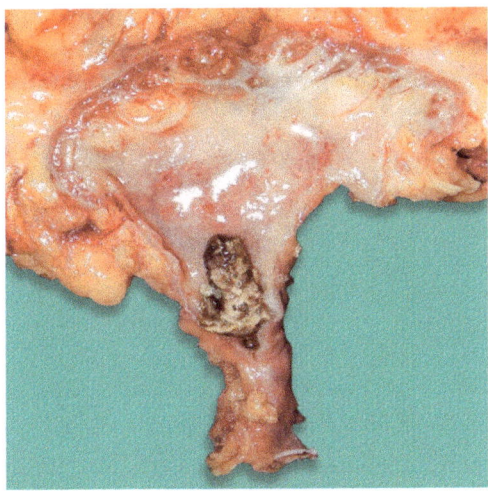

Figure 1: Nephrectomy specimen.

1. **Is it an antemortem or postmortem specimen?**
   Ans. Mostly antemortem as this is the treatment for the condition—nonfunctioning kidney; looks like an adult kidney.

2. **How this patient would have presented with?**
   Ans.
   - Flank pain off and on
   - Recurrent episodes of fever—UTI, leading to pyelonephritis, pyonephrosis
   - Silent—with incidental detection on USG

3. **Is it the correct treatment?**
   Ans. Yes, because if there is a nonfunctioning kidney, nephrectomy is the treatment.

4. **How is the specimen cut open?**
   Ans. Generally, the specimen is cut open from the convex border.

5. **Is there any suspicion of squamous metaplasia/carcinoma in this case? How and where do you check?**
   Ans. It is checked by grossly inspecting the mucosa at the impaction site of the stone. In microscopy, it is checked by taking cuts at the mucosa where the stone was impacted.

SPECIMEN 2: XANTHOGRANULOMATOUS PYELONEPHRITIS

Description

The specimen showing grossly dilated PCS lined by yellowish white slough-like material present at the interface of calyx and parenchyma (**Fig. 2**). Focal areas of necrosis present in the calyx and two large brownish stones present in the dilated pelvis. The diagnosis is xanthogranulomatous pyelonephritis (XGPN).

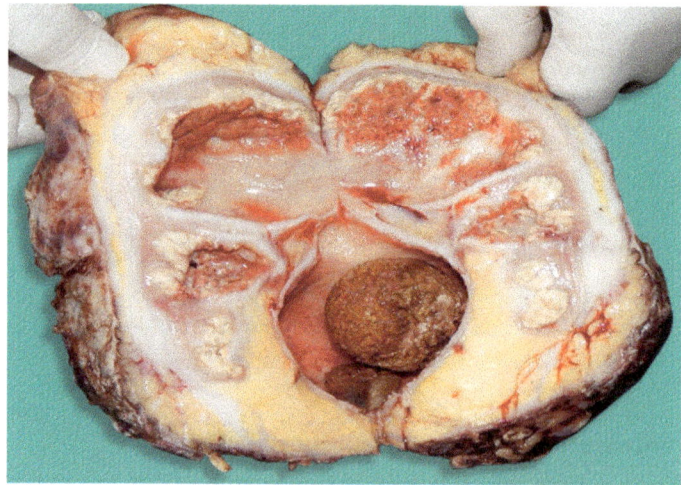

Figure 2: Dilated pelvicalyceal system.

1. **What is XGPN?**

   Ans. It is a form of chronic pyelonephritis of kidney, which is usually because of stone causing infection. Condition causes destruction of parenchyma which gets replaced by granulomatous tissue. Parenchyma shows yellow color deposits (due to lipid laden macrophages), which is a hallmark of the disease. Xantho is a Greek word meaning yellow and because microscopy shows granuloma and hence the name given is xanthogranulomatous pyelonephritis.

2. **Which organisms will cause this condition?**

   Ans. Common organism is *E.coli* in about 60–70% cases, next common is *Proteus*. However, other organisms such as *Enterococcus faecalis*, *Klebsiella*, and *Pseudomonas* can also cause this condition.

3. **What are the etiological factors? Why every chronic pyelonephritis does not end in XGPN?**

   Ans. Obstruction along with infection is the main factor causing XGPN. Other proposed factors are abnormal lipid metabolism, lymphatic blockage, altered immunological competence, renal ischemia, altered host response, incomplete antibiotic response, etc. So multiple factors are proposed.

4. **How this patient would have presented with?**

   Ans. Typically, middle-aged women, recurrent episodes of UTI, long history of flank pain, fever with rigors, kidney lump, unilateral, enlarged, poor or nonfunctioning, and pyonephrotic kidney, and persistent positive urine culture are some of the presenting features.

5. **Can this be diagnosed or suspected on investigations?**

   Ans. Typically on CT intravenous urogram—triad of enlarged kidney, staghorn or large stone, and poor or nonfunctioning kidney is a hallmark of XGPN. CT also can show multiple cavities which can be seen in the specimen ,which are actually abscess cavities. Capsule is thick and perinephric fat can show severe fat stranding. Often it can be mistaken for renal cell carcinoma (RCC).

SPECIMEN 3: AUTOSOMAL DOMINANT POLYCYSTIC KIDNEY DISEASE

Description

The nephrectomy specimen shows marked renomegaly with bosselated surface (**Fig. 3**). On bisection, there is a replacement of renal parenchyma by multiple variable sized thin-walled cysts filled with clear to dirty brown fluid. The diagnosis is adult polycystic kidney disease (ADPKD).

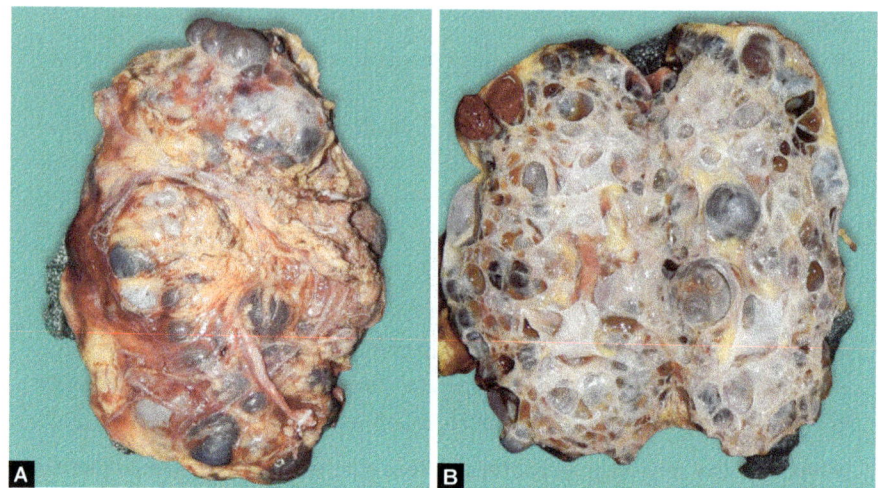

Figures 3A and B: Nephrectomy specimen shows marked renomegaly.

1. **Is this an antemortem or postmortem specimen?**

   Ans. It can be antemortem, even if both kidneys are put together; still it can be antemortem as nephrectomy is the treatment for the condition.

2. **Why you think nephrectomy is done in this case?**

   Ans. This could be to create a space before renal transplant. However, other indications of nephrectomy are hematuria, bleeding in cyst, persistent pain, stones with recurrent UTI, and tumor formation.

3. **How this patient would have presented with?**

   Ans. Chronic dull aching pain, off and on, fever, hematuria, clot colic, hypertension, or as chronic kidney disease (CKD) symptoms such as malaise, fatigue, edema feet, puffiness of face, breathlessness, and asymptomatic lump.

   The patient could be asymptomatic, and nephrectomy is done just to create space for transplantation.

4. **What are the complications of nephrectomy done for ADPKD?**

   Ans.
   - Intraoperative difficulty due to big size of kidney
   - Usually dissection planes are easy, there is large retroperitoneal raw area, which may cause persistent oozing and serous secretion causing persistent high drainage from drain.
   - There could be chemical peritonitis due to cystic fluid contents spilled during the surgery.
   - Prolonged paralytic ileus – due to extensive retroperitoneal dissection
   - If patient is diagnosed with end-stage renal disease (ESRD), then bleeding during dialysis is also a possibility.

5. **If this patient is for transplant, whom and how will you accept as related donor?**

   Ans. Criteria to take related donor in autosomal dominant polycystic kidney disease (ADPKD) are spouse, as it is unlikely that both have ADPKD.
   - Ask history—if disease has come from mother's side or father's side; unaffected parent and his or her relations can be accepted as donor.
   - For sibling—if age >40 years and no cysts on CT IVP, then that donor can be accepted; if <40 years, then genetic testing is to be done (**Flowchart 1**).

6. **What are the implicated genes? How is the transmission?**

   Ans. The implicated genes are *PKD1* on chromosome 16 and *PKD2* gene on chromosome 4. The latest gene implicated is *GANAB* which is located on chromosome 3. An additional new gene is *DNAJB-11*. It is autosomal dominant in 90% cases, and 10% cases are new mutations.

7. **What is pro-PKD score?**

   Ans. The pro-PKD score is a prognostic index which utilizes both genetic and clinical data to prognosticate the survival in diseased individuals.

8. **What are the associated extrarenal manifestations with ADPKD?**

   Ans. Berry aneurysms, diverticulosis, aortic aneurysms, hernias, and cysts in other organs.

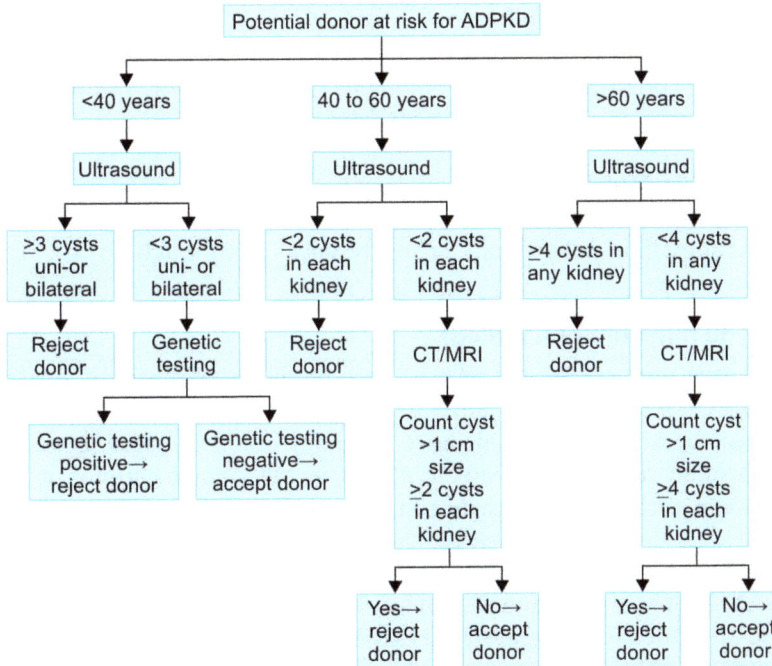

Flowchart 1: Potential donor evaluation in a person with family history of ADPKD.

SPECIMEN 4: ANGIOMYOLIPOMA WITH HEMATOMA

Description

Bisected nephrectomy specimen displaying replacement of upper and mid pole of kidney by uncircumscribed yellowish adipocytic mass with large hematoma extending into perinephric fat (**Fig. 4**). Most likely, the condition is hemorrhage in the angiomyolipoma (AML).

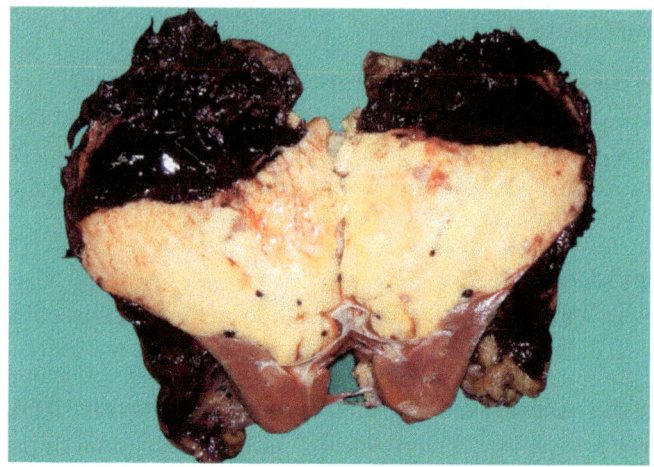

Figure 4: Bisected nephrectomy specimen.

1. **Why do you say it is AML?**

   Ans. It is a large tumor, yellow in color, and homogeneous in nature, suggesting the presence of fat. No areas of necrosis; only in the upper pole, hematoma is seen. Hence, AML with bleeding in tumor.

2. **What is the origin of the AML?**

   Ans. It originates from perivascular epithelioid cells. It is monoclonal in origin rather than polyclonal. Previously, it was also thought to be a form of hamartoma.

3. **Why you think tumor has bled?**

   Ans. Large tumors (usually >4 cm) have tendency of bleeding. AML is composed of three parts, mature adipose tissues, smooth muscles, and vessels. The abnormal vessels have tendency to form microaneurysms, which often ruptures and bleed. AML can bleed in the tumor, it can rupture in perinephric space, or can cause severe hematuria.

4. **How this patient would have presented with?**

   Ans. Acute flank pain due to sudden bleeding, sudden appearance of lump or sudden increase in size of existing lump, sudden breathlessness, fainting, and giddiness.

5. Is it the correct surgery that they have done?

Ans. When a patient presents with severe bleeding, then often nephrectomy is required especially of the tumor of this size. However, if bleeding is stopped, patient is hemodynamically stable, then nephron preserving surgery can be attempted. On CT scan, if normal renal parenchyma is adequate, then exploration with sos hypothermia and all attempts to preserve renal tissue should be done. However, in acute stage, this may not be possible and lifesaving nephrectomy may be required.

SPECIMEN 5: LARGE ANGIOMYOLIPOMA

Description

Bisected nephrectomy specimen with large exophytic unencapsulated yellowish lobulated mass replacing middle and upper pole renal parenchyma (**Fig. 5**). Renal PCS is mildly dilated. Most likely diagnosis is a large AML.

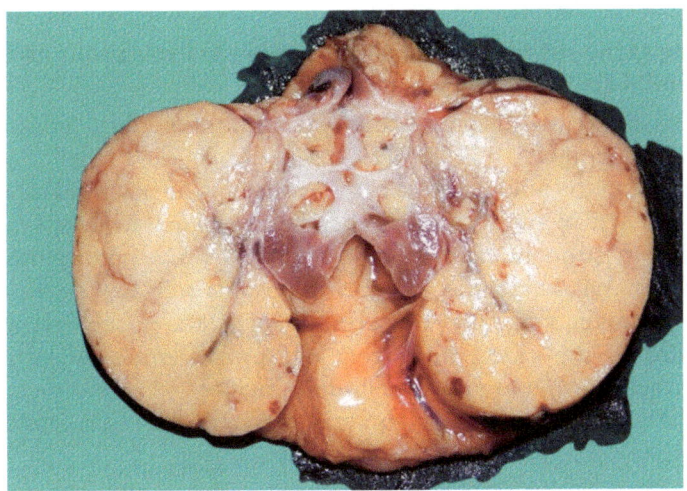

Figure 5: Nephrectomy specimen with large exophytic unencapsulated mass.

1. How this patient would have presented with?

Ans. Chronic dull aching pain, asymptomatic, or as a part of tuberous sclerosis (TSC) complex

2. What is tuberous sclerosis?

Ans. It is an autosomal dominant genetic disorder due to mutation of *TSC1* and *TSC2* genes. Various organs affected are kidneys, brain, eyes, skin, heart, pancreas, lungs, and liver. A TSC patient can have hypopigmented patches on face, epilepsy, facial angiofibromas, retinal hamartoma, and liver AML. Often patient has associated epilepsy, mental retardation, and behavioral problems.

3. **If asymptomatic, would you have done surgery?**

    Ans. Such large AMLs (>4 cm) require treatment. Since it is a benign condition, all attempts to preserve nephrons should be the objective. Angiography and embolization can be done if there is a feeder vessel, then it is an ideal case of angioembolization. However, if embolization is not possible, partial nephrectomy can be done. Since this is a big but exophytic tumor, proper hypothermia can be done, and tumor margins can be identified and excised. If PCS gets injured, that can be repaired. However, sometimes, due to technical difficulty and possibility of very small left out renal mass, nephrectomy can be done.

4. **You said—"because it is >4 cm, you wish to treat", why so?**

    Ans. It is shown that AMLs >4 cm have high chances of bleeding and hence it is better to treat them electively as if bleeding occurs, that time, they land up in lifesaving nephrectomy, while in elective setting, renal preservation surgery can be done.

5. **Looking at the cut-open specimen, how sure are you about AML? Any differential diagnosis?**

    Ans. The differential diagnoses are lipoma of perinephric fat or a low-grade liposarcoma.

    In 50% of the angiographies, AML will show aneurysmal dilatation of vessels. Size of aneurysms is directly proportional to risk of rupture. Also, tumor strongly expresses estrogen and progesterone receptors suggesting that hormones play an important role in growth of the tumor. Estrogen receptors are present in all the cases, however in one-third of the cases, androgen and progesterone receptors are also present. AML's are not so common before puberty but common in middle aged women. In pregnancy there can be rapid growth and rupture.

SPECIMEN 6: RCC (CLEAR CELL)

Description

Bisected radical nephrectomy specimen showing replacement of upper and mid pole parenchyma by partially exophytic grayish pink mass with focal golden yellow areas with cystic changes and areas of hemorrhage and necrosis (**Fig. 6**). Tumor grossly extends into renal sinus and renal vein.

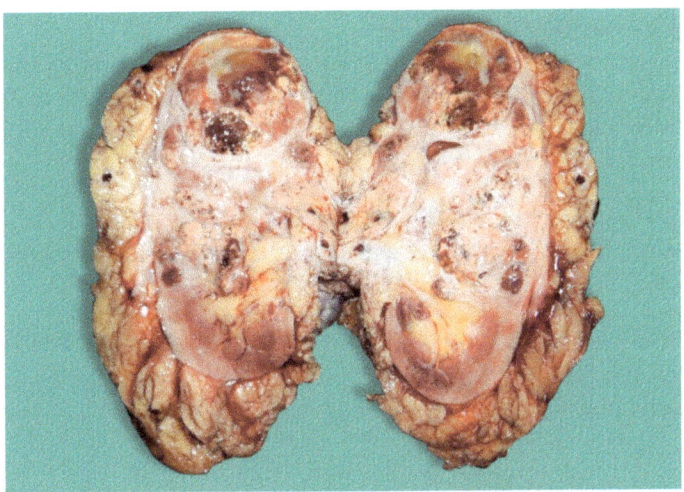

Figure 6: Bisected radical nephrectomy specimen.

1. **Why do you say it RCC and not TCC?**

   Ans. Tumor is more peripherally located with golden yellow areas.
   In TCC, tumor originates either from pelvis or calyx and then grows outside. Here in this specimen, upper calyx and middle calyx appear normal and compressed. Tumor appears to be growing outside as well inside. It has also extended in renal sinus. Hence it appears to be RCC.

2. **How would you differentiate RCC and TCC on IHC?**

   Ans. Immunohistochemistry (IHC) markers positive in RCC are CD10, PAX8, CD9, AMACR, and CK7 (in papillary type 1). IHC markers positive in TCC are p-63 and GATA-3 and Uroplakin.

3. **How this patient would have presented with?**

   Ans. Recurrent episodes of painless hematuria, clots in urine, clot colic, vague flank pain, general symptoms such as loss of weight/appetite, and other symptoms of paraneoplastic syndrome such as fever, cachexia, hepatic dysfunction, hypercalcemia, and anemia.

4. **From where does RCC originate?**

   Ans. Origin of RCC is proximal convoluted tubules.

5. **What are the different types of RCCs you know?**

   Ans. Various types are—clear cell, which is very common, papillary, chromophobe, and other variant morphologies.

6. **How do you grade clear cell RCC?**

   Ans. Previously, the grades were described as Fuhrman grade. However, from the year 2014, ISUP grading is common. It is based on nucleolar size. It is only for clear cell and papillary RCC. Nuclear grade is not applicable for chromophobe RCC.

7. **How much ureter will you remove in RCC?**

   Ans. As much as easily possible, usually upper one-third of the ureter is removed.

8. **Why complete ureter is not removed here as in TCC upper tract?**

   Ans. Because RCC is not a tumor arising from urothelium. Hence it is immaterial how much ureteric length you remove.

SPECIMEN 7: RCC (CHROMOPHOBE)

Description

Bisected radical nephrectomy specimen displaying well-circumscribed partially exophytic mass present at the junction of mid and lower pole of renal parenchyma (**Fig. 7**). Tumor is brownish with areas of hemorrhage and necrosis, and central scarring is visible. Grossly tumor is abutting on sinus fat likely to be RCC.

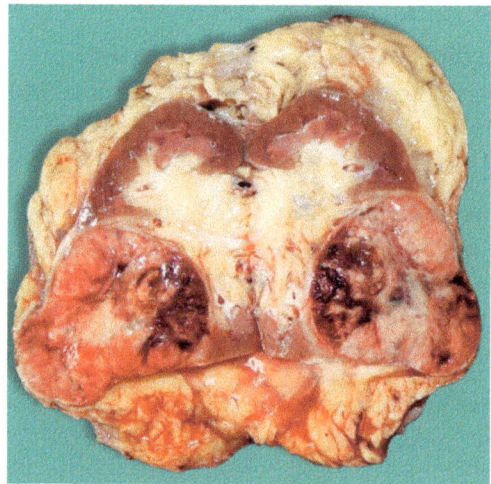

Figure 7: Radical nephrectomy specimen displaying well-circumscribed partially exophytic mass.

1. **Why do you say it is likely to be chromophobe RCC?**

   Ans. The tumor has brownish tan color. So, it can be a chromophobe RCC or oncocytoma.

2. **If you get report as chromophobe RCC after radical nephrectomy, what will you do? How does it differ from clear cell RCC?**

   Ans. Prognosis of chromophobe RCC is far better than any other type of RCCs. 5-year survival of T2 disease after radical nephrectomy is almost 95%. Very small percent have metastasis (about <10%). Hence follow-up will not be that aggressive.

3. **How this can be differentiated from oncocytoma?**

   Ans. Often preoperative, on gross specimen and microscopically it can be mistaken for oncocytoma. Differentiating features are—these tumors are Hale's colloidal iron positive and CK-7 positive.

SPECIMENS 8 AND 9: ONCOCYTOMA

Description

Specimen 8: Bisected radical nephrectomy specimen displaying well-circumscribed partially exophytic yellowish brown mass with central myxoid scar present at the junction of upper and mid pole renal parenchyma (**Fig. 8**).

Specimen 9: Bisected radical nephrectomy specimen displaying brown tan tumor in the upper pole with central scar and focal area of hemorrhage (**Fig. 9**). Diagnosis is likely to be Oncocytoma.

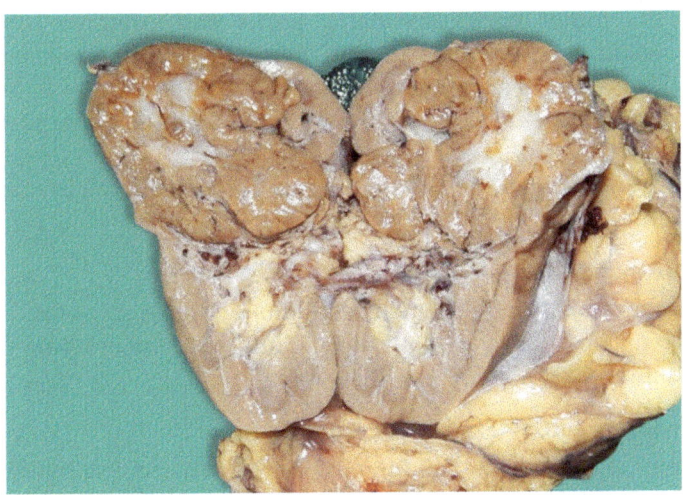

Figure 8: Specimen well-circumscribed partially exophytic yellowish brown mass.

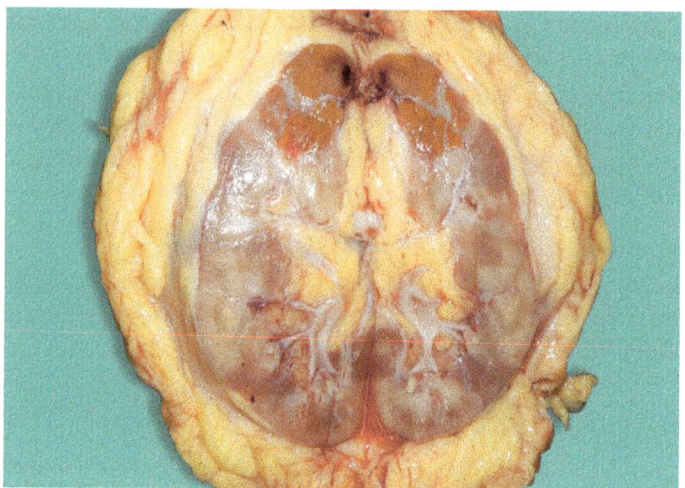

Figure 9: Specimen displaying brown tan tumor.

1. **What are the characteristics of oncocytoma on gross specimen?**

   Ans. It is a well circumscribed brownish tumor with central stellate scar predominantly in larger tumors.

2. **What are the characteristics of central scars? Why are they formed?**

   Ans. The central scar represents the myxoid degeneration of the tumor.

   As the tumor grows outside, it grows and outgrows its blood supply, leading to necrosis, which then leads to myxoid degeneration, eventually leading to a scar.

   It is present in about 50–60% of cases generally when large tumors are seen.

   The scars can be appreciated on the CT scan as well as the gross specimen.

3. **Can it be malignant?**

   Ans. Oncocytoma is a benign condition. However, some of the oncocytomas can have element of RCC and pure oncocytoma can be locally infiltrative.

4. **What is treatment of large oncocytoma?**

   Ans. Since it is a benign condition, nephron preserving surgery is the ideal treatment. However, often preoperatively, it is difficult to diagnose the condition. In large oncocytoma, even if biopsy is done, it cannot rule out the element of RCC, especially chomophobe RCC at some other place. Often it is postoperatively diagnosed after radical nephrectomy is done.

5. **How do you differentiate chromophobe RCC and oncocytoma on histology?**
   Ans. Hale's colloidal iron staining is negative in oncocytoma, while it is positive in chromophobe RCC. The other differentiating features in IHC are CK-117 (c-kit) (positive) and CK-7 (negative).

SPECIMEN 10: RCC (PAPPILARY)

Description

Bisected radical nephrectomy specimen shows replacement of mid pole parenchyma by partially exophytic, multifocal yellow mass with areas of hemorrhage, and necrosis with variegated cut surface (**Fig. 10**). Tumor grossly extends into upper pole calyx and renal sinus. The diagnosis is likely to be RCC.

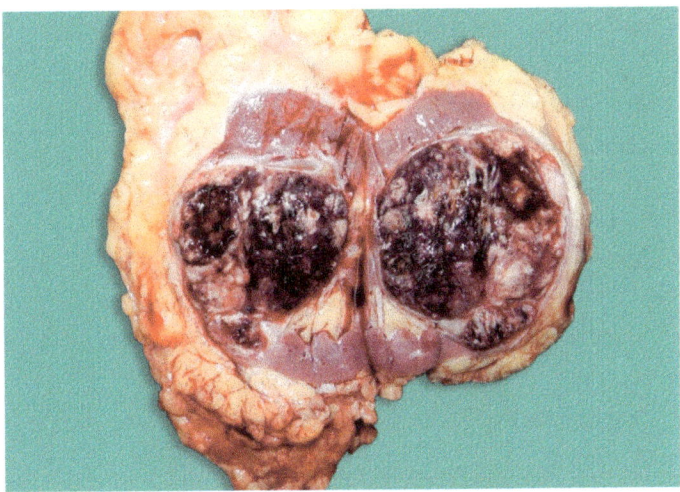

Figure 10: Specimen shows replacement of mid pole parenchyma.

1. **What are the features of papillary RCC on gross specimen?**
   Ans. Grossly, the tumor appears pink to yellow in color, with areas of hemorrhage and necrosis.

2. **What are the stages of RCC?**
   Ans.

Stages	Description
TNM staging:	
T	T1
T1a	Tumor confined to kidney, <4 cm
T1b	Tumor confined to kidney, >4 cm but <7 cm
T2	Limited to kidney >7 cm
T2a	Tumor confined to kidney, >7 cm but not >10 cm
T2b	Tumor confined to kidney, >10 cm
T3	Tumor extension into major veins or perinephric tissues, but not into ipsilateral adrenal gland or beyond Gerota's fascia
T3a	Tumor grossly extends into the renal vein or its segmental (muscle-containing) branches, or tumor invades perirenal and/or renal sinus fat but not beyond the Gerota's fascia
T3b	Spread to infra diaphragmatic IVC
T3c	Spread to supra diaphragmatic IVC or invades the wall of the IVC
T4	Involves ipsilateral adrenal gland or invades beyond Gerota's fascia
N	
N0	No nodal involvement
N1	Metastatic involvement of regional lymph node(s)
M	
M0	No distant metastases
M1	Distant metastases
Stage grouping:	
Stage I	T1 N0 M0
Stage II	T2 N0 M0
Stage III	T3 or N1 with M0
Stage IV	T4 or M1

The distinction between N1 and N2 is discontinued.

Contiguous involvement of the ipsilateral adrenal gland is considered T4 while noncontiguous involvement is considered M1.

3. **How is papillary RCC from outcome point of view in comparison to clear cell RCC?**
   Ans. Papillary RCC had better outcome in patients without metastasis, however, this is not true if metastasis are present. In subclassification,

type 1 papillary RCC had similar prognosis as clear cell RCC and type 2 papillary RCC has poor prognosis.

4. **What is type 1 and type 2 papillary RCC?**

   Ans. Type 1 papillae are covered with a single layer of cuboidal cells with foamy macrophages often present in coarse papillae.

   It has basophilic cytoplasm and is classified as a low-grade tumor.

   Type 2 papillae show pseudostratification and are covered with large cells with abundant eosinophilic cytoplasm and nuclei with prominent nucleoli (grade 3 or more).

5. **What do you mean by multicentric origin of RCC?**

   Ans. Papillary RCC—there can be multiple foci of RCC either in the same kidney or in the opposite kidney.

6. **What are the syndromes associated with papillary RCC?**

   Ans. Birt-Hogg-Dubé syndrome, familial leiomyomatosis syndrome, familial papillary carcinoma, etc. These are more common with type 2 papillary RCC.

Table showing Gross morphological features of different types of RCC

Clear cell RCC	Grossly, clear cell RCCs characteristically contain solid yellow areas with variable amounts of cystic change, haemorrhage and necrosis.
Papillary RCC	Papillary RCCs are grossly solid, with or without cystic change or encapsulation, and are often reddish-brown in colour with a soft friable cut surface showing frequent necrosis and haemorrhage. They frequently have a well demarcated pseudocapsule.
Chromophobe RCC	Grossly chromophobe RCC are well circumscribed - brown tan mass with central myxoid scar and usually confined to kidney.
Tubulocystic RCC	Tubulocystic RCC has characteristic 'bubble wrap' appearance grossly, due to the presence of fibrotic stroma separating cystic spaces
Oncocytoma	Mahogany colour, well circumscribed, occasional central scar and rarely with necrosis
Collecting duct RCC	Partially cystic, white grey appearance and often exhibit invasion into the renal sinus
Medullary RCC	Tan/white poorly defined capsule, extensive haemorrhage and necrosis
MiT family RCC	Yellowish tissue often studded by haemorrhage and necrosis

Table showing IHC markers for different types of renal masses.

	Clear RCC	Papillary RCC	Chromophobe RCC	Collecting duct ca	Xp11.2 RCC	MTSCCC	Oncocytoma
CK7	0–37%	80–87%	83%	NA	17%	79–100%	0–10%
HMWCK	0–13%	33%	-	29–67%	NA	15–33%	10%
Vimentin	87%	100%	-	100%	65–70%	55–100%	-
CD10	94–100%	67–93%	0–72%	25%	100%	9–50%	12–58%
AMACR	4–68%	80–100%	0–29%	0–18%	100%	92–100%	2–25%
E-cadherin	0–14%	13–31%	100%	75%	66%	93%	47–100%
KIT	0–5%	0–13%	82–100%	0–53%	NA	NA	58–100%
RCC Ma	72–85%	87–95%	0–91%	-	100%	7–92%	-
PAX2	92%	87%	0–83%	0–100%	0–100%	75–100%	88–100%
PAX8	98%	87%	83%	100%	100%	100%	87–95%
CAIX	100%	57%	-	40–100%	40%	-	-
CD82 (KAII)	2–23%	-	78–87%	NA	NA	NA	0–7%

SPECIMEN 11: RADICAL NEPHROURETERECTOMY

Description

Bisected nephroureterectomy specimen showing, entire ureter with bladder cuff. It shows whitish infiltrative growth arising from renal pelvis and lower calyx and infiltrating into peripelvic tissue and renal parenchyma. Most likely diagnosis is urothelial carcinoma arising from renal pelvis and lower calyx (**Fig. 11**).

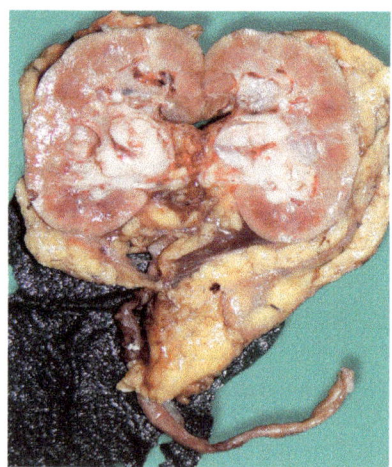

Figure 11: Specimen showing whitish infiltrative growth arising from renal pelvis and lower pole calyx.

CHAPTER 24: Renal Pathology | 299

1. **Is it antemortem specimen?**

   Ans. Yes, because nephroureterectomy is the treatment for this condition.

2. **What is the characteristic of cut open specimen of TCC upper tract? What things you will check after removal of kidney on table?**

   Ans. Urothelial carcinoma arises from pelvicalyceal mucosa. On cutting open the specimen, we see the location of tumor, gross configuration of the tumor, and color of the tumor. Also, check whether the tumor grossly extends into the peripelvic tissue or adjoining renal parenchyma.

3. **Suppose you do nephrectomy thinking as RCC and 4 days later, histopathology comes as TCC, what will you do?**

   Ans. In that case, patient needs ureterectomy with bladder cuff at earliest. It is to be done as per the convenience of the patient. Earliest it can be done as soon as report comes, or it can be done later but should not be delayed too much. No definitive duration as such.

4. **How much bladder cuff you will remove? Why?**

   Ans. No definitive guidelines as such but around 1 cm bladder cuff is sufficient. Oncological objective is to remove whole unilateral urothelial system in continuity. Ureteric muscle and epithelium continue for about 1 cm around the orifice and hence bladder cuff is removed.

5. **What are the chances of bladder tumor recurrence after nephroureterectomy?**

   Ans. There is a wide variation in percentage of patients who will get tumor recurrence in bladder. Some have reported 25% and some 60%. In general, accepted tumor recurrence rate is about 25–35%. This recurrence is due to two factors—field change and other is due to spillage of cancer cells in bladder during surgery. It is shown that single instillation of mitomycin-C significantly reduces bladder tumor recurrences. Two methods are suggested—instilling mitomycin and clamping the catheter for about 1–2 hours, by then ureter is either clipped or ligated. Mitomycin C should be completely removed before opening bladder for cuff excision. Other method suggested is to instill mitomycin C at the time of catheter removal. This is also found to be equally effective. The exact mechanism by how it prevents is not known.

6. **In a tumor like this, will you remove the lymph nodes?**

   Ans. Lymph node dissection is necessary. The template of the dissection is described by Kondo et al. which is for kidney and upper ureter (**Fig. 12**).

7. **Will you do check cystoscopy in follow-up?**

   Ans. Since the incidence of bladder tumor is high, all such patients require regular check cystoscopy at every 6 months for the first 2 years and annual check cystoscopy up to 5 years after that.

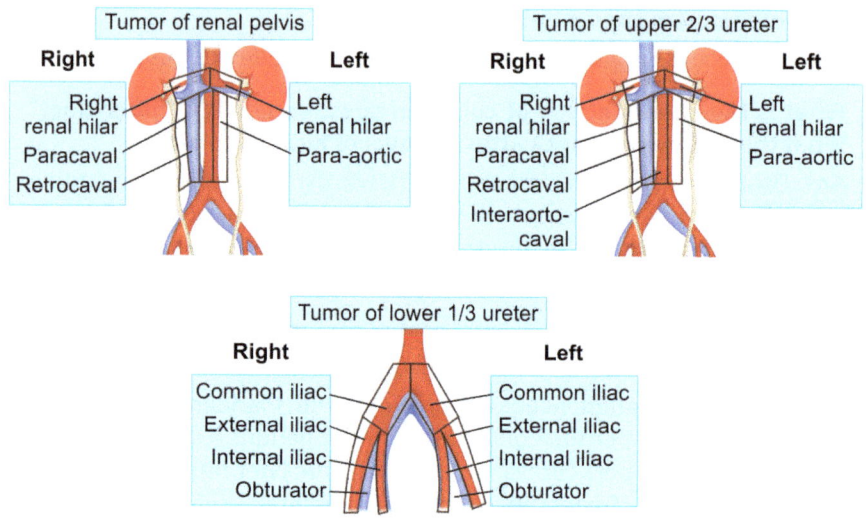

Figure 12: Template of dissection.

8. **How this patient would have presented?**

   Ans. The likely presentation could be recurrent episodes of hematuria, flank pain, and weight loss.

SPECIMEN 12: WILMS' TUMOR

Description

Bisected radical nephrectomy specimen showing uncircumscribed soft pinkish-white lobulated mass involving and replacing upper and mid pole renal parenchyma (**Fig. 13**). Mass shows areas of hemorrhage and necrosis

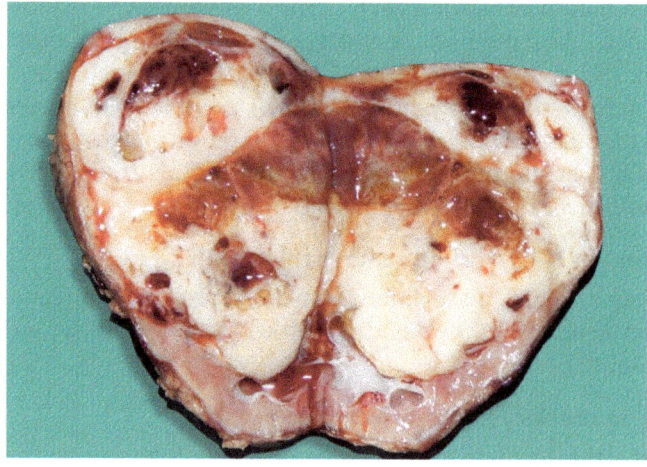

Figure 13: Specimen showing areas of hemorrhage and necrosis with cystic changes.

with cystic changes. Tumor grossly appears to be limited to the kidney. Likely diagnosis is wilms tumor.

1. **How this patient would have presented with?**

   Ans. Patient may notice lump in abdomen, pain, hematuria, nausea, vomiting, fever, breathlessness, headache (due to hypertension), general cachexia, weakness, loss of weight, and not thriving well.

2. **What are the types of Wilms' tumor?**

   Ans. There are two variants. One is conventional Wilms' tumor and other is cystic nephroblastoma.

3. **What is favorable histology and unfavorable histology?**

   Ans. In favorable histology, there is no or minimal focal anaplasia whereas in unfavorable histology, there is diffuse anaplasia. However, focal anaplasia may also lead to chemotherapy resistance.

4. **What is triphasic nature of tumor?**

   Ans. If all three elements, viz., blastemal, epithelial, and mesenchymal components are present in variable degree. Then it is a triphasic tumor Tumor could be predominantly monophasic, biphasic or it could be purely monophasic. It was thought that triphasic component makes favorable histology and monophasic denotes the unfavorable histology. However, the favorable or unfavorable is decided by nuclear anaplasia. Majority of the times, the triphasic components have less nuclear anaplasia and hence make a favorable histology.

5. **What is origin of Wilms' tumor?**

   Ans. Nephrogenic blastemal cells

6. **What are the syndromic associations associated with Wilms' tumor?**

   Ans. WAGR syndrome, Denys–Drash syndrome, and Beckwith Wiedemann syndrome

7. **Why the name Wilms' is given to this tumor?**

   Ans. This tumor was first described by Thomas Rance in 1814. However, in 1899, Carl Max Wilms, General Surgeon and Pathologist, gave a detailed description. Since then, it is called as Wilms' tumor.

8. **Why this occurs in children?**

   Ans. It occurs due to a mutation of *WT1* gene.

9. **Can it occur in adults?**

   Ans. Yes, it can occur in adults.

10. What are the differential diagnoses in renal tumors in pediatric population?

Ans. Neuroblastoma, clear cell sarcomas, and congenital mesoblastic nephroma.

11. What is the difference between Wilms' tumor of adult and children from clinical point of view?

Ans. In adults, the tumor tends to be more aggressive.

12. What are the stages of this tumor?

Ans. Tumors are staged according to two systems—NWTS, which is largely followed, and SIOP system.

The NWTS staging system:

Stages	Description
Stage 1	• Tumor is limited to the kidney and completely excised • The tumor is not ruptured before or during removal • No residual tumor apparent beyond the margins of excision
Stage 2	• Tumor extends beyond the kidney but is completely excised • No residual tumor is apparent at or beyond the margins of excision • Tumor thrombus in vessels outside the kidney is stage II if the thrombus is removed en bloc with the tumor
Stage 3	Residual nonhematogenous tumor is present and confined to abdomen: • Lymph nodes in the renal hilum, the periaortic chains, or beyond are found to contain a tumor • Diffuse peritoneal contamination by the tumor • Implants are found on the peritoneal surfaces • Tumor extends beyond the surgical margins either microscopically or grossly • Tumor is not completely resectable because of local infiltration into vital structures
Stage 4	Hematogenous metastasis or lymph node metastasis
Stage 5	Bilateral renal involvement

This system relies on surgical and pathological evaluation of a tumor in patients not submitted to the preoperative chemotherapy.

The SIOP staging system:

Stages	Description
Stage 1	• Tumor is limited to kidney and is completely resected (resection margins "clear") • The tumor may be protruding into the pelvic system and "dipping" into the ureter (but it is not infiltrating their walls) • The vessels of the renal sinus are not involved • Intrarenal vessel involvement may be present
Stage 2	• The tumor extends beyond kidney or penetrates through the renal capsule and/or fibrous pseudocapsule into perirenal fat but is completely resected (resection margins "clear") • The tumor infiltrates the renal sinus and/or invades blood and lymphatic vessels outside the renal parenchyma but is completely resected • The tumor infiltrates adjacent organs or vena cava but is completely resected
Stage 3	• Incomplete excision of the tumor, which extends beyond the resection margins • Any abdominal lymph nodes are involved • Tumor rupture before or intraoperatively • The tumor has penetrated through the peritoneal surface • Tumor thrombi present at resection margins of vessels or ureter, transected or removed piecemeal by surgeon • The tumor has been surgically biopsied (wedge biopsy) prior to preoperative chemotherapy or surgery
Stage 4	Hematogenous metastases (lung, liver, bone, brain, etc.) or lymph node metastases outside the abdominopelvic region
Stage 5	Bilateral renal tumors at diagnosis

This system is based on findings at post chemotherapy tumor nephrectomy and the microscopic examination of the whole sample.

13. What surgery will you do? Will you approach this tumor laparoscopically?

Ans. Generally, radical nephrectomy is required. However, in case of solitary kidney with tumor or bilateral Wilms, kidney preserving surgery can be considered. Important aspect during surgery is that tumor handling and dissection should be minimal so as not to tear the capsule, tumor, and to prevent the spillage as it will upstage the disease.

In a solitary kidney tumor or a bilateral tumor, the chemotherapy can be given after confirming it with a biopsy.

CHAPTER 25

Bladder and Ureter Pathology

SPECIMEN 13: CYSTECTOMY

Description

Opened up cystoprostatectomy specimen displaying multifocal polypoidal pinkish-white growth completely covering the bladder mucosa (**Fig. 1**). Prostate shows enlarged median lobe. Prostatic urethra appears uninvolved. The likely diagnosis is muscle invasive bladder tumor.

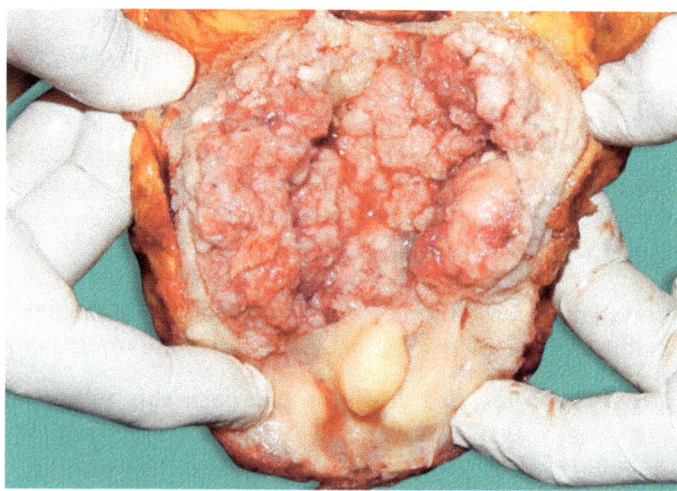

Figure 1: Cystoprostatectomy specimen.

1. **Can it be an antemortem specimen?**
   Ans. This can be antemortem as this is the classical treatment for bladder tumor which ascribes to the structures removed during radical cystectomy.

2. **What must be the stage of this cancer? In short, in which stage will you do radical cystectomy?**

   Ans. Stage of this tumor is likely to be T2. However, even in T3 or T4 disease, cystectomy is required, which could be radical or palliative cystectomy.

3. **What are the types of bladder carcinoma?**

   Ans. Most common is papillary followed by squamous cell carcinoma (SCC) and other variants of urothelial malignancy such as micropapillary, adenocarcinoma, and neuroendocrine tumors.

4. **How this patient could have presented with?**

   Ans. Recurrent episodes of hematuria, passage of clots or fleshy masses, frequency, dysuria, clot retention, flank pain, features of obstructed kidneys, etc.

5. **What structures are removed during cystectomy?**

   Ans. Refer to Operative Urology section.

6. **Why is prostate removed in all cases? Can you do prostate sparing radical cystectomy?**

   Ans. Prostate removal is a part and parcel of cystectomy and hence it is also called as cystoprostatectomy. Prostate cannot be spared as otherwise you have to take incision at bladder neck, also bladder and trigone urothelium is in continuation in prostatic urethra, and hence from oncological point of view, prostate also must be removed.

   The combined incidence of prostatic urethral involvement, prostatic ducts involvement by the malignancy, direct extension of the malignancy, and simultaneous adenocarcinoma prostate is around 30–35% in such cases.

7. **What is the difference between squamous cell carcinoma of bladder and squamous differentiation of TCC?**

   Ans. The primary squamous cell carcinoma (SCC) is associated with chronic irritation such as stone, schistosomiasis, and radiation. The primary SCC has a poorer prognosis, response to chemotherapy is less in primary SCC.

8. **How do you stage urachal carcinoma?**

   Ans. Sheldon staging system:

   T1—no invasion beyond the urachal mucosa (in situ)
   T2—invasion limited to the urachus

T3—local extension to the (1) bladder, (2) abdominal wall, and (3) viscera other than the bladder

T4—metastasis to (1) regional lymph nodes and (2) distant sites

9. **What are the indications of urethrectomy?**

    Ans. The indications are positive urethral margin and concomitant urethral tumor.

10. **How are the dissected lymph nodes processed to examine the lymph node status?**

    Ans. All the material which has been received in the pathology is supposed to be processed to get the maximum lymph node yield. After the lymph nodes resected are sent in formalin, they are kept in formalin for 24 hours for proper fixation. After that, they are processed in alcohol/acetone. This causes dissolution of all the fat. After that, it is processed in xylene and then impregnated with wax. The counting is done under microscope after staining the tissue section.

11. **What do you consider as an adequate lymph node dissection?**

    Ans. In the standard lymph node dissection, the adequate lymph node sampling is considered when the lymph nodes are at least 16 in number, equally distributed on both sides.

12. **What are the absolute contraindications of neobladder?**

    Ans. Absolute contraindication is positive surgical margin, clinically T4 disease, permanently compromised renal function, and severe hepatic dysfunction.

SPECIMEN 14: NEPHROURETERECTOMY WITH CYSTECTOMY

Description

Opened up specimen of nephroureterectomy with cystoprostatectomy (**Fig. 2**). Renal cortex is thinned out with grossly dilated pelvicalyceal system (PCS) and ureter. Bladder shows large polypoidal growth involving right lateral wall with right vesicoureteric junction (VUJ) and lower ureter involvement. The likely diagnosis invasive TCC at the VUJ.

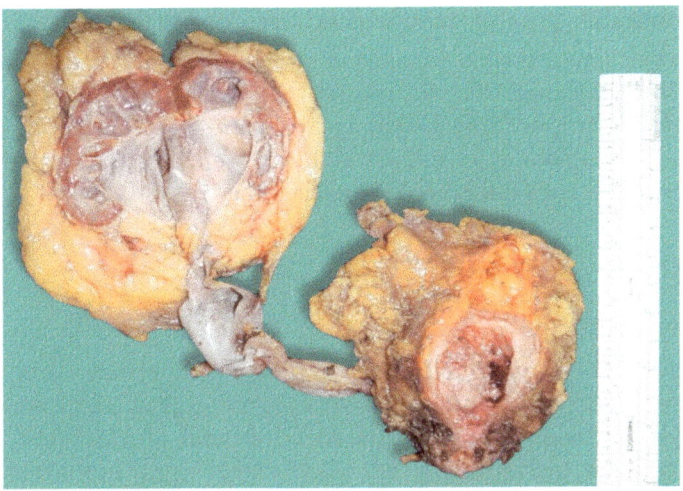

Figure 2: Specimen of nephroureterectomy with cystoprostatectomy.

1. **Is it an antemortem or postmortem specimen?**

   Ans. It is likely to be an antemortem specimen as this is the surgery done for the condition.

2. **Why you think kidney and bladder are removed in toto?**

   Ans. Bladder tumor is situated on right later wall, involving ureterovesical junction (UVJ) and tumor also appears to be extending in the ureter. Hence, he needs full nephroureterectomy with cystectomy. Generally, because urothelium should not be disrupted and come in touch with surrounding structures and to avoid spillage, it is removed as one single specimen. However, if proper precautions are taken, ureter, where there is no tumor, can be ligated on each side and cut.

3. **If suppose UVJ and ureter was not involved, would you have done the same surgery?**

   Ans. Cut open specimen of kidney appears to have variable thickness of parenchyma and dilated PCS and ureter. HN, HU in such situation is often due to involvement of muscle near ureteric orifice which causes obstruction. Nephrectomy in such situation is decided by functioning of the kidney. Not every hydroureteronephrosis due to extensive bladder carcinoma requires nephrectomy.

4. **What diversion you think could have been done in this case?**

   Ans. Since prostate is seen, this is a male patient. Bladder tumor is on right lateral wall. Although he will have solitary kidney, choice of diversion depends on various factors such as GFR, age, and his acceptability to conduit or neobladder. In solitary kidney, if other ureter is also dilated, then end cutaneous ureterostomy is also a valid option.

SPECIMEN 15: DISTAL URETERIC TUMOR

Description

Bisected radical nephroureterectomy specimen with bladder cuff shows mildly dilated PCS system and upper and mid ureter (**Fig. 3**). Lower ureter shows single pinkish-white broad-based polypoidal growth. Rest of the ureteric mucosa is hemorrhagic. The likely diagnosis is urothelial cancer arising from the lower ureter.

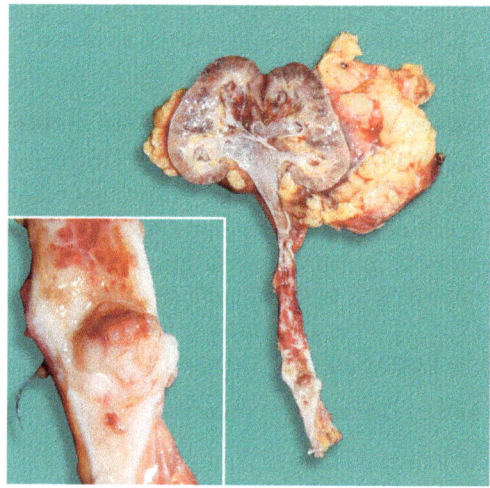

Figure 3: Bisected radical nephroureterectomy specimen.

1. **How this patient would have presented with?**

   Ans. Pain, dull aching or repeated episodes of colic, off and on hematuria, passage of serpentine clots, and recurrent episodes of urinary tract infection.

2. **Is it the correct treatment?**

   Ans. The tumor appears to be in the upper ureter about 10 cm from pelvi-ureteric junction (PUJ) and the treatment for the tumor at this location is nephroureterectomy with bladder cuff excision.

3. **If you suspect a tumor in the ureter on CT IVP, what will you do next?**

   Ans. Ureteroscopy to see the appearance of the tumor and if possible, to take the biopsy.

4. **How will you take biopsy?**

   Ans. The biopsy can be taken with the help of basket; if it is a papillary tumor, it can be obtained with the help of forceps. Small tumor can be cut with the help of a laser. If it is not possible, then take a barbotage cytology.

5. **In distal ureteric tumor, why nephroureterectomy is done?**

   Ans. A distal ureteric mass which is high grade, invasive, locally advanced or if lymphnodes are involved then nephroureterectomy is required. Also, in a high grade tumor which is a field change disease there are high chances of ispsilateral upper ureteric and pelvic involvement, hence it is advisable to do nephroureterectomy.

6. **What are treatment options of distal ureteric tumor?**

   Ans. Distal ureteric tumors can be managed by excision (distal ureterectomy including the intramural ureter) and reimplantation, or endoscopic means. If the tumor is low garde and localized on imaging studies. Sometimes in a solitary kidney this option can be offered in a high grade disease.

CHAPTER 26

Penile Mass

SPECIMEN 16: RADICAL PENECTOMY

Description

An opened up radical penectomy specimen displaying whitish infiltrative growth present at the base of penis and extending into penile shaft and perineal skin and soft tissue with extensive tumor necrosis (**Figs. 1A and B**).

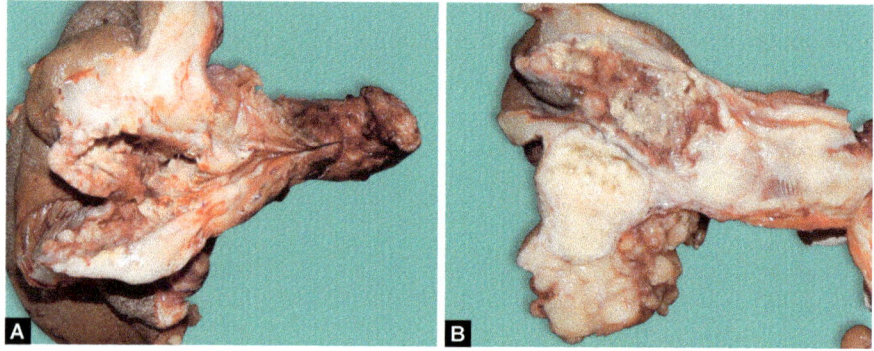

Figures 1A and B: Radical penectomy specimen displaying whitish infiltrative growth.

1. **What is the origin of the tumor? Is it urethral tumor or penile tumor? From where is it arising?**

   Ans. It is a penile tumor. It is arising from the urethral cutaneous lesion of the perineal urethrostomy which has extended to the base and mid penile shaft.

2. **What are the structures removed in radical penectomy?**

   Ans. Entire stretch of penile length from glans to the pubic bone, corporeal bodies are removed in totality, they are shaved off from pubic bones till a point at corporal arteries seen arising from common penile artery. Urethral margin of about 1 cm away from the tumor margin is secured from the bulbar urethra.

3. **Can it be urethral tumor? If so, what is the treatment?**
   Ans. It can be urethral tumor. Urethral tumors arising from distal urethral are squamous in nature but are very rare. Urethral tumors arising from proximal urethra are urothelial in nature. In that case, full urethrectomy is required up to bulbomembranous (BM) junction. Origin of urothelium beyond BM junction and proximal to it is different. If tumor has gone into the surrounding structures, then radical penectomy with complete urethrectomy is the treatment of choice.

4. **In radical penectomy, will you remove both testes?**
   Ans. It is not necessary to remove testes. Penile cancer and urethral cancer do not spread to testes. However, if perineal urethrostomy is done, then he has to lift scrotum to pass urine. Removal of testes will have all side effects of androgen deprivation.

5. **How to evaluate the lymph node status in a case of Ca penis?**
   Ans. On palpation, any groin node >1.5 cm should be considered significant.
   Whenever the groin nodes are clinically significant, a CT groin and pelvis is warranted.
   The groin needs to be evaluated by CT or MRI, especially in patients having obesity, undergone previous groin surgery or chronic lymphedema due to any other cause.

6. **What is the utility of FNAC of groin lymph node?**
   Ans. All clinically significant groin lymph nodes can be subjected to fine needle aspiration cytology (FNAC). Positive FNAC is helpful as the clinician can plan a complete groin node dissection (superficial + deep). But a negative FNAC means nothing and will have to rely on frozen section of superficial nodes or further operative decision. USG-guided FNAC increases the yield of FNAC with sensitivity of 39% as shown by Kroon et al.

7. **What is dynamic scintigraphy?**
   Ans. Tc-99m labeled sulfur colloid is injected on the previous day before the procedure. Also, 1 mL of methylene blue is injected intradermally 5 minutes before the skin incision peritumorally. The activity is confirmed using handheld gamma camera probe and blue dye. The nodes showing high activity and/or blue color are removed and separately sent for frozen section.

SPECIMEN 17: PARTIAL PENECTOMY

Description

Partial penectomy specimen displaying whitish growth involving prepuceal skin and infiltrating into glans with tumor necrosis and destruction of glans penis (**Figs. 2A and B**).

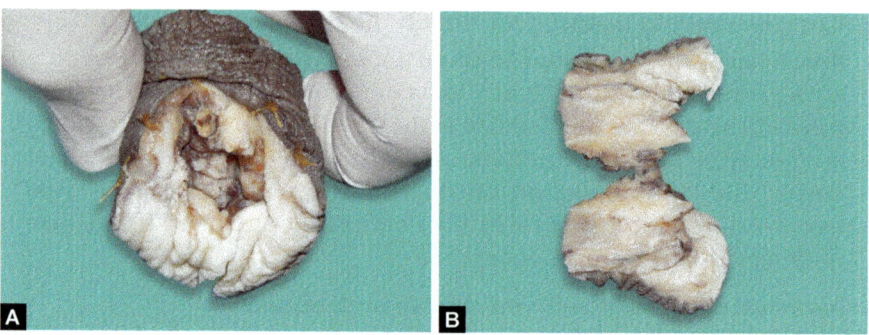

Figures 2A and B: Partial penectomy specimen displaying whitish growth.

1. **From where the Ca penis originates?**

   Ans. Most common site is coronal sulcus and prepuce, followed by glans, followed by shaft of penis.

2. **What are different types of Ca penis?**

   Ans. Squamous cell carcinoma [not otherwise specified (NOS)], adenosquamous carcinoma, basaloid carcinoma, verrucous carcinoma, and clear cell carcinoma.

3. **Which are premalignant conditions of Ca penis?**

   Ans. Leukoplakia, penile warts, lichen sclerosis (BXO), Bowen's disease, erythroplasia of Queyrat, Bushke-Lowenstein tumor, cutaneous horn, and condyloma acuminate.

4. **What are differential diagnoses of lesion on penis shown in specimen?**

   Ans. Chancroid and penile cancer.

5. **From where do you take biopsy?**

   Ans. In suspected case of Ca penis, biopsy has to be taken as multiple quadrants, edge biopsy from representative area.

   Multiple, because often there is necrosis and if you take one biopsy, report may not be accurate as it may either show necrosis or details may not be appreciable.

   Edge, because the tumor activity is maximum at edge and also comparison with normal tissue can be done.

   Representative area because, in Ca penis many areas have ulceration, fungation, necrosis, and infection. If biopsy taken from such areas may not be representative of pathology, area which does not have all these and which is most likely representative of underlying pathology should be chosen for biopsy.

6. **What specific features you would like to see on biopsy sample?**

   Ans. Type of tumor, grade of tumor, depth of invasion, lymphovascular invasion (LVI), and perineural invasion.

7. **In this specimen of partial penectomy, what specific features you wish to know in microscopic examination?**

   Ans. Type of tumor, grade of tumor, depth of invasion, LVI and perineural invasion, urethral involvement, margins of urethra and skin and corporal involvement. HPV related changes can be diagnosed on immunohistochemistry. Squamous cell carcinoma with HPV-related changes has better prognosis.

8. **What are the indications for groin node dissection in a case of N0 groin?**

   Ans. If the tumor is T1G3 or higher stage, T1G2 with high-risk features (LVI present), then groin node dissection is needed even if clinically or radiologically groin nodes are not present.

9. **In which cases will you not do partial penectomy?**

   Ans. Clinically, when the induration is up to the base of the penis, penile stump adequate for voiding in upright position is unlikely.

10. **If clinically lymph nodes are palpable and fixed, then will you go for radical penectomy or a partial penectomy?**

    Ans. The decision of partial or radical penectomy depends on the local extent of the disease irrespective whether lymph nodes are palpable or not. If locally tumor is present only in the distal portion, then partial penectomy is advised.

CHAPTER 27

Testicular Mass

SPECIMEN 18: TESTICULAR TUMOR

Description

Bisected specimen of high inguinal orchidectomy shows complete replacement of testicular parenchyma with pinkish lobulated mass with areas of necrosis (**Fig. 1**). Cord structures are visualized and appear to be normal.

1. **How this patient would have presented with?**

   Ans. Painless swelling and heaviness in scrotum. Many times, they present due to symptoms of metastasis such as abdominal mass, pain, backache, cough, hemoptysis, breathlessness, and dyspnea.

2. **Why inguinal orchiectomy is done?**

   Ans. Scrotal skin lymphatic drainage is different than testicular lymphatics and hence during surgery, if there is contamination, tumor cells will go to inguinal lymph nodes. Radical inguinal orchiectomy is done.

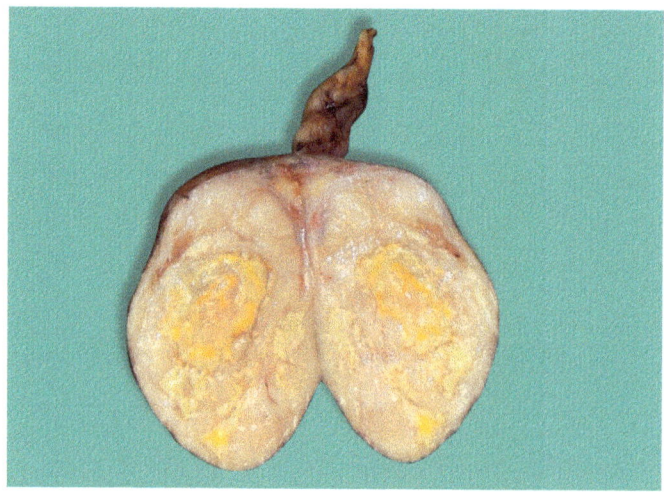

Figure 1: Small testicular carcinoma.

3. **What are different types of testicular tumors?**

   Ans. Testicular tumors can be classified into:
   - Primary testicular neoplasms:
     - Germ cell tumors
     - Non-germ cell tumors
   - Secondary testicular neoplasms
   - Paratesticular neoplasms
   According to World Health Organization (WHO) 2016 classification:
   - **Germ cell tumors:**
     - Intratubular malignant germ cell neoplasia (ITGCN; carcinoma in situ)
     - Classic seminoma (syncytiotrophoblastic)
     - Spermatocytic seminoma
     - Embryonal carcinoma
     - Yolk sac tumor
     - Trophoblastic tumors
     - Choriocarcinoma
     - Teratoma
     - Dermoid cyst
     - Tumors of more than one histologic type (mixed forms)
   - **Non-germ cell tumors:**
     - Pure forms:
       - Leydig cell tumor
       - Sertoli cell tumor
     - Granulosa cell tumor
     - Gonadoblastoma
     - Incompletely differentiated sex cord/gonadal stromal tumors
     - Mixed forms
   - **Metastasis:**
     - Most commonly from primary malignancy of prostate followed by lung, GI tract, melanoma, and kidney
   - **Lymphoid and hematopoietic tumors:**
     - Lymphoma
     - Plasmacytoma
     - Leukemia
   - **Paratesticular tumors:**
     - Tumors of the tunica, epididymis, spermatic cord, supporting structures, and appendices
     - Soft tissue tumors

4. **Can you differentiate type of tumor on gross cut open specimen?**

   Ans. On gross cut open specimen, we can differentiate between seminomatous and nonseminomatous germ cell tumor. Seminomatous tumors are more homogenous, have pinkish gray, soft, with minimum of necrosis as compared to nonseminomatous germ cell tumors.

Nonseminomas are nonhomogenous and have more necrosis with some cystic areas found.

5. What is the role of contralateral testicular biopsy in a known case of Ca testis?

Ans. The indications for contralateral biopsy are:
- On USG, dense microcalcifications may prompt us to do a testicular biopsy which has to be done by a high inguinal approach using Chevassu maneuver.

6. What is the ideal time to do biomarkers?

Ans. All the biomarkers should be done post-orchiectomy.

7. Increased incidence of ca testis is associated with?

Ans. Increased incidence of ca testis is associated with male reproductive disorders like hypospadias, cryptorchidism and subfertility. Broadly this symptom complex is known as testicular dysgenesis syndrome.

8. What percentage of germ cell tumors (GCT) are extra gonadal?

Ans. About 5% germ cell tumors are extra gonadal and arise from midline anatomic locations in retroperitoneum and mediastinum.

9. How is mediastinal NSGCT different from gonadal NSGCT?

Ans. Mediastinal GCT's have poorer prognosis and are less chemosensitive. They are more likely to have a Yolk sac tumor and hence alpha fetoprotein is elevated. Five year survival is about 45%.

10. What is germ cell tumor neoplasia in situ (GCNIS)?

Ans. GCNIS consists of undifferentiated germ cell that appear like a seminoma and are located in the basal region of the seminiferous tubule. These tubule have a decreased or absent spermatogenesis. GCNIS does not have a prognostic significance if found in the orchidectomy specimen.

11. What is a spermatocytic tumor?

Ans. Sermatocytic tumor was previously called as spermatocytic seminoma and subclassified as a subtype of Seminoma, but now it is considered as a separate entity. It does not arise from GCNIS and not associated with testicular dysgenesis syndrome. The peak incidence of this tumor occurs in the sixth decade. These tumors do not stain for OCT3/4, PLAP and PAS. This tumor has a very high cure rate unless it is a anaplastic or sarcomatoid variant.

12. Does choriocarcinoma also arise from testis?

Ans. Yes, choriocarcinoma can arise from the testis. It is a rare and aggressive tumor and is associated with high levels of HCG. They spear by hematogenous route and involve lung liver and brain. On microscopy it is associated with syncytiotrophoblasts and cytotrophoblasts. High levels of HCG can cause hyperthyroidism and elevated androgen levels. After starting chemotherapy these tumors can have spontaneous hemorrhage which can be life-threatening.

13. **What is growing teratoma syndrome?**

    Ans. A third of metastatic tumors after chemotherapy in NSGCT are Teratomas. At metastatic sites these teratomas may grow uncontrollably and invade the adjacent structures this is known as the growing teratoma syndrome.
    On rare Occasion these teratomas may transform into somatic malignancies like rhabdomyosarcoma, adenocarcinoma or primitive neuroectodermal tumor.

CHAPTER 28

Adrenal Mass

SPECIMEN 19: ADRENAL TUMOR

Description

Specimen consists of adrenal gland with mass (**Fig. 1**). On bisection, well circumscribed, pinkish tan homogenous mass with normal adrenal stretched out over the mass and shows hemorrhage.

1. **What is the suspected diagnosis?**

   Ans. This appears a pheochromocytoma because it has pinkish tan homogenous appearance with minimum of necrosis. It will turn to dark yellowish brown with exposure to formalin.

2. **What are the other common tumors of adrenal?**

   Ans. Adrenal adenoma, myelolipoma, adrenocortical carcinoma, neuroblastoma, and schwannoma. Myelolipoma on gross appearance is

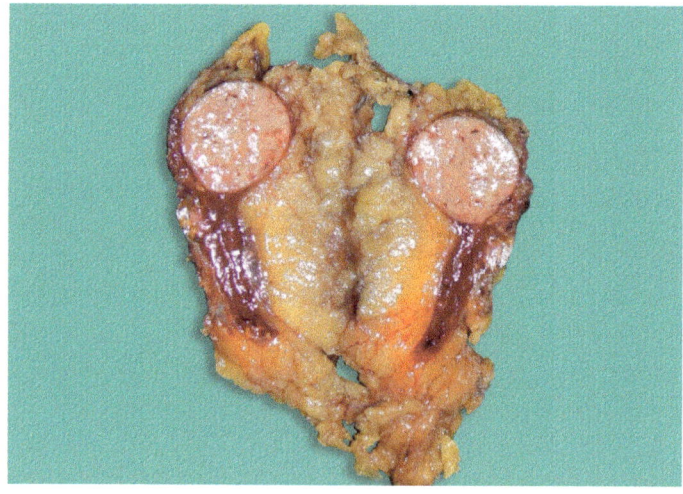

Figure 1: Specimen showing adrenal gland with tumor.

similar to fat, and adrenal adenoma also appears pinkish without any necrosis, however it will not turn to dark yellowish brown on exposure to formalin. Functional adrenal tumors such as Conn's syndrome or Cushing's syndrome on gross specimen appear like adrenal adenoma.

3. **How would this patient have presented?**

    Ans. The patient would have presented with uncontrolled hypertension, frequent headaches, giddiness, palpitation, seizures, etc.

4. **What is the characteristic appearance of pheochromocytoma on microscopic examination?**

    Ans. Tumor cells are arranged in small nests known as Zellballen bodies.

5. **Are there any histological criteria to diagnose metastatic pheochromocytoma?**

    Ans. The malignant pheochromocytoma is diagnosed only by the presence of metastasis. Markers which may suggest malignant nature are p53, Bcl-2 expression, and Mib-1 mitotic index; but these are not confirmatory.

6. **What are the histological criteria for diagnosis of adrenocortical carcinoma known as?**

    Ans. Weiss criteria; they are high nuclear grade, atypical mitotic figures, eosinophilic tumor cell cytoplasm, diffuse architecture, necrosis, venous invasion, sinusoidal invasion, and capsular invasion.

    Tumor size >6.5 cm, tumor weight >50 g, and on microscopic examination, increased mitotic activity, atypical mitosis, and Ki-67 index >4% suggest poor prognosis.

7. **What percentage of adrenal adenoma are metabolically active?**

    Ans. Seven percent of the adrenal adenomas may be metabolic active.

8. **What is neuroblastoma?**

    Ans. Neuroblastoma is a malignant tumor arising from neural crest which give rise to adrenal medulla and sympathetic ganglia. It is the most common solid extra-cranial tumor of childhood.

9. **What is the difference between renal and adrenal oncocytoma?**

    Ans. Renal oncocytomas are benign, but adrenal oncocytoma can be malignant on 50% of the occasions. Adrenal oncocytomas are rare and only about 50 cases have been reported in literature so far.

10. **What are the oncological principles of Resection of a ACC?**

    Ans. 1. Follow no touch technique
    2. Intact peritoneum on the anterior surface of adrenal gland should be preserved

3. En-Block resection with wide margin of surrounding fat should be done
4. Strict preservation of the tumor capsule
5. Exclude rest of the peritoneal cavity with mops and pads.
6. Minimizing blood and fluid spill into the peritoneal cavity.
7. Extraction of specimen in bag in case of laparoscopic surgery
8. Change of gloves, gown and instrument for closure of the wound.

11. How would you prepare a non-functional adrenal incidentaloma for surgery?

Ans. The preparation has to be same as pheochromocytoma. Around 5% pheochromocytoma are non functional at evaluation but may have blood pressure fluctuations during the surgery.

CHAPTER 29

Prostatic Pathology

SPECIMEN 20: RADICAL PROSTATECTOMY

Description

Radical prostatectomy specimen with intact bilateral seminal vesicles (SVs) (**Figs. 1A to F**). Grossly, there is no capsular breach evident in the specimen. Apex and bladder base grossly appear intact. Specimen shows bilateral SVs with segments of vas on each side.

1. **How do you process this specimen?**

    Ans. The specimen is first received in 10% buffered formalin and kept in formalin for 18–24 hours for fixation. After fixation, the specimen is measured and outer surface is inked with India ink. After fixing the ink, a thin slice of 2 mm is taken from the apex and base region to look for the margins. Rest of the specimen is serially sectioned with slice thickness of 4–5 mm. Whole prostate is embedded and after processing, the sections are evaluated as a whole mount (**Figs. 2A and B**).

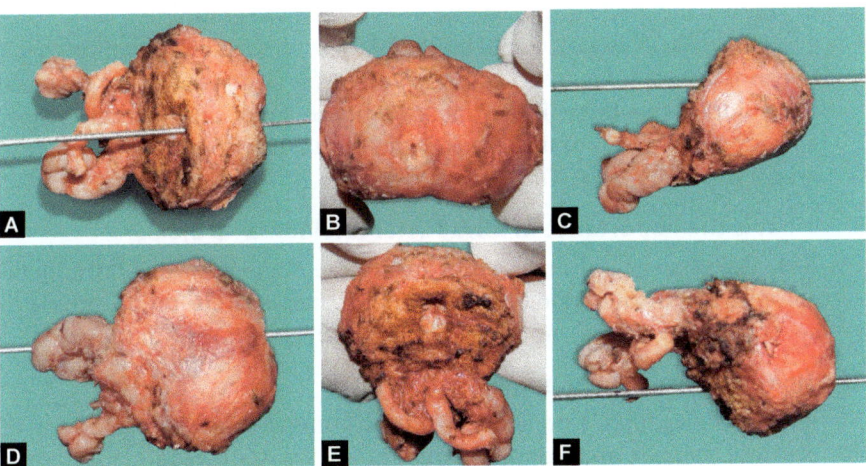

Figures 1A to F: Radical prostatectomy specimen.

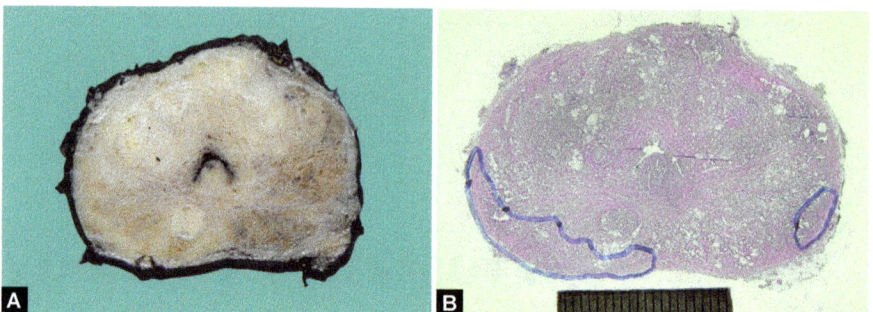

Figures 2A and B: (A) Prostatic hyperplasia in human prostate tissue; (B) Histology specimen of the same.

2. **What is Gleason's grade? What is grade group?**

    Ans. Gleason's grade is described by Gleason and that takes into consideration of morphology/pattern of the glands.

    Gleason's score is summation of primary Gleason's grade and second most common Gleason's grade.

    Grade group is divided into five categories depending on the Gleason's score:
    - Group 1: 3 + 3
    - Group 2: 3 + 4
    - Group 3: 4 + 3
    - Group 4: Any 8
    - Group 5: Any 9 and 10

    Note: The grade grouping (ISUP-2014) for prostate biopsy and specimen is different. In prostate specimen, highest and second common grade is taken for summation. For example in a specimen if the most common grade in 4, second most common grade is 3 and there is a small quantity of grade 5, the grade group will be 4 + 3 = 7 (Grade group 3).

    However, in biopsy, the highest and the worst grade (even though if it may not be second common grade) is taken for summation. For example in a biopsy specimen if the most common grade in 4, second most common grade is 3 and there is a small quantity of grade 5, the grade group will be 4 + 5 = 9 (Grade group 5).

3. **What is the importance of intraductal carcinoma (IDC)?**

    Ans. The presence of malignancy inside the ducts indicates intraductal ca, and it indicates poor prognosis, does not secrete much prostate-specific antigen (PSA), and is associated with germline mutations.

4. **What is extracapsular extension?**

    Ans. Extracapsular extension is tumor going behind the confines of prostatic capsule and extending into the periprostatic connective tissue. It can be focal (1–2 high-power field) or multifocal (>2 high-power field on two different sections).

5. **How are the seminal vesicles (SVs) involved in Ca prostate?**

   Ans. The SVs can be involved by:
   - Direct invasion from the base of the prostate
   - Extraprostatic extension with infiltration in SV walls
   - Invasion through ejaculatory ducts
   - Vascular lymphatic spread

6. **What is the importance of LVI and PNI?**

   Ans. LVI is lymphovascular invasion and PNI is perineural invasion. In some studies, PNI has shown to be a poor prognostic factor, but in multivariate analysis, it is considered to be of questionable factor.

7. **What is the significance of bladder neck involvement?**

   Ans. It is considered like extraprostatic extension.

8. **What is margin positivity in Ca prostate?**

   Ans. If the tumor is touching the ink margin, it is considered as margin positive. It can be true margin positivity or iatrogenic. In iatrogenic margin positivity, there will be no evidence of capsule.

9. **How do you estimate tumor volume in a specimen?**

   Ans. Tumor area is evaluated under scanning microscope and volume is measured by image analysis.

10. **What is PIRADS scoring?**

    Ans. PIRADS is Prostate Imaging Reporting and Data System. It is based on multiparametric MRI.

11. **In which persons should PSA screening be done?**

    Ans. PSA screening should be done in:
    - Men >50 years of age
    - Men >45 years of age with family history of prostate cancer
    - Men of African descent >45 years
    - BRCA mutations >40 years

    Do not screen if life expectancy <15 years.

SECTION 4

Miscellaneous

CHAPTER 30

Chemotherapy in Urological Malignancies

INTRODUCTION

Knowledge of the chemotherapeutic regimen is essential for all the urologists as this enables them to discuss out the relevant options with the medical oncologist. Also, this may help them deliver certain drugs.

CHEMOTHERAPY FOR BLADDER CANCER

Intravesical agents for nonmuscle-invasive bladder cancer (NMIBC):
Agents that can be used are as follows:
- Mitomycin
- Gemcitabine
- BCG

Mitomycin C
- *Dose*: 40 mg in 20 mL sterile water
- Instill via catheter
- *Dwell time*: 1-2 hours
- *Perioperative regimen*: Single instillation within 24 hours of transurethral resection of bladder tumor (TURBT)
- *Induction regimen*: Weekly for 6 weeks
- *Maintenance regimen*: To start 6 weeks after induction. Monthly for 10 months

Indications
- Intermediate risk NMIBC
- Bacillus Calmette-Guérin (BCG) ineligible, intolerance, or unresponsive.

Contraindications
- Hypersensitivity to mitomycin
- Gross hematuria

- Bladder perforation
- Urinary tract infection (UTI)

Gemcitabine

- *Dose*: 2,000 mg diluted in normal saline up to 90 cc
- Instill via catheter using 50 mL syringe—two syringes
- *Dwell time*: 1–2 hours
- *Perioperative regimen*: Single instillation within 24 hours of TURBT
- *Induction regimen*: Weekly for 6 weeks
- *Maintenance regimen*: To start 6 weeks after induction. Monthly for 10 months

Indications

- Intermediate risk NMIBC
- BCG ineligible, intolerance, or unresponsive

Contraindications

- Hypersensitivity to gemcitabine
- Gross hematuria
- Bladder perforation
- UTI

BACILLUS CALMETTE-GUÉRIN (BCG)

Intravesical BCG is used as an immunomodulator in NMIBC.

Mechanism of Action

Bacillus Calmette–Guérin attaches to the urothelium through fibronectin and integrins. The antigen 85 complex plays a central role in synthesizing major components of the inner and outer leaflets of the mycobacterial outer membrane and binds fibronectin. BCG is then internalized by urothelial cells and captured by the first line of innate immune response cells. Antigen presentation and cytokine release result in major histocompatibility complex (MHC) II upregulation and of interleukin (IL)-6, IL-8, and granulocyte-macrophage colony-stimulating factor (GM-CSF). Immune cells including granulocytes, CD4 and CD8 T cells, natural killer (NK) cells, and macrophages get activated. TH-1 cytokines, including interferon gamma, IL-1, IL-12, IL-18, IL-23, and tumor necrosis factor (TNF)-alpha are produced by these immune cells.

The immunological complexity of live-attenuated mycobacteria is necessary to trigger immune responses required to clear and control tumor cells locally in the bladder.

Indications
- HGT1 disease
- CIS (carcinoma in situ)

Various strains used are Danish strain, Frappier strain, Pasteur strain, Japanese strain, Connaught strain, and Tice strain.

Dose and Schedule
About 120 mg is the standard dose but 80 mg can also be used depending on the side-effect profile of the patient. But many reports have suggested that 80 mg has same efficacy and less side effects.
- *Schedule*: After 2-4 weeks of TURBT, instillation of induction course is done.
- 1 dose every week for 6 weeks is given.
- After that, maintenance protocol is weekly instillation for 3 weeks on 3rd month, 6th month, and then every 6 months up to 3 years with check cystoscopy (Lamm regimen).

Contraindications
Absolute Contraindications
- Immunocompromised patients
- Immediately after transurethral resection
    - Personal history of BCG sepsis
    - Gross hematuria (intravasation risk)
    - Traumatic catheterization (intravasation risk)
    - Total incontinence (patient will not retain agent)

Relative Contraindications
- Urinary tract infection (intravasation risk)
- Liver disease (precludes treatment with isoniazid if sepsis occurs)
- Personal history of tuberculosis
- Poor performance status
- Advanced age

Cleveland Clinic Approach to BCG Toxicity
Grade 1: Moderate Symptoms <48 Hours
- Mild or moderate irritative voiding symptoms, mild hematuria, fever <38.5°C
- *Assessment*: Possible urine culture to rule out bacterial urinary tract infection

Symptom Management
- Anticholinergics, topical antispasmodics (phenazopyridine), analgesics, and nonsteroidal anti-inflammatory drugs

Grade 2: Severe Symptoms and/or >48 Hours
- Severe irritative voiding symptoms, hematuria, or symptoms lasting >48 hours
- All investigations for grade 1, plus the following: Urine culture, chest radiograph, liver function tests (LFTs).

Management
- Consider dose reduction to one half to one third of dose when instillations are started. Treat culture results as appropriate.

Antimicrobial Agents

Administer isoniazid and rifampin, 300 mg/day and 600 mg/day, orally until symptom resolution. Do not use monotherapy. Observe for rifampin drug-drug interactions (e.g., warfarin).

Grade 3: Serious Complications (Hemodynamic Changes, Persistent High-grade Fever)
- Allergic reactions (joint pain and rash)
- Perform all investigations for grades 1 and 2, plus the following:
  - Isoniazid, 300 mg/day and rifampin, 600 mg/day, for 3-6 months depending on response
  - Solid organ involvement (epididymis, liver, lung, kidney, bone, joint, and prostate)
  - Isoniazid, 300 mg/day; rifampin, 600 mg/day; ethambutol, 15 mg/kg/day single daily dose for 3-6 months
  - BCG is almost uniformly resistant to pyrazinamide, so this drug has no role.
  - Consider prednisone, 40 mg/day, when response is inadequate or for septic shock (never given without effective antibacterial therapy)

CHEMOTHERAPY FOR MUSCLE INVASIVE BLADDER CANCER

It can be given as:
- Neoadjuvant chemotherapy
- Adjuvant chemotherapy
- Palliative chemotherapy

Neoadjuvant Chemotherapy
- *Regimen*: Gemcitabine and cisplatin (GC)
- Indications:
  - Muscle invasive bladder cancer
  - N0 M0
  - Planned cystectomy
  - Eastern Cooperative Oncology Group (ECOG) 0 or 1

- Exclusion:
  - Major comorbidities
  - Renal insufficiency [glomerular filtration rate (GFR) <60 mL/min]
  - Variant histology such as adenocarcinoma, small cell carcinoma, and pure squamous carcinoma
  - Significant hearing loss
- Blood test at baseline:
  - *Complete hemogram*: Hemoglobin (Hb), total leukocyte count (TLC), differential leukocyte count (DLC), platelet count, serum creatinine, Sr. bilirubin, alkaline phosphatase, and alanine aminotransferase (ALT)
- Drug and dosage:
  - *Gemcitabine*: 1,250 mg/m^2/dose in 250 mL normal saline (NS) over 30 minutes to be given on days 1 and 8.
  - *Cisplatin*: 70 mg/m^2/dose on day 1
    - Prehydrate with 1,000 mL NS over 1 hour
    - Cisplatin to be given 500 mL NS with 20 mEq potassium, 1 g magnesium sulfate, and 30 g mannitol over 1 hour
      - Each cycle is 21 days' duration. Hospital visit required on day 1 and day 8 for drug injection
      - Maximum four cycles prior to surgery
      - Re-imaging to be done after two cycles
      - Repeat blood investigation on days 1 and 8 of each cycle
- Dose modification gemcitabine:
  - *Full dose to be given if:* Absolute neutrophil count >1 × 10^9/L and platelet count >100 × 10^9/L
  - Dose reduction to 75% if absolute neutrophil count between 0.5 and 1 × 10^9/L and platelet count between 75 and 100 × 10^9/L
  - If the count is less than the above dose should be delayed or omitted.
- Dose modification cisplatin:
  - If GFR >60 mL/min—100% of the dose, i.e., 70 mg/m^2 should be given
  - If GFR is between 45 mL/min and 60 mL/min, the dose should be split: 35 mg/m^2 on day 1 and day 8
  - If GFR is <45 mL/min, dose should be omitted or consider carboplatin.
- Using carboplatin:
  - Carboplatin can replace cisplatin when the GFR is <45 mL/min.
  - *Dose*: 5 AUC (area under the curve) = 5 × (GFR + 25) single dose on day 1
  - So if the GFR is 40 dose of carboplatin will be (5 × 65) = 325 mg

Advantage of Neoadjuvant Chemotherapy

- Benefits in T2, T3, and T4
- European Organisation for Research and Treatment of Cancer (EORTC) randomized multi-institutional trial using MVAC (methotrexate/vinblastine/doxorubicin/ cisplatin) as three cycles of neoadjuvant therapy in $T_2 G_3$, T_3, T_{4a}, N_0-N_x, and M_0 disease.

- Showed only a 5.5% (nonsignificant, $p = 0.075$) survival difference at 3 years favoring the chemotherapy arm (55.5%) compared to nonchemotherapy arm (50%)
- Although small, this difference in survival has been shown to be maintained even at longer follow-up of 5 and 8 years (50% vs. 44% and 43% vs. 37%, respectively) and even attained statistical significance.
- Medical Research Council (MRC)/EORTC trail (RCT: 976 patients) with three cycles of MVAC f/b versus surgery versus radical cystectomy showed at 4 years, 15% reduction in risk of death in neoadjuvant group.
- Southwest Oncology Group (SWOG) trail (RCT: 317 patients):
  - Neoadjuvant MVAC versus radical cystectomy
  - 38% were T_0 in neoadjuvant group
  - Risk of death decreased by 33%

Disadvantages

- Benefit is 5–7%. So, 9–95% patients, it is not necessary.
- Some patients can get toxicity and bone marrow depression and patient may become inoperable.
- Not all patients respond, so unnecessary delay in surgery

Adjuvant Chemotherapy for Urothelial Bladder Cancer

Indication

- To be given 90 days within radical cystectomy
- Pathological stage PT3–T4
- Node positive N1-3
- Margin positive disease
- M0
- ECOG 0–1

The regimen and duration remain the same. That is 4 cycles of 21 day duration. If the 4 cycles were not completed as neoadjuvant the remaining given as adjuvant.

Palliative Chemotherapy for Bladder Cancer

Indication

- M + disease
- Gross residual disease
  First-line regimen remains the same.
  - MVAC regimen for bladder cancer
  - Drugs:
    - Methotrexate
    - Vinblastine
    - Doxorubicin (adriamycin)
    - Cisplatin

- Dose and regimen: It is a 28-day cycle.
  - Methotrexate: 30 mg/m² on day 1, 15, 22—intravenous (IV) push
  - Vinblastine: 3 mg/m² on days 2, 15, 22—IV in 50 mL NS over 15 minutes
  - Doxorubicin: 30 mg/m² on day 2—IV push
  - Cisplatin: 70 mg/m² on day 2—to be given 500 mL NS with 20 mEq potassium, 1 g magnesium sulfate, and 30 g mannitol over 1 hour

Dose Modification

- For methotrexate, vinblastine, and doxorubicin if neutrophil count:
  - Between 1 and 1.5×10^9/L—reduce to 66%
  - $<1 \times 10^9$/L—delay first dose until recovery or 1 week and omit other doses
- *For renal dysfunction*: Cisplatin to be modified as above.
  - For methotrexate
  - Creatinine clearance 61-80 mL/min—75% dose
  - Creatinine clearance 51-60 mL/min—70% dose
  - Creatinine clearance 10-50 mL/min—30-50% dose
  - Creatinine clearance <10 mL/mim—omit
- Single-dose cisplatin when used as a trimodality agent, when used with radiation.
  - Cisplatin 40 mg/m² weekly for 5-7 weeks

Drugs that are used along with bladder cancer chemotherapy regimen:
- Dexamethasone 4 mg PO BD: 2-3 days
- Dimenhydrinate 50-100 mg PO 1 STAT then SOS
- *Lorazepam*: 1 mg SOS
- *Prochlorperazine*: 10 mg PO SOS
- MVAC is less preferred to GC due to increased toxicity. There was a great risk of febrile neutropenia with MVAC.
- Now dose dense MVAC is available which has better tolerability

IMMUNOTHERAPY FOR BLADDER CANCER

Pembrolizumab

Indication

- Metastatic bladder cancer
- Second line post-cisplatin based first line
- First line in platins ineligible
- ECOG 0-2
- Normal hepatic and renal function

Exclude

- Patient with autoimmune disease
- Patient on immunosuppression or steroids

Baseline tests: Complete blood count (CBC) and differential, platelets, creatinine, alkaline phosphatase, ALT, total bilirubin, lactate dehydrogenase (LDH), sodium, potassium, thyroid-stimulating hormone (TSH), morning serum cortisol, and chest X-ray.

Repeat before each cycle is 21 days in duration.

Dose: Pembrolizumab 2 mg/kg/dose (maximum = 200 mg) IV with 50 mL NS using a 0.2 micron inline filter.

Cycle and duration: 3 weekly up to a maximum of 35 cycles or 2 years

Toxicity: Severe immune reactions, enterocolitis, intestinal perforation or hemorrhage, hepatitis, dermatitis, neuropathy, endocrinopathy, as well as toxicities in other organ systems

CHEMOTHERAPY FOR CARCINOMA PROSTATE

- Docetaxel-based chemotherapy
- For hormone naïve disease:
    - *Dose*: 75 mg/m² in 250 mL NS over 1 hour, if the total dose is >220 mg, then use 500 mL NS
    - *Cycle*: Six cycles
    - Each cycle is 21 days.
    - Steroid to be given during the day of injection
    - Dexamethasone per orally 8 mg BD for 3 days
    - *Baseline tests*: CBC and differential, platelets, bilirubin, ALT, alkaline phosphatase
    - Tests to be repeated before each cycle
    - Non-polyvinyl chloride (PVC) or diethylhexyl-phthalate (DEHP) IV sets should be used.

Dose modification due to hematological alteration (**Table 1**):

TABLE 1: Dose modification due to hematological alteration.

ANC × 10⁹	Platelet × 10⁹	Dose
>1.5	>90	Full dose
1.0–1.5	70–90	75% of the total
<1	<70	Delay

(ANC: absolute neutrophil count)

Dose modification due to hepatic dysfunction (**Table 2**)

TABLE 2: Dose modification due to hepatic dysfunction.

Bilirubin	Alkaline phosphatase	ALT and AST	Dose
Up to upper limit of normal (ULN)	2.5 × ULN	1.5 × ULN	Full dose
Up to ULN	2.6–5 × ULN	1.6–5 × ULN	75% of the total dose

(ALT: alanine aminotransferase; AST: aspartate aminotransferase)

If bilirubin > upper limit of normal (ULN) or alkaline phosphatase >5 times normal and aspartate aminotransferase (AST)/ALT >5 times normal withhold the drug and consult a hepatologist.

Docetaxel for Hormone Refractor Prostate Cancer

- Dose remains the same but the number of cycles can be up to 10.
- Tab prednisolone 10 mg OD or 5 mg BD to be added for the entire duration of the treatment.
- To prevent cutaneous toxicity and onycholysis of the hands, patients can be given frozen gloves (special gloves like 'Elasto Gel' glove which can be frozen and worn during docetaxel chemotheraphy) to wear 15 minutes before the infusion and up to 15 minutes after the infusion.

Cabazitaxel and Prednisolone for Hormone Refractory Prostate Cancer

- *Dose*: 25 mg/m² in 250 mL NS over 1 hour
- *Cycles*: 10
- Each cycle is 21 days.
- Prednisolone 10 mg OD or 5 mg BD to be continued. Till all cycles of Chemo are continued
- Dexamethasone PO 8 mg BD for 3 days
- *Baseline tests*: CBC and differential, platelets, bilirubin, ALT, creatinine, sodium, and potassium
- Tests to be repeated before each cycle
- Non-PVC or DEHP IV sets should be used
- Premedication:
    - Dexamethasone 8 mg IV 45 minutes prior to infusion over 15 minutes
    - Diphenhydramine 50 mg IV and ranitidine 50 mg IV over 20 minutes—to be give 30 minutes prior to infusion.

Exclusion Criteria

1. ECOG > 2
2. Poor cardiac function. Ejection fraction <50% at baseline
3. If lever functions are altered. Bilirubin, AST, and ALT >1.5 times the normal

Dose modification for hematological reasons (**Table 3**):

TABLE 3: Dose modification for hematological reasons.		
ANC × 10^9	Platelet × 10^9	Dose
>1.5	>90	Full dose
1.0–1.5	70–90	75% of the total
<1	<70	Delay

(ANC: absolute neutrophil count)

ADJUVANT THERAPY FOR RENAL CELL CARCINOMA

International Metastatic Renal Cell Carcinoma Database Consortium Risk Classification

- <1 year from time of diagnosis to systemic therapy
- Hemoglobin less than lower limit of normal <10 g%
- Corrected calcium greater than ULN
- Karnofsky performance status <80
- Absolute neutrophil count > ULN
- Thrombocytosis > ULN
- *Low risk*: No features
- *Intermediate risk*: 1–2 features
- *Poor prognosis*: Defined if at least three out of six risk factors are present (minimum of three poor-risk features required)

Drugs for Advanced Clear Cell Renal Cell Carcinoma

- Favorable risk:
  - First line
    - Pembrolizumab + Axitinib
    - *Alternative*: Sunitinib and pazopanib
- Intermediate and poor risk:
  - Pembrolizumab + Axitinib, ipilimumab, and nivolumab
  - *Alternative*: Cabozantinib, sunitinib and pazopanib

  In patient who have received immunotherapy as first line any of the above-mentioned tyrosine kinase inhibitor (TKI) can be used.

Patients who have received prior TKI:
- Nivolumab and cabozantinib can be used standard of care and axitinib can be used as an alternative

Sunitinib

- Can be used in any risk of IMDC (International Metastatic Renal Cell Carcinoma Database Consortium) and any histology with advance renal cell carcinoma (RCC)
- ECOG > 2
- Exclude if poor cardiac status, ejection fraction (EF) <55%
- Exclude is severe hypertension
- *Base line test*: CBC and differential, platelets, bilirubin, ALT, creatinine, sodium, potassium, bilirubin, alkaline phosphatase, urine analysis, and TSH
- Test to be repeated before every cycle
- *Each cycle*: 6 weeks, to be continued till disease progression or toxicity
- *Dose and cycle*: 50 mg OD for 4 weeks and then 2 weeks off
- If patient shows progression during the 2 week off period, 37.5 mg daily can be considered.

- In case of toxicity, the dose can be reduced to 37.5 mg and then to 25 mg
- Dose modification:
  - *Hematological*: ANC <1 × 10⁹/L and platelet <75 × 10⁹/L : Delay the cycle
  - *Cutaneous toxicity*: For grade 1-2 continue full dose, for grade 3-4 delay till the toxicity subsides to grade 1-2
  - *Cardiac toxicity*: If there is <10% decrease in EF then it can be continued. But if absolute fall in EF is >15%, then hold the drug, between 10% and 15% if the EF is below the lower limit of normal then hold drug.
  - *Sunitinib-induced hypothyroidism*: Fatigue is common symptom, TSH should be done before each cycle. Patients with TSH >20 mU/L, symptomatic, and prior cardiac condition need to be treated.
  - For age <50 years and with cardiac illness and >50 without cardiac illness, start with levothyroxine 25–50 µg/day orally.
  - For age >50 years and with cardiac illness, start with levothyroxine 12.5–25 µg/day orally.

Pazopanib

- It can be used in any risk of IMDC and any histology with advance RCC
- ECOG > 2
- Exclude if poor cardiac status, EF < 45%
- Exclude is severe hypertension.
- Exclude is moderate-to-severe liver impairment.
- *Baseline test*: CBC and differential, platelets, bilirubin, ALT, creatinine, sodium, potassium, total protein, albumin, bilirubin, alkaline phosphatase, urine analysis, and TSH
- Test to be repeated before every cycle
- *Dose*: 800 mg/day per orally empty stomach
- Each cycle 4 weeks—to be taken orally. No gap between cycles.
- Dose can be reduced to 400 mg and then 200 mg.
- Dose modification:
  - *Hematological*: ANC <1 × 10⁹/L and platelet <75 × 10⁹/L: Delay the cycle
  - *Cutaneous toxicity*: For grade 1-2, continue full dose, for grade 3-4 delay till the toxicity subsides to grade 1-2
  - In moderate-to-severe liver dysfunction, delay the cycle.

Cabozantinib

- For metastatic RCC
- Can be used in any risk of IMDC and any histology with advance RCC
- ECOG > 2
- Second-line therapy after first-line TKI
- Exclude is severe hypertension

- *Baseline test*: CBC and differential, platelets, bilirubin, ALT, creatinine, sodium, potassium, bilirubin, alkaline phosphatase, urine analysis, TSH, and uric acid
- Test to be repeated before every cycle
- *Dose*: 60 mg daily per orally continuous
- Does reduction to 40 mg in case of mild-to-moderate hepatic dysfunction
- Consider dose reduction with severe diarrhea
- Consider temporary suspension of the drug if systolic blood pressure (BP) >200 mm Hg or diastolic BP >110 mm Hg.

Axitinib

- For metastatic RCC
- It can be used in any risk of IMDC and any histology with advance RCC
- ECOG > 2
- Second-line therapy after first-line TKI
- Exclude is severe hypertension
- Exclude in severe cardiac disease EF <40%
- *Baseline test*: CBC and differential, platelets, bilirubin, ALT, creatinine, sodium, potassium, bilirubin, alkaline phosphatase, urine analysis, TSH, and uric acid
- Test to be repeated after each cycle
- *Cycle*: 4 weeks = 1 cycle
- *Dose*: 5 mg twice a day to increase to 10 mg twice a day per orally
- Dose reduction to 2–4 mg in case of intolerance
- Consider dose reduction with severe diarrhea
- Consider temporary suspension of the drug if systolic BP >200 mm Hg or diastolic BP >110 mm Hg.
- Consider 50% dose reduction in moderate hepatic dysfunction

Everolimus

- For metastatic RCC
- Can be used in any risk of IMDC and any histology with advance RCC
- Second-line therapy after first-line TKI
- Exclude if major surgery in the past 4 weeks
- Exclude if pulmonary compromise or pneumonitis
- Exclude if on other immunosuppression
- Exclude if intolerant to mechanistic target of rapamycin (mTOR) inhibitors
- *Baseline test*: CBC and differential, platelets, bilirubin, ALT, creatinine, sodium, potassium, bilirubin, alkaline phosphatase, urine analysis, TSH, uric acid, random blood sugar (RBS), calcium, chest X-ray, O_2 saturation, total cholesterol, and triglycerides (TGs)
- *Prior to each cycle*: Hb and CBC
- *Dose*: 10 mg per orally on empty stomach or after a fat-free meal
- *Cycle*: Each cycle 4 weeks

- *Dose reduction*: Can be done to 5 mg OD and then to 5 mg on alternate days
- Dose modification:
  - *Hematological*: ANC <1 × 10⁹/L and platelet <75 × 10⁹/L: Delay the cycle
  - *Cutaneous toxicity*: For grade 1-2 continue full dose, for grade 3-4 delay till the toxicity subsides to grade 1-2
  - *In moderate-to-severe liver dysfunction*: Child Pugh A—7.5 mg/day can be decreased to 5 mg/day if not tolerated
  - Child Pugh B—5 mg/day can be decreased to 2.5 mg/day if not tolerated
  - Child Pugh C—2.5 mg/day
- *Stomatitis prophylaxis*: Dexamethasone mouthwash 0.1 mg/mL four times a day.
  - Start from day 1 to can continue up to 16 weeks

Temsirolimus

- For metastatic RCC
- Can be used in any risk of IMDC and any histology with advance RCC
- Second-line therapy after first-line TKI
- Exclude if major surgery in the past 4 weeks
- Exclude if pulmonary compromise or pneumonitis
- Exclude if on other immunosuppression
- Exclude if intolerant to mTOR inhibitors
- *Baseline test*: CBC and differential, platelets, bilirubin, ALT, creatinine, sodium, potassium, bilirubin, alkaline phosphatase, urine analysis, TSH, uric acid, RBS, calcium, chest X-ray, O_2 saturation, total cholesterol, and TGs
- Repeat tests before next cycle
- *Premedication*: Diphenhydramine 25-50 mg IV 30 minutes prior to infusion
- *Dose*: 25 mg IV in 250 mL in NS in non-DEHP tubing and bag over 30 minutes to 1 hour, once a week
- *Cycle*: 4 weeks
- Dose adjustment:
  - *Hematological*: ANC <1 × 10⁹/L and platelet <75 × 10⁹/L: Delay the cycle
  - *Cutaneous toxicity*: For grade 1-2 continue full dose, for grade 3-4 delay till the toxicity subsides to grade 1-2
  - No data for moderate-to-severe hepatic dysfunction

Ipilimumab and Nivolumab

- For metastatic RCC, first-line treatment for intermediate- or poor-risk advanced RCC

- Any histology
- ECOG > 2
- Good hepatic and renal dysfunction
- Access to center with expertise to manage reactions of immune checkpoint inhibitors
- Exclude patients with central nervous system (CNS) metastasis
- Exclude patient with autoimmune disease
- *Baseline test*: CBC and differential, platelets, bilirubin, ALT, creatinine, sodium, potassium, bilirubin, alkaline phosphatase, urine analysis, TSH, uric acid, RBS, calcium, chest X-ray, and morning serum cortisol
- Repeat before each cycle.
- *Premedication*: Diphenhydramine 25–50 mg IV 30 minutes prior to infusion, acetaminophen 375–975 PO, and hydrocortisone 25 mg IV 30 minutes prior to treatment
- *Induction phase*: Nivolumab 3 mg/kg in 100 mL NS over 30 minutes and ipilimumab 1 mg/kg in 50 mL NS over 90 minutes (0.2 micron inline filter)
- *Cycle*: Every 3 weeks for four cycles
- *Maintenance phase*: Start 3 weeks after induction: Nivolumab 3 mg/kg in 100 mL NS over 30 minutes. To be repeated every 2 weeks till disease progression.
- *Or*: Nivolumab 6 mg/kg in 100 mL NS over 30 minutes. To be repeated every 4 weeks till disease progression.
- Immune-mediated reaction can be severe and fatal. May develop months after discontinuation of therapy. Enterocolitis, intestinal perforation or hemorrhage, hepatitis, dermatitis, neuropathy, endocrinopathy, pneumonitis, as well as toxicities in other organ systems may occur.

Pembrolizumab and Axitinib
- First line for low-risk metastatic clear cell RCC
- Dose 200 mg every 3 weeks and axitinib 5 mg BD
- To continue till disease progression
- Total of 35 cycles were used in keynote 426 study
- About 94% patients had tumor reduction
- Superior to sunitinib in terms of depth of tumor shrinkage

CHEMOTHERAPY IN SQUAMOUS CELL CARCINOMA OF PENIS

Cisplatin and 5 Fluorouracil
- Locally advanced disease
- No hearing impairment
- ECOG > 2
- Adequate bone marrow function
- Creatinine clearance >50 mL/min

- *Baseline test*: CBC and differential, platelets, bilirubin, ALT, creatinine, sodium, potassium, and bilirubin
- Repeat before each test
- Premedications:
    - Ondansetron 8 mg PO daily 30 minutes before cisplatin each day
    - Dexamethasone 12 mg PO daily 30 minutes before cisplatin each day
    - Dexamethasone 4 mg PO daily 12 hours after cisplatin each day
    - *Days 4 and 5*: Dexamethasone 4 mg PO BID
    - Dimenhydrinate, prochlorperazine, metoclopramide, and lorazepam SOS
    - Five fluorouracil (FU) 1,000 mg/m² over 24 hours in 1,000 mL 5% dextrose for 4 days
- Cisplatin 25 mg/m² in 500 mL NS over 30 minutes for 3 days
- Dose modification due to hematological alteration 5 FU (**Table 4**):

TABLE 4: Dose modification due to hematological alteration for 5 flurouracil (FU).

ANC × 10^9	Platelet × 10^9	Dose
>1.5	>100	Full dose
<1.5	<100	Delay for 1 week

(ANC: absolute neutrophil count)

- In case of stomatitis and diarrhea >grade 4, reduce the dose of 5 FU to 3 days.

CHEMOTHERAPY IN TESTICULAR CANCERS

Carboplatin Single Agent Adjuvant for Seminoma

- *Indication*: Stage 1 high-risk seminoma
- *Exclusion*: Creatinine clearance <50 mL/min and deafness
- *Baseline test*: CBC, TLC, DLC, renal function test, and LFT
- Repeat CBC, TLC, DLC on days 14 and 21
- *Dose*: 7 AUC = 7 × (GFR + 25) in 250 mL NS over 30 minutes
- *Cycle and duration*: 28 cycle × two cycles
- *Toxicity*: Nephrotoxic and ototoxic. May give acute hypersensitivity reaction.

BEP PROTOCOL

BEP stands for bleomycin, etoposide and cisplatin.

Indication

- Stage I nonseminomas and metastatic germ cell tumors
- For IGCCCG (International Germ Cell Consensus Classification Group) good risk: Three cycles

- For IGCCCG intermediate risk seminomas/nonseminomatous germ cell tumor (NSGCT) or NSGCT poor risk—four cycles BEP
- Eligibility criteria to deliver adjuvant BEP:
  - NSGCT stage 1 with vascular invasion (50% risk of relapse)
  - RPLD histology s/o of >5 nodes involved, any node >2 cm, extranodal extension
- *Low-risk metastatic*: Four cycles BEP: Primary testis/retroperitoneal with no nonpulmonary visceral metastases, mediastinal seminoma. Markers S1
- *Intermediate risk metastatic*: Primary testis/retroperitoneal with no nonpulmonary visceral metastases, mediastinal seminoma. Markers S2.
- *High-risk metastatic*: Mediastinal primary or nonpulmonary visceral metastasis or S3 markers

Note: Consider sperm banking prior to starting chemotherapy

Relative Contraindications
- Poor renal function
- Poor hematological function (anemia and cytopenia)
- Poor pulmonary reserve
- Hearing impairment

Baseline tests (repeat prior to each cycle): CBC and differential, platelets, liver enzymes (including LDH), creatinine, sodium, potassium, magnesium, calcium, AFP, serum human chorionic gonadotropin (hCG), random glucose, baseline pulmonary function tests (PFTs).

Cycles and Duration
- All cycles are 21 days
- *Adjuvant setting*: Two cycles
- *Low-risk metastatic*: Three cycles
- *Intermediate- and high-risk metastatic*: Four cycles
- *Premedication*: 1 L NS over 20 mEq potassium and 2 g magnesium sulfate over 1 hour.
- *Cisplatin*: 20 mg/m^2/day, on day 1–5, in 100 mL NS over 30 minutes: Day 1–5
- *Etoposide*: 100 mg/m^2/day, on day 1–5, in 1,000 mL NS over 1 hour (use a non-PVC or non-DEHP IV set)
- *Bleomycin* 30 units IV in 50 mL NS over 10 minutes on day 1, to be repeated every week up to the tolerable dose.
- *Hydrocortisone*: 100 mg IV STAT, before bleomycin
  Note: GM-CSF to be given if patient has not recovered ANC till day 5 or have neutropenic fever.

Toxicity

- *Bleomycin*: Causes pulmonary toxicity, total dose to be restricted to <270 units. Hydrocortisone decreases the risk of fever associated with bleomycin. Chest examination, chest X-ray should be done before each cycle. PFT can be repeated if symptomatic. Oxygen can cause toxicity so FIO_2 should be restricted to 30–40%. Anesthetist should be informed and these patients can be identified by a tag or bracelet.
- *Etoposide*: Acute hypersensitivity reaction can be seen, also extravasation leads to severe skin reaction.
- *Cisplatin*: Nephrotoxicity can occur. Keep the patient well-hydrated do not use nephrotoxic drugs such as aminoglycosides if patient develops infection. Cisplatin causes ototoxicity also.

EP REGIMEN (ETOPOSIDE AND CISPLATIN)

In this regimen, bleomycin is removed. The dose and duration of etoposide and cisplatin remain the same.

Indication

- Good-risk seminomatous germ cell tumor (SGT) or NSGCT
- S1 markers
- Pure seminoma
- Four cycles to be given and in adjuvant settings, three cycles

TIP PROTOCOL (PACLITAXEL, IFOSFAMIDE, AND CISPLATIN)

TIP Regimen can also be Used in CA Penis as a Primary Treatment

- *Indication*: Relapsed germ cell tumor
- *Baseline test*: Hb CBC, TLC, DLC, serum creatinine, serum sodium, serum potassium, RBS, serum bilirubin, serum glutamic oxaloacetic transaminase (SGOT), serum glutamic pyruvic transaminase (SGPT), and serum albumin
- This is a highly emetogenic protocol, so antiemetics drugs have to be used.
- Prior to paclitaxel:
  - Injection dexamethasone 20 mg IV in 50 mL NS over 15 minutes, 45 minutes prior to paclitaxel. Diphenhydramine 50 mg IV and ranitidine 50 mg IV in 50 mL NS over 20 minutes, 30 minutes prior.

Cycle and Duration: 21-day Cycle, Repeat 4 Cycles

- Day 1: Injection paclitaxel 175 mg /m^2 in 500 mL NS over 3 hours using a non-PVC and non-DEHP tubing.

- Days 2-6:
    - *At 0 hours*: Injection cisplatin 20 mg/m²/day IV in 100 mL NS over 30 minutes
    - *At 0.5 hours*: Injection Mesna 300 mg/m²/day IV in 100 mL D5 over 15 minutes
    - *At 0.75 hours*: Injection ifosfamide: 1,200 mg/m²/day IV in 500 mL D5 ½ NS over 1 hour
    - *From 1.75 to 9 hours*: Hydration with D5 ½ NS IV at the rate of 250 mL/h for 8 hours
    - *At hours 5 and 9*: Injection Mesna 300 mg/m²/day IV in 100 mL D5 over 15 minutes
    - *At 9 hours*: Hydration with D5 ½ NS IV at the rate of 250 mL/h for 8 hours
- *Day 9*: Start filgrastim for 5-7 days

Dose modification for paclitaxel is given in **Table 5**.

TABLE 5: Dose modification for paclitaxel.

ANC × 10⁹	Platelet × 10⁹	Dose
>1.0	>90	Full dose
>1	<90	Delay

(ANC: absolute neutrophil count)

Dose modification for ifosfamide is given in **Table 6**.

TABLE 6: Dose modification for Ifosfamide.

ANC × 10⁹	Platelet × 10⁹	Dose
>1.0	>75	Full dose
>1	<75	Delay

(ANC: absolute neutrophil count)

Toxicity

- *Hematological*: Neutropenia
- Nephrotoxicity
- Hepatic dysfunction may occur due to paclitaxel.
- Arthralgia and myalgia can be treated with paclitaxel. It can be treated with prednisolone 10 mg BD, T. gabapentin 300 mg BD to TDS.
- Neuropathy can occur due paclitaxel and cisplatin.

Hypersensitivity Reaction Secondary to Paclitaxel

- *Mild symptoms*: Rash and itching: Complete paclitaxel infusion under close observation.
- *Moderate symptoms*: Rash, flushing, dyspnea, mild hypotension: Stop paclitaxel, give hydrocortisone and diphenhydramine.

- Start infusion again at the rate of 20 mL/h for 5 minutes and increase 10 mL/h every 5 minutes till 60 mL/h.
- *Severe symptoms (respiratory distress, hypotension, generalized urticaria, angioedema)*: Discontinue paclitaxel, give hydrocortisone and diphenhydramine. Add epinephrine and bronchodilators.

VEIP PROTOCOL (VINBLASTINE, IFOSFAMIDE, AND CISPLATIN)

Indication

Relapse After Chemotherapy for Gonadal and Extragonadal Germ Cell Tumor

- *Baseline test*: Hb CBC, TLC, DLC, serum creatinine, serum sodium, serum potassium, RBS, serum bilirubin, SGOT, SGPT, and serum albumin
- *Cycle and duration*: 21-day cycle × 4
- *Prehydration*: D5 ½ NS 1,000 mL with magnesium sulfate 2 g over 2 hours.
- Schedule:
    - *At 0 hours*: Vinblastine 0.11mg /kg IV in 50 mL NS over 15 minutes on day 1–2
    - *At 0.5–1 hours*: Cisplatin 20 mg/m²/day IV in 100 mL NS over 30 minutes on day 1–5
    - *At 1–1.25 hours*: Injection Mesna 300 mg/m²/day IV in 100 mL D5 over 15 minutes on day 1–4
    - *At 1.5–2.5 hours*: Ifosfamide 1,500 mg/m² IV in 500 mL D5W—1/2 NS over 1 hour on day 1–4
    - *At 6.5 hours*: Injection Mesna 300 mg/m²/day IV in 100 mL D5 over 15 minutes on day 1–4
    - *At 10.5 hours*: Injection Mesna 300 mg/m²/day IV in 100 mL D5 over 15 minutes on day 1–4

Mesna 720 mg/m² PO in carbonated beverage at after injection ifosfamide can replace the injection.

CHEMOTHERAPY FOR NEUROENDOCRINE TUMORS OF GENITOURINARY SYSTEM

Regimen Includes Cisplatin and Etoposide

Indication
- Small cell tumor of bladder
- Small cell tumor of prostate
- Poorly differentiated CA prostate—poorly hormone responsive and low prostate-specific antigen (PSA) secretion.

Baseline tests: CBC and differential, platelets, creatinine, bilirubin, ALT, alkaline phosphate, albumin, and INR

Repeat Before Each Cycle

Premedication
- 1,000 mL of NS over 1 hour prior to cisplatin. Injection hydrocortisone 100 mg IV STAT and injection diphenhydramine 50 mg IV prior to etoposide

Schedule
- Injection cisplatin 25 mg/m^2/day IV in 100 mL NS over 30 minutes from day 1–3
- Injection etoposide 100 mg/m^2/day in 500 mL NS in over 45 minutes (using a non-PVC and non-DEHP lines)
- If cisplatin cannot be given, injection carboplatin 5 AUC [5 × (25 + GFR)] should be used.

Duration and Cycle: 6 Cycles 21 Days Each
Dose modification for hematological reasons is given **Table 7**.

TABLE 7: Dose modification for hematological reasons.

ANC × 10^9	Platelet × 10^9	Dose
>1.5	>90	Full dose
1.0–1.5	75–90	75% of the total
<1	<75	Delay

(ANC: absolute neutrophil count)

Toxicity
- Neutropenia
- Nephron and ototoxicity
- Hypersensitivity reactions

CHEMOTHERAPY FOR ADRENOCORTICAL CARCINOMA

Drugs: Doxorubicin, Etoposide, Cisplatin, and Mitotane
Indication: Metastatic ACC
- *Baseline test*: CBC and differential, platelet, electrolytes, creatinine, calcium, magnesium, random glucose, phosphate AST, ALT, gamma-glutamyl transferase (GGT), alkaline phosphatase, bilirubin, albumin, 24-hour urinary cortisol, or serum cortisol.

Schedule
Premedicate with hydrocortisone and diphenhydramine
- Doxorubicin 40 mg/m^2/day IV push on day 1

- Injection cisplatin 40 mg/m²/day IV in 100 mL NS over 30 minutes from day 1–2
- Injection etoposide 100 mg/m²/day in 500 mL NS in over 45 minutes (using a non-PVC and non-DEHP lines)

Cycle and Duration: 28-day Cycle for 4–6 Times

- Mitotane 2 g daily in four divided doses, escalate by 1 g/day every 1–2 weeks till maximum tolerated dose.
- Dose-limiting factor is nausea and vomiting.
- *Cortisone*: 25 mg every morning and 12.5 mg in evening
- Fludrocortisone 0.1 mg every morning
- To continue till progression

CHEMOTHERAPY FOR WILMS' TUMOR

Chemotherapy

Post nephrectomy stage 1 wilms tumor in a child <2 years, tumor weighing <550 g and favorable histology does not merit chemotheraphy.

The following are the indications for chemotherapy and regimen required:
1. Stage 1 unfavorable histology, >2 years of age, >550 g tumor size: Vincristine, dactinomycin × 18 weeks
   If chromosomal abnormality detected doxorubicin to be added. If anaplastic histology radiotherapy to be added.
2. Stage 2 : Favorable histology (FH): Vincristine, dactinomycin × 18 weeks
   FH with chromosomal abnormality: Vincristine, dactinomycin, doxorubicin × 24 weeks
   Focal anaplasia: Radiation therapy (RT) + Vincristine, dactinomycin, doxorubicin × 24 weeks
   Diffuse anaplasia: RT + Vincristine, dactinomycin, doxorubicin, cyclophosphamide, and etoposide
3. Stage 3: Favorable histology (FH): Vincristine, dactinomycin × 18 weeks with sos RT
   If chromosomal abnormality present: RT + Vincristine, dactinomycin, doxorubicin, cyclophosphamide, and etoposide
   Focal anaplasia: Radiation therapy (RT) + Vincristine, dactinomycin, doxorubicin × 24 weeks
   Diffuse anaplasia: RT + Vincristine, dactinomycin, doxorubicin, cyclophosphamide, and etoposide
4. Stage 4: Favorable histology :+ Vincristine, dactinomycin, doxorubicin × 24 weeks with sos RT
   Anaplasia present: RT + Vincristine, dactinomycin, doxorubicin, cyclophosphamide, and etoposide

5. Stage 5: Neo-adjuvant chemotherapy
   - Preoperative chemotherapy before nephrectomy is indicated in:
     - Wilms' tumor in a solitary kidney
     - Synchronous bilateral Wilms' tumor
     - Extension of tumor thrombus in the inferior vena cava above the level of the hepatic veins
     - Tumor involves adjacent structures
     - Inoperable Wilms' tumor
     - Pulmonary compromise resulting from extensive pulmonary metastases

Chemotherapy Regimens for Wilms' Tumor (Table 8)

- Preoperative chemotherapy includes doxorubicin in addition to vincristine and dactinomycin unless anaplastic histology is present; in such cases, chemotherapy then includes treatment with regimen I.
- Newborns and all infants younger than 12 months who will be treated with chemotherapy require a 50% reduction in chemotherapy dose compared with the dose given to older children.
- Dosing for infants (younger than 12 months) is calculated per kilogram of weight, not body surface area.
- This reduction diminishes the toxic effects reported in children in this age group enrolled in NWTS (National Wilms Tumor Study) studies while maintaining an excellent overall outcome.
- Liver function tests in children with Wilms' tumor are monitored closely during the early course of therapy because of hepatic toxic effects

TABLE 8: Chemotherapy regimens for Wilms' tumor.

Regimen name	Regimen description
Regimen EE-4A	Vincristine, dactinomycin × 18 weeks postnephrectomy
Regimen DD-4A	Vincristine, dactinomycin, doxorubicin × 24 weeks; baseline nephrectomy or biopsy with subsequent nephrectomy
Regimen I	Vincristine, doxorubicin, cyclophosphamide, etoposide × 24 weeks postnephrectomy
Regimen M	Vincristine, dactinomycin, doxorubicin, cyclophosphamide, and etoposide with subsequent radiation therapy
Regimen UH1	Vincristine, doxorubicin, cyclophosphamide, carboplatin, and etoposide × 30 weeks + radiation therapy
Regimen UH2	Vincristine, doxorubicin, cyclophosphamide, carboplatin, etoposide, vincristine, and irinotecan × 36 weeks + radiation therapy

(sinusoidal obstructive syndrome, previously called veno-occlusive disease).
- Dactinomycin or doxorubicin should not be administered during radiation therapy.
- Patients who develop renal failure while undergoing therapy can continue receiving chemotherapy with vincristine, dactinomycin, and doxorubicin.
- Vincristine and doxorubicin can be given at full doses; however, dactinomycin is associated with severe neutropenia.
- Postoperative radiation therapy to the tumor bed is required when a biopsy is performed or in the setting of local tumor stage III.

CHAPTER 31

Operative Notes

HYPOSPADIAS

DISTAL HYPOSPADIAS

Distal Tubularized Incised Plate (TIP) Repair (Snodgrass repair)

Steps (Figs. 1A to G)

1. Circumcising skin incision 2 mm below the meatus
2. U incision along the visible junction of the glans wings to the urethral plate

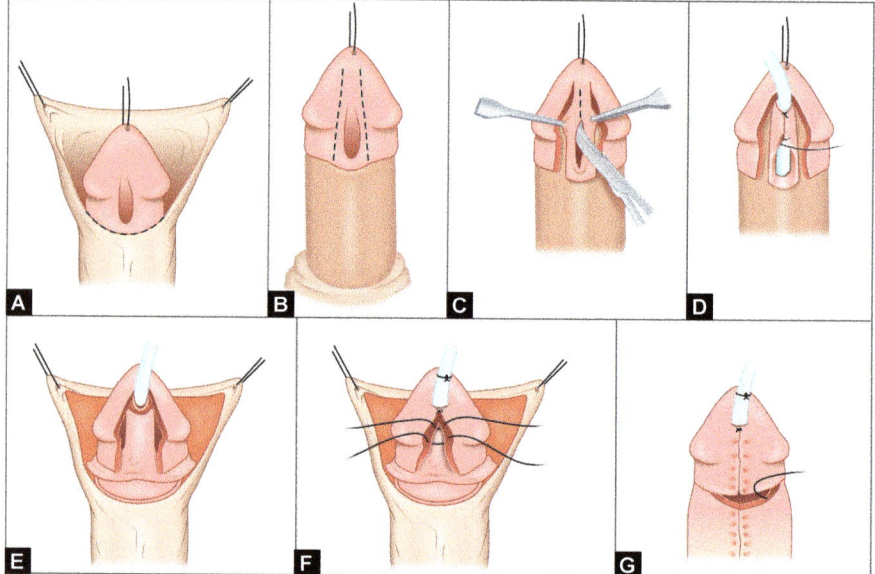

Figures 1A to G: Tubularized incised plate repair.

- Incision made in midline of the urethral plate extending to the underlying corpora
- The urethral plate is tabularized over the catheter from distal to proximal direction with the first stitch is about 3 mm proximal to the end of the urethral plate, creating an oval opening
- The neourethra is covered with a dartos flap
- Glansplasty creating the neomeatus and continuing down to the corona
- Circumcision completed

PROXIMAL REPAIR

The transverse preputial island flap (TPIF) is described in **Figure 2**.

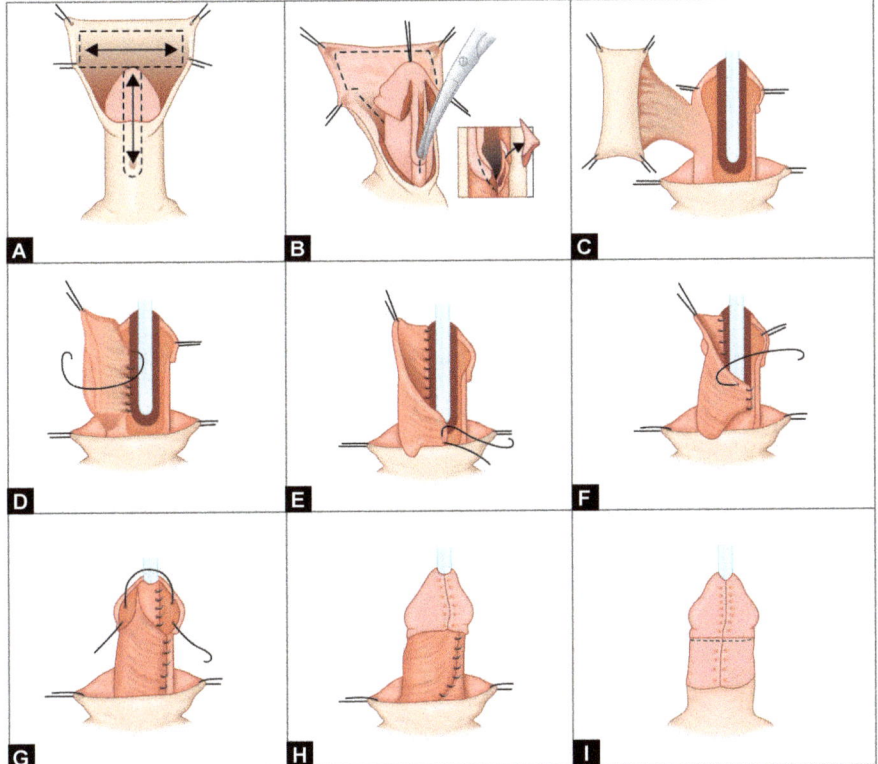

Figures 2A to I: The onlay island flap (OIF) technique. (A) Planned incisions to harvest transverse preputial flap and urethral plate. (B) Isolation of preputial flap on vascularized pedicle. *Inset*, preparation of meatus for anastomosis, including excision of stenotic or hypoplastic meatal tissue. (C) Initiation of anastomosis of onlay flap and urethral plate. (D) Proximal approximation at the native urethra. (E) Completion of the neourethra channel. (F) Application of second layer of barrier coverage. (G-I) Glansplasty and skin closure.

Two Stage Repair

The management of proximal hypospadias with severe ventral penile curvature is majority shifting towards two-stage repair. This can be divided as:

1. **Two-staged repair with pedicle flap (Figs. 3A to I)**
   The Byars flap surgery which uses dorsal preputial skin with its vascular pedicle to be transposed ventrally to form further scaffold for neo-urethra as a part of first stage. The second stage involves tubularization of urethra using standard Thiersch-Duplay technique.

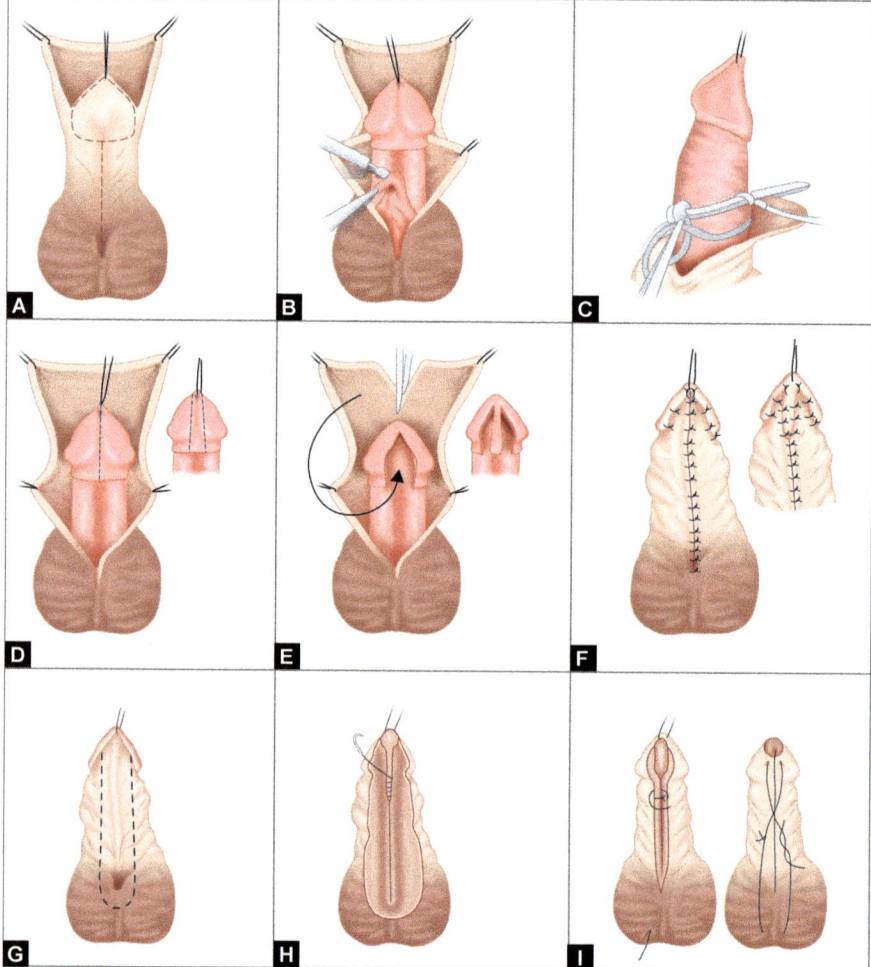

Figures 3A to I: (A and B) Penis degloved upto penoscrotal junction removed any tissue causing chordee. (C) Artificial erection test for assessing chordee. (D) Midline glans incision taken. (E) Dorsal inner preputial skin incised in midline to form Byars flaps. (F) The dorsal skin is transposed ventrally and secured. (G) Tubularization U-shaped incision taken using Thiersch-Duplay principle. (H and I) Multiple layers urethroplasty done including dartos or tunica vaginalis flap

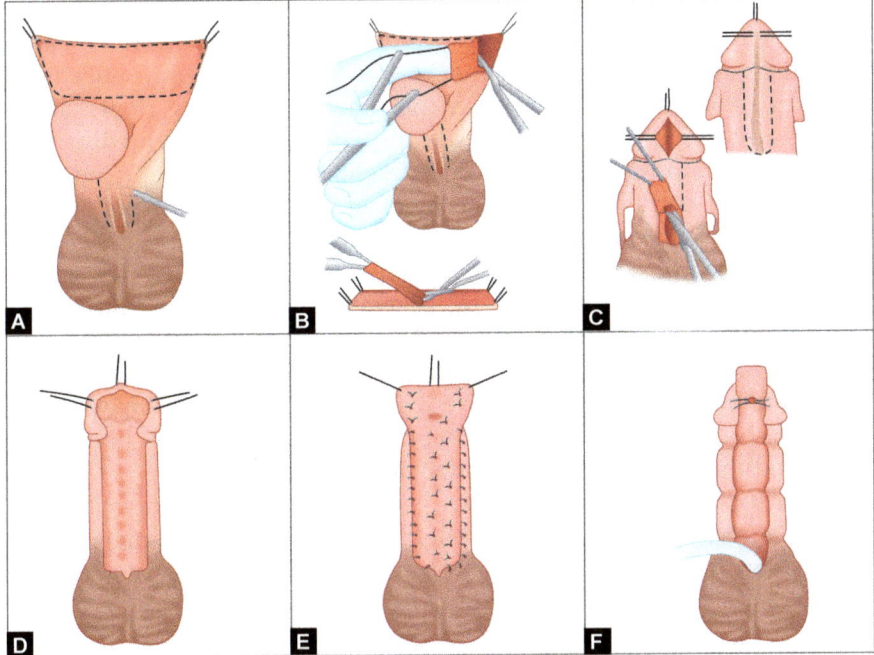

Figures 4A to F: Bracka two stage repair. (A and B) Inner preputial skin graft is marked and harvested. (C) Penis degloved and abnormal penile urethra excised. (D) Adequate mobilization of glans wings. (E) The graft quilted to the base (F) Compression dressing placed over the graft.

2. **Two-staged repair with free graft (Figs. 4A to F)**
   It uses free graft like inner preputial skin, buccal mucosa or post-auricular skin graft as urethral replacement. In this repair, first the penile curvature is corrected, and the urethral plate is divided, creating bed for the graft. After 6 months, the send stage is performed. This second stage involves U-shaped incision and tubularization of urethra using standard Thiersch-Duplay technique.
- Bracka two stage repair with buccal mucosal graft.
- Two stage hypospadias repair using Byar's flap (**Figs. 3A to I**): The second stage consists of tubularization of the urethral plate after 6 months of first stage to ensure adequate graft uptake.

COMPLICATIONS

Early Postoperative Complications

1. Tissue ischemia is involved in creating edema, delayed healing, and fibrosis. Ischemia of the tissue can result in formation of fistula and stricture. Ischemia of island flaps, which rely on diffusion of nutrients from tissue beds and their delicate blood supply, leads to marginal wound

necrosis and later wound contraction. Treatment is initially conservative. However, clear cut demarcated eschar formation will require debridement.
2. Bleeding and hematoma: Intraoperative hemostasis and effective compression dressing usually prevent postoperative bleeding. Hematoma will distort tissue planes, interfere with perfusion of flaps, predispose to infection and breakdown of repair. Significant hematoma needs to be identified and controlled. Placement of drain can be done. Small hematomas can be managed conservatively.
3. Wound infection: Traumatized poorly perfused tissues and free graft predispose to infections. They are generally gram negative and from perimeatal tissue of urethra. Urinary tract infections (UTI) can occur in the catheterized patient when organisms migrate along the indwelling catheter. Infections need aggressive management as they delay wound healing and predispose to fistula formation. Devitalized tissue should be debrided and subcutaneous collection drained.
4. Wound separation: The reasons for wound separation are hematoma, postoperative erection, suturing under tension, trauma or manipulation by patient. If defect is small, it will close with secondary intention. Additional sutures should not be placed.

Late Postoperative Complications

1. Meatal stenosis: It is the most common complication, related to technical problem of urethral meatus during surgery.
2. Urethrocutaneous fistula: Second most common complication. Etiology is related to decrease vascular supply, infection, and hematoma. Distal urethral obstruction either due to crusting or meatal stenosis may also lead to fistula formation. Overlapping of suture lines, poorly absorbable sutures and improper tissue handling predispose to fistula. Small fistulas without inflammation close spontaneously. Large fistulas require delayed surgery after a period of 6 months. Fistulous tract needs to be probed or outlined during excision. The origin of fistula, when identified, can be closed with 7-0 sutures. Large fistulas will require trap door or island flap, tunica vaginalis flap, scrotal dartos flap or buccal mucosa flaps.
3. Urethral stricture: They tend to form at anastomotic suture line and apparent usually after 3 months of surgery. Patient will present with splaying of stream, urethral fistula, and urinary retention. In tubularized pedicle flaps, stricture maybe secondary to redundant neourethra.
4. Urethral diverticulum: Usually seen 6 months after surgery and present with thin stream, post-void dribbling and UTI. They usually result from lack of supporting spongiosum, a larger caliber of urethra and distal obstruction. A localized saccular diverticulum can be excised and reduced onto position. A tunica vaginalis or dartos flap maybe employed. Urethral plication procedure has been advocated by a few.

5. Meatal retrusion: Commonly seen after meatal advancement and glanuloplasty incorporated (MAGPI) in urethra, which is immobile. The defect is usually cosmetic. However, revision maybe done.
6. Persistent chordee: It is due to improper intraoperative assessment, corporal disproportion or development of urethral fibrosis. Depending upon severity, a proper dissection of neourethra, resection of scar, mobilization of bulbar urethra and proper correction is required.

ANTERIOR URETHRAL STRICTURES

Reconstruction of anterior urethral strictures can be:
1. Excision and reanastomosis
2. Substitution urethroplasty
    a. Partial substitution
    b. Total substitution

Excision and reanastomosis: More dependable and safe technique involving excision of entire area of fibrosis and a spatulated, tension free, ovoid anastomosis. It is useful for stricture from 1 to 5 cm. It is necessary to mobilize the bulbar, penoscrotal or membranous urethra, depending upon the site of anastomosis. However, when the length of stricture precludes primary anastomosis, then various substitution grafts need to be utilized.

Flaps and grafts have a higher success rate than tubularized grafts. Tubularized flaps have better results than tubularized grafts. The grafts utilized in urethral anastomosis are:
- Split thickness skin graft
- Full thickness skin graft from posterior auricular and inguinal region
- Buccal mucosa graft
- Bladder mucosa
- Number of genital skin islands based on dartos fascia of penis
- Scrotal skin flaps

Vascularity of flap, non-hirsute skin and mechanics of flap transfer need to be evaluated. The skin islands can be oriented transversally or longitudinally and are usually placed on lower scrotum or perineum. The penile skin can be utilized to produce circular skin islands and spiral skin islands as long as 15 cm. The mechanism of flap transfer dictates the outcome. A flap can be used as an alternative to graft or in addition to a graft. Skin flap should not be used in balanitis xerotica obliterans (BXO) as there is very high recurrence rate for stricture. A graft maybe utilized as an onlay or as tubularized flap. The flap should be properly tailored and adequate size to prevent diverticulum formation. The flaps which are raised on penile, perineal and scrotal skin are reasonable options for long strictures. Epilation of flaps can be planned 10-12 weeks in advance, if the hair bearing scrotal skin is being utilized. Buccal mucosa is the tissue of choice for strictures associated with BXO and graft technique is better than tubularized graft. Few cases of skin flap based island technique have been reported in association with BXO.

GRAFTS

- Mesh graft [Schreeter and Noll (1989)]: Placed over the dartos fascia, tunica or corpora. Second stage tubularization is difficult.
- Monsieur: Urethra opened dorsally and sutured to underlying triangular ligament or corpora or both.
- Barbagli: Urethrostomy through dorsal wall, graft placed between edges of stricture and sutured to underlying corpora.
- Ventral onlay with spongioplasty: Lateral onlay with quilting to ischiocavernosus
- Dorsal dartos fascia based flap – Duckett: Thin island is mobilized transversally
- Dorsal transverse island flap
- Urethral longitudinal skin island flap: Orandi's dartos fascial flap placed longitudinally in lateral urethrotomy incision
- Ventral longitudinal island flap (Jordan): The longitudinal island is used for inversion upto external urethral meatus
- Ventral transverse island flap: Based on penile dorsal fascia
- Strictures of fossa navicularis and external urinary meatus (EUM):
  o Blandy: Random penile skin island advanced to a meatotomy defect.
  o Cohney: Penile skin transverse random flap advanced into meatotomy defect
  o Brannen: Midline flap
  o De Sy: Ventral longitudinal island flap
  o Jordan: Ventral skin island based transversally, transposed on its pedicle into meatotomy defect.

URETHRAL STRICTURES

- **Penile urethral strictures**
- Substitution urethroplasty:
  o Especially for BXO
  o Always dorsal buccal mucosa graft (BMG) inlay done
  o Ventral BMG not possible because of lack of support of spongiosum ventrally
  o Anastomotic repair not done due to penile shortening and chordee formation
- **Bulbar urethral stricture**
- Substitution urethroplasty:
  o Dorsal BMG:
    – It can be dorsal inlay repair with circumferential dissection of urethra
    – Dorsolateral repair with only one side mobilization of urethra

- Ventral Onlay:
    - For proximal bulbar stricture
    - The graft is support by spongioplasty.
  - Double faced BMG:
    - Dorsal inlay + ventral onlay
    - For near obliterative repair

Substitution Buccal Mucosa Graft Urethroplasty

- *Anesthesia*: General anesthesia with nasal intubation and throat packing
- *Position*: Lithotomy
- Perineal midline incision
- Subcutaneous tissue separated
- Bulbospongiosum opened in midline
- Urethra dissected circumferentially for dorsal inlay and only one side for dorsolateral repair
- Distal extent of stricture identified with 16 Fr PUC
- Urethra incised dorsally/dorsolaterally till the proximal extent of the stricture
- BMG harvested
- BMG graft anastomosed with the proximal extent of stricture
- BMG quilted to the cavernosum
- Urethra anastomosed with the BMG on both sides.
- 16 Fr PUC passed
- Hemostasis achieved
- Spongioplasty done and incision closed

PROGRESSIVE PERINEAL URETHROPLASTY

- It was described by Webster and colleagues in 1983.
- *Indication*: Urethral stricture caused by pelvic fracture related urethral injury
- Timing of surgery—at least 3 months after initial injury

Preopeartive assessment:
- Uroflowmetry (if able to void)
- Urine culture
- Micturating cystourethrogram (MCU)-Retrograde urethrogram (RGU) (Up and down-o-gram)
- Urethroscopy with suprapubic cystoscopy
- Documentation of erectile function
- Penile Doppler (assessment of vascularity)

Position: Dorsal lithotomy with lower limbs well supported and padded at bony prominences
- Suprapubic catheter must be in situ (if not, suprapubic cystotomy is required)

Principles: Koraitim's Golden triad
- Complete excision of callus
- Lateral fixation of mucosa of ends
- Tension free anastomosis

STEPS

Incision and Dissection of Distal Urethra

1. Incision: Midline perineal/lambda shaped incision is made
2. Subcutaneous tissue is divided
3. Bulbospongiosus muscle is divided in midline raphe till perineal body and then reflected off the spongiosum
4. Looping of bulbar urethra is done followed by circumferential mobilization till suspensory ligament distally and obliterated segment proximally
5. Bulb is mobilized from the perineal body followed by division of urethra distal to obliteration (as guided by Foley's catheter or sound) (3 cm urethral length gain)
6. Fibrous tissue is trimmed till healthy edges are seen.
7. Bleeding from spongiosum maybe controlled with gentle pressure or application of Bulldog clamp
8. Haygroove's dilator is passed from suprapubic tract and palpated in perineum to identify proximal urethra
9. Incision is made on the tip of dilator/sound till lumen is visible
10. Excision of all callus is done till healthy tissue and supple urethra is seen
11. Beware of vessels at 11 o'clock and 1 o' clock position
12. At this point verumontanum should be visible
13. Check whether approximation of urethral ends is possible or not.

Crural Separation (2 cm Urethral Length Gain)

1. Done if proximal urethra cannot be identified by palpation of sound or ends of urethra are far apart
2. The corpora can be split over 4–6 cm in the midline and intercrural plane
3. This allows the urethra to lie between the crura rather than on the surface of the crura
4. Beware—not to enter corpora and injure the dorsal penile vessels
5. This maneuver is sufficient in 50% cases to reduce tension on anastomosis

Inferior Pubectomy (2 cm Urethral Length Gain)

1. Done if access remains restricted despite corporal splitting or the urethra cannot be anastomosed without tension
2. Corpora are separated fully to expose the pubic periosteum and it can be incised with diathermy done to bone

3. Inferior half of pubic symphysis can be excised using a hammer, chisel and bone rongeur (or similar instrument)
4. This will allow tension free anastomosis in 10–15% cases

Supracorporal Rerouting of Urethra (2 cm Urethral Length Gain)

- Required rarely, when despite previous maneuvers, anastomosis is under tension
- Distal urethra is rerouted above the corpora on one side after creating a tunnel
- Ensure adequate channel and not to leave any bony spike

ANASTOMOSIS

- Proximal and distal urethral ends are spatulated
- 4-0 or 5-0 absorbable suture are used (polyglactin or PDS)
- Lateral fixation of mucosa of proximal end is done
- Six sutures are placed through the full thickness of the proximal urethra at 2, 4, 6, 8, 10, and 12 o'clock positions
- Ensure epithelium with adequate bit of the surrounding tissue in each suture to make sure the sutures hold
- The sutures are then passed through the distal end of the urethra and tied "parachute" style
- 14 Fr or 16 Fr per urethral catheter is inserted either after posterior sutures are tied or after completion of anastomosis
- Suprapubic catheter should be changed

Closure

- The wound is then closed in layers (bulbocavernosus, subcutaneous tissue and skin)
- Obliterate all the dead space as far as possible to reduce the risk of hematoma formation
- If dead space cannot be obliterated by suture, then a wound drain should be left in place
- This is usually necessary in those patients who have had a wedge pubectomy or rerouting of the urethra
- Sterile dressing is applied and catheters are strapped

Postoperative Care

- IV antibiotics for 48 hours to 5 days
- Elastic compression stockings
- LMWH if needed in high risk patients

- Pericatheter urethrogram and catheter removal after 2-6 weeks (as per institutional protocol)
- Baseline uroflow at catheter removal and later at 6 months
- SPC can be removed after 1 week if voiding satisfactory

COMPLICATIONS

1. Related to patient positioning:
   a. Compartment syndrome
   b. Neuropraxia, with motor deficits
   c. Rhabdomyolysis
   d. Deep vein thrombosis and pulmonary thromboembolism
2. Recurrence of stricture/obliteration:
   Causes:
   a. Inadequate proximal exposure
   b. Inadequate scar excision
   c. Spatulated urethra <30 Fr
   d. Non tension free repair
3. Ischemic stenosis of anterior/bulbar urethra
4. Incontinence
5. Wound infection
6. Erectile dysfunction

VESICOVAGINAL FISTULA REPAIR

Vaginal Repair

It has the following advantages:
- Reduced operative time
- Minimal blood loss
- The bladder is untouched or not opened separately
- Concomitant prolapse surgery maybe done
- Local flaps can be easily placed
- Quicker postoperative recovery

Abdominal Repair

Advocated when there is:
- Associated complex fistula involving other organs in addition to vesicovaginal fistula (VVF)—involving ureter, rectum, colon.
- Procedures requiring augmentation cystoplasty—tubercular fistula and postradiation
- Large fistulas > 5 cm with multiple failed attempts

Vaginal repair (by Shlomo Raz): After proper positioning of the patient, cystoscopy is done to assess VVF. Urethral catheter maybe placed and episiotomy performed, if required. If concomitant vaginal surgery is required, it is done before the repair is started. After infiltration, fistula tract, and bladder are separately cannulated with Foley's catheter and vagina marked in U, J or Mercedes Benz shaped incision. Fistula is not excised as it may lead to bleeding. It may extend to the bladder opening and the tissue of chronic fistula may add some strength to vagina. Vagina is adequately mobilized to create two flaps. The fistula is closed with interrupted sutures in vertical or transverse fashion, incorporating bladder wall and fistula tract. Second layer is for imbrication of perivesical fascia approximately 5 mm from first suture layer and at 90 degrees angle from the first suture line. Interpositional peritoneal or Martius flap is advanced below vaginal mucosa to reach the area of closure. Then, vaginal wall flaps are advanced over the fistula. Excess vaginal tissue is excised and closed by running suture. Bladder needs to be checked for integrity before vaginal closure. Grafts which can be used vaginally are Martius flap, Martius with overlying skin and peritoneal flap, gluteus muscle flap, tensor fascia lata and gracilis flap.

Latzko repair (1942): This technique involves extension of vaginal epithelium around the fistula and closure of epithelium, i.e., colpocleisis, with several layers of absorbable sutures join anterior to posterior wall to obliterate the vagina. Vaginal shortening may occur by this method.

Webster has reported results with vaginal cuff excision. Here, fistula tract is isolated and excised leaving funnel shaped defect between bladder and vagina. This defect is closed in several layers with absorbable sutures.

Abdominal approach (O' Conner 1950) suprapubic, intra- or extraperitoneal approach: Bladder is exposed either intra- or extraperitoneally and opened. Cystostomy is extended upto the VVF. VVF tract is excised. Dissection is continued in vesicovaginal space and vagina dissected off the VVF beyond the VVF tract. Vagina is closed with absorbable sutures. Flap of peritoneum is placed and bladder is closed in routine manner.

Transvesical approach: Here, bladder is not bivalved but opened at anterior vaginal wall. VVF tract is excised. Vagina is mobilized from the bladder and they are closed separately. Posterior wall of bladder maybe brought down as flap. The flaps which can be utilized are:
- Bladder
- Myocutaneous flap of rectum, sartorius, gracilis
- Omentum
- Peritoneal flaps

Bladder mucosa as free graft has also been utilized for VVF repair. Vascularized ileal segment can also be utilized for simultaneous bladder and vaginal augmentation and closure.

Complications:
1. Fistula recurrence
2. Injury to surrounding structures including ureters
3. Decreased vaginal size and length leading to dyspareunia.

NEPHRECTOMY

PREOPERATIVE EVALUATION

1. Cardiovascular systems is stressed due to position, blood loss and other causes such as limited excursion of diaphragm.
2. Cross-sectional imaging to evaluate the vasculature and other anatomical landmarks.
3. Contralateral kidney function
4. Treatment of active urinary infection

Site verification: Confirming the side of surgery, marking of surgical site and documentation is important.

Subcostal flank approach: It is suitable for pediatric patients.

Supracostal approach: Either above 11th/12th rib popularized by Turner. It is effective in radical and partial nephrectomy. It also begins from lateral border of sacrospinalis up to lateral border of ipsilateral rectus abdominis muscle. Care should be taken to avoid damage to pleura.

Thoracoabdominal approach: Ideal for large renal and suprarenal masses and tumors with inferior vena cava (IVC) thrombus. It can extend from 8th rib to contralateral rectus abdominis muscle or upto pubic symphysis.

Disadvantages: Morbidity, postoperative discomfort, possible injury to spleen rare complications: Hemidiaphragm paralysis, injury to costal cartilage leading to annoying clicking sensation.

Anterior midline approach: It is used for renal trauma and associated intraperitoneal injury, endovascular surgery and bilateral renal procedures. Incision is between xiphoid process and symphysis pubis. Entire bowel needs to be reflected depending upon side, to permit access to renal axis.

Chevron incision: Ideal for renovascular surgeries, IVC thrombectomy. Incision extends between tips of both 11th ribs parallel to coastal margin.

INDICATIONS FOR SIMPLE NEPHRECTOMY

- Nonfunction of kidney due to obstruction, infection, trauma.
- High grade VUR with non-functioning kidney with recurrent UTI
- Nephrectomy for functional obstruction due to intractable symptoms such as bleeding, pain, hypertension and intractable infection.
- Pretransplant nephrectomy for ADPKD for refractory hypertension, hematuria, large size obviating transplant.

STEPS

1. Posterior layer of renal fascia is dissected from posterior abdominal wall.
2. Anterior layer is dissected from peritoneum.
3. Gerota fascia incised and perirenal fat dissected.
4. Attention to aberrant vessels should be given.
5. Aspiration of pelvis contents will be necessary at times.
6. Adrenal glands are spared.
7. Superior attachment to spleen, liver, pancreas is freed.
8. Inferior attachment of ureter and gonadal vein are taken care of and divided.
9. Hilar structures are dissected and divided.
10. The specimen is delivered out and the incision closed in layers after keeping a drain in the wound.

PARTIAL NEPHRECTOMY

Indications

- Malignant tumors 4–7 cm
- Benign diseases like caliectasis with parenchymal atrophy
- Infected calyceal diverticulum
- Segmental renal injury
- Benign renal tumors

Relative Contraindications

- <20% nephron mass is retained
- Diffuse encasement of renal pedicle by tumor
- Diffuse involvement of pelvicalyceal system
- Renal vein/IVC involvement
- Adjacent organ invasion
- Regional lymphadenopathy

Procedures

- Lateral position
- 11th rib cutting incision
- Dissect hilum and loop renal artery and vein
- Identify tumor location with the help of intraoperative USG
- Mark the tumor location and do not remove perinephric fat over the tumor
- Clamp the renal vessels and surround the kidney with ice slush to decrease the core renal temperature
- *Simple enucleation*: Renal occlusion is not necessary. Tumor is excised with adequate margin. Frozen section of deep margin is optional. Hemostasis is achieved. Pelvicalyceal system checked for injury. Horizontal mattress sutures are used for closure

- *Wedge resection*: 1 cm margin used to take a wedge shaped incision and tumor is removed with blunt and sharp dissection. Bleeding vessels are controlled. PCS injury is checked for. Renal defect reconstructed using bolster and pledges. Fibrin glue may or may not be used. Renal vessels are unclamped and checked for bleeding.
- *Segmental nephrectomy*: IV mannitol and furosemide are used. Vascular control is taken. If possible, segmental artery is isolated and dissected. Line of ischemia can be observed by selective clamping if possible. Renal cooling done to 20°C for 15 minutes. With blunt and sharp dissection, whole kidney mobilized. Hemostasis is achieved. PCS is repaired with horizontal mattress sutures. Pedicle is declamped. Double-J stent is inserted over guidewire and kept for 4 weeks.

Complications

Intraoperative

1. Hemorrhage: Though surgeries previously required transfusion, transfusion rate is now 3–15% and hemorrhage is common for neoplastic conditions.
   a. Arterial hemorrhage:
      i. Accurate knowledge of renal anatomy
      ii. Accessory renal artery in 25%
      iii. Avoiding injury to gonadal, adrenal and inferior phrenic arteries
   b. Venous anatomy
      i. Multiple renal veins in 1%
      ii. Extensive collateral vessels maybe seen in IVC thrombosis, renal malignancies and AV malformations

Preoperative embolization: It was supposed to theoretically reduce the blood loss, though not documented in most studies. Possible benefits include shrinkage of arterialized tumor. In anticipated difficult hilar dissection when anatomical approach to arteries is difficult (larger hilar tumor, bulky nodal disease, encasement of artery) and ability to ligate the renal vein before the renal artery. However, postinfarction syndrome (flank pain, nausea, vomiting) is seen in three-fourths of patients and at times increased edema secondary to renal infarction makes dissection difficult.

Other complications are:
1. Postoperative ileus
2. Acute renal failure due to accidental embolization of contralateral kidney
3. Accidental embolization of other organs such as spinal cord.
4. Occasionally associated with embolization of tumor thrombus causing sudden death. Mortality rate is 3.3%
- Avulsion of the lumbar veins must be avoided as they are thin walled and retract into paraspinal muscles. Compression is effective at times a bolster with figure of 8 suture will help in tamponade of vein.

- *Hematomas*: They are common when large potential spaces are left behind. Verification of dry surgical bed is necessary as healthy person may loose >25% of volume before having symptoms.
- *Splenic injury*: Common in obese, increasing age, large left kidney in upper polar regions. Incidence is 2–26% (2% in donor nephrectomy).
- *Mechanism*: Inadequate exposure
- Excessive retraction on spleen
- Direct injury during dissection of large tumors
- *Prevention*: Early and complete division of renocolic and lienorenal attachments.
- Splenorrhaphy, coagulation, hemostatic products, wrapping with mesh and splenectomy maybe necessary.
  Vaccination of pneumococcus, *Haemophilus* and meningococcal infection are advocated after splenectomy. Sepsis is more serious after splenectomy.
- *Pancreatic injuries*: Incidence is 1%. It is seen during Kocher's maneuver on right side and injury to tail on left side.
  Risk factors:
- Previous surgery
- Inflammation and difficult dissection at hilum
  Simple injury can be tackled with nonabsorbable suture and dissection of distal pancreas. Help of GI surgeons should be taken. Postoperative increase in amylase and lipase levels can be managed by nasogastric tube and parenteral alimentation. Fluid collection suggestive of pancreatitis and leak may require intervention. Octreotide to decrease pancreatic output is suggested.
- *Duodenal injuries*: Simple injuries maybe closed with two layer technique and reinforced with omentum. Larger injuries should involve GI surgeons, feeding jejunostomy and specialized attention.

COMPLICATIONS OF PARTIAL NEPHRECTOMY

1. Positive margin: Negative margin dictates oncologic efficacy of surgery. However, thickness of margin kept beyond tumor does not predict negative margin. Frozen section of shaved margin is widely used but is impractical in oncologic efficacy.
2. Bleeding: It can be intraoperative or immediately postoperative or upto several weeks following surgery.
3. Urine leak: Urinary fistula is defined as urinary leakage persisting for >4 weeks. Careful closure of collecting system, proper identification of calyceal injury, ureteral drainage, drainage of surgical site, prevention of infection can prevent urinary leak. Retrograde instillation of methylene blue, use of tissue glue and two-layered closure with imbricated suture that keep parenchyma over defect are useful. Early leak is treated conservatively with treatment of infection and relieving any obstruction

(stenting). Delayed leak beyond 48 hours should be investigated by CT urogram and proper repositioning of drain. Placement of drain for any urinoma, antibiotics, treatment of any blood clots or debris in collecting system may be required.
4. Renal dysfunction: Functional renal outcome depends upon length of arterial clamping, amount of parenchyma resected, intraoperative blood pressure variation, fluid resuscitation and aggressive handling of patient with diabetes, hypertension, cardiovascular disease, solitary kidney have increased risk.

RADICAL NEPHRECTOMY

It involves complete removal of kidney with ipsilateral adrenal gland. Complete lymphadenectomy consists of lymph nodes removal from diaphragm to aortic bifurcation as dissected by Robson.

Many a times, adrenal gland is spared and lymphadenectomy done in selected cases.

Indications

Renal tumors are not amenable for partial nephrectomy. Adrenalectomy is indicated when there is:
- Large, upper polar tumor
- Extrarenal extension
- Adrenal mass on imaging

Regional lymphadenectomy is done:
- When there are enlarged lymph nodes on imaging
- Presence of tumor necrosis on imaging
- Tumor size >10 cm
- Extrarenal extension
- Invasion of extrarenal organ

STEPS

1. Anesthesia: General anesthesia
2. Position: Lateral
3. Incision: 11th rib cutting incision
4. Incise skin, subcutaneous and muscles
5. Identify 11th rib, elevate the periosteum and cut the rib, taking care of pleura
6. Do not open the Gerota's fascia
7. Identify the ureter and hook it
8. Dissect the kidney all around
9. On right side, reflect peritoneum and duodenum medially
10. Identify renal artery, ligate and cut
11. Identify IVC, renal vein, ligate and cut

12. On left side, reflect peritoneum medially
13. Identify renal artery and renal vein
14. Ligate artery followed by renal vein, the renal vein can be ligated above insertion of adrenal vein into renal vein
15. Ligate and cut the ureter
16. Check hemostasis
17. Points of help: Renal artery is identified just behind the renal vein. However, in difficult dissection, it can be dissected in interaortocaval region at its origin from the aorta. Identification of artery can be done lateral to IVC and in difficult cases after entire mobilization of renal tumor posteriorly, vein should be palpated and if flaccid, ligated twice. Gonadal vein can be ligated but is spared by many surgeons. Many a times, en bloc ligation of pedicle can be done after placement of long vascular Satinsky clamps. The risk of AV fistula with en bloc ligation is not evident from various series.
18. Regional lymphadenectomy

For right sided tumor, paracaval, precaval, retrocaval and interaortocaval lymphatic tissue is cleared cranially from diaphragm 4 cm above right renal vein and caudally upto bifurcation of IVC. Laterally it is upto anterior border of aorta. Care should be taken about lumbar veins and lymphatic trunks on left side as they drain into cisterna chyli and thoracic duct. On left side, lymphatic dissection extends from anterior surface of aorta to medial surface of IVC and lower extent upto iliac crest, superior extent is upto origin of SMA. Interaortocaval nodes are dissected if they are palpable.

PYELOPLASTY

There are various ways in which pyeloplasty can be done. Different techniques are described below.

DISMEMBERED PYELOPLASTY

1. It is most universally applicable surgery allowing excision of abnormal ureteropelvic junction (UPJ). However, it is not suited for associated proximal ureteric strictures and small intrarenal UPJ. After surgical exposure of UPJ and proximal ureter, area of excision should be marked with fine sutures. Reduction pyeloplasty is excision of redundant portion of enlarged pelvis keeping 1.5 cm distal to renal margin. The proximal ureter is spatulated on its lateral aspect and the apex brought upto the inferior dependent margin of cut renal pelvis. The ureteral plate is brought upto the superior aspect of cut pelvis. Anastomosis should be dependent, water tight, tension free, full thickness, mucosa to mucosa and adequate lumen of 8 Fr or more. Accessory vessels can be transposed posteriorly.
2. *Y-V Plasty (Foley's)*: A "V"-shaped incision on lateral aspect of ureter is converted into a 'Y', keeping one wall intact. It is of little value in presence

of accessory vessels and a large pelvis. The "V'" flap is based on the medial aspect of the pelvis and ureter and brought down to the spatulation of the proximal ureter ('Y').
3. *Culp-DeWeerd spiral flap*: It is suitable for large extrarenal pelvis with long segment of upper ureter which is narrow and strictured. Flap is outlined with broad base obliquely on most dependent part of pelvis. The base of flap is between the renal parenchyma and ureteral insertion lateral to the UPJ. The length of flap is determined by length of defect and it is important to maintain vascularity of the flap. The anastomosis is performed with inverted sutures.
4. *Scardino spiral flap*: It is similar to vertical flap except that the base is positioned more vertically on the dependent part of renal pelvis. Side and length of the flap are determined by length of the ureter to be bridged. Incision is carried out through the proximal ureter and flap is rotated down to the most inferior aspect of the ureterotomy.
5. *Intubated anastomosis*: It is useful for multiple strictures in the ureter in association with PUJ obstruction. It may be combined with vertical or spiral flap if length of stricture is long.

    Internal stenting is necessary as ureterotomy heals by secondary intention. Diverting nephrostomy also allows for antegrade radiological studies 6 weeks postoperatively.
6. *Ureterocalycostomy*: The kidney is mobilized to gain access to the lower pole. Lower pole parenchyma must be excised to expose lower calyx which is anastomosed to ureter over a stent and indwelling nephrostomy. A full set of circumferential sutures is securely placed in anastomosis covered with perineal or omental flap.

COMPLICATIONS

1. Hematoma
2. Urinoma
3. Urinary ascites secondary to stent migration
4. Transient ileus
5. Retroperitoneal hematoma
6. Prolonged drainage of urine from anastomotic leakage may require Foley's catheterization and repositioning of drain and percutaneous nephrostomy (PCN). It may be due to stent migration or clot obstruction. Urinoma may occur in spite of meticulous suturing and stent placement and can be detected by persistent drain output and checked by drain creatinine. Position of drain needs to be checked radiologically and repositioning done if required. CT scan with IV contrast maybe required to check for urine leak. It can be managed by Foley's catheter drainage, percutaneous drainage of urinoma and PCN. Restricturing at UPJ after stent removal at 4–6 weeks of surgery may be relieved by treatment of infection or restenting. Conservative treatment with balloon dilatation maybe tried.

SURGERIES FOR VUR

PRINCIPLES OF ANTIREFLUX SURGERY

1. Treatment and proper management of causes of vesicoureteric reflux
2. Mobilization of distal ureter and preserving its blood supply
3. Creating an intravesical tunnel in a ratio of 5:1
4. Attention to entry point of the ureter in the bladder
5. Angle, direction and point of entry of ureter in the bladder has to be properly decided.
6. Mucosa to mucosa anastomosis of ureter and bladder, adequate vascular packing should be done

APPROACHES

1. Intravesical
2. Extravesical
3. Combined

Also, on the basis of neomeatus in relation to hiatus—suprahiatal or infrahiatal

Preoperative cystoscopy is necessary to detect subtle anomalies, inflammatory changes, ureterocele and diverticulum.

Incision: Pfannenstiel, Gilvernet, paramedian, midline
- The ureters need to be dissected with maximum care to prevent injury to their blood supply. Intravesical technique—the bladder is opened on the anterior wall taking care not to extend incision into the bladder neck.
- Mucosa of the bladder needs to be handled carefully.
- The ureters are cannulated to maintain their proper caliber.
- A circumscribing incision is made and ureter mobilized by sharp dissection.
- Submucosal tunnel maybe supra or subhiatal.

RADICAL PROSTATECTOMY

It has been reported 150 years ago (Kuschler 1886, Young 1905). It remains the gold standard as other modalities are never curative and cancer can develop in remaining tissue.

Advantages:
- Possibility of cure in properly selected patients with minimal damage, if properly performed.
- Accurate tumor staging by pathological examination.
- Treatment failure is readily identified.
- Morbidity and mortality has been significantly low.
- Other modalities of treatment can be successfully applied in case of recurrence.

Surgical morbidity depends on:
- Surgical experience
- Age and comorbidities
- Anatomy of prostate and pelvis
- Preoperative modalities such as radiotherapy

Survival, continence and potency are priorities of patient, known as trifecta.

SURGICAL APPROACH

Open Abdominal Surgery

This approach has lower risk for rectal injury. Prostatic excision and neurovascular preservation decrease the risk of positive surgical margins.

Laparoscopy

It is associated with less bleeding, better visualization, decreased postoperative pain and early recovery. Extraperitoneal and transperitoneal approach has been described. Earlier reported complications of thermal injury, rectal, ureteral and vascular injury and other complications are comparable to open surgery and better in high volume centers.

Robotic Surgery

No superiority has been seen between open, laparoscopic or robotic surgery, both functionally and oncologically. However, it is associated with lower transfusion rate, shorter hospital stays and lower positive surgical margins. Long-term surgical control is better documented for open prostatectomy and surgical experience helps in decreasing complications is well documented.

Perineal Approach

It requires a surgeon familiar with this approach. It is associated with less blood loss.

Disadvantages:
- Access for pelvic lymphadenectomy is not there.
- Increased rate of rectal injury and fecal incontinence.

SURGICAL TECHNIQUE

It involves removal of prostate, seminal vesicle and modified pelvic lymph node dissection. Pelvic lymph node dissection is optional for low risk metastasis and patient can have an option of not proceeding with radical prostatectomy if lymph nodes are positive on frozen section.

Steps

1. Bilateral pelvic lymphadenectomy
2. Dissection and opening of endopelvic fascia
3. Suture ligation of DVC
4. Dissection of urethra at the apex and its transection
5. Dissection of prostate from neurovascular bundle
6. Transection of prostatic pedicle
7. Transection and resection of bladder neck
8. Dissection of seminal vesicle and transection of vas deferens
9. Vesicourethral anastomosis

An anterior or posterior approach can be used depending on surgeon preference.

COMPLICATIONS

Intraoperative Complications

1. Bleeding: Most commonly encountered during division of DVC. Rate of blood transfusion is variable, from 2 to 21% with average blood loss of 300 mL to 2 L. Factors responsible for control of bleeding include knowledge of proper anatomy of DVC, endopelvic fascia and puboprostatic ligaments.
2. Cancer control: Primary objective of radical prostatectomy is to completely excise the cancer, and end points for cancer control are:
   a. Surgical margin
   b. Detectable serum prostate-specific antigen (PSA)
   c. Local recurrence
   d. Metastasis
3. Rectal injury: Common in patients with previous radiation, transurethral resection, bleeding at the time of prostatic biopsy. Salvage RP has highest rate of 6–15%. Following division of posterior urethra, rectourethralis muscle and Denonvilliers fascia is encountered. If this is not divided properly, traction of prostate can result in shearing of Denonvilliers fascia and injury. Hence, dissection of Denonvilliers fascia must be complete and done by sharp dissection. Excessive bleed will prevent seeing the tissue planes clearly. Simple rectal injury can be treated with resection of devitalized tissue and two-layered closure. Presence of large injury or soiling should lead to temporary diverting colostomy. Rectourethral fistula following rectal injury is seen in 15–43% and greatest risk is in patients with unrecognized injury and irradiation.
4. Ureteric injury: It can occur at the level of bladder neck dissection or during lymphadenectomy. In patient with large median lobe, ureteric orifices can be damaged if not visualized during bladder neck transection. On rare occasion, injury to ureter can occur during seminal vesicle dissection.

Early Postoperative Complications

1. Urinary leak: True incidence is not known as small leaks are never diagnosed. It was reported that intraoperative blood loss resulting in hematoma could cause disruption of vesicourethral anastomosis, leading to urinary leak. It usually settles with adequate catheter retropubic drainage. Pelvic suction drains can be used in addition to gravity drainage. It is important to ensure that tip of the drain is not abutting or migrated into anastomosis. The patient may have catheter blockage due to a bladder clot leading to a leak. Leak persisting for >10 days is a cause of concern. Complete disruption of anastomosis is rare and healing occurs in anastomosis over a catheter. However, postoperative bladder neck contracture is common in these patients. Cross-sectional imaging should be done in patients with fever and percutaneous drainage of pelvic collections should be done.
2. Loss of catheter: Occasionally, Foley's catheter may fall out following RP in early postoperative period. It is unwise to attempt reinsertion of catheter. Use of cystoscopy under anesthesia is safest. If one is unable to get across the anastomosis, then suprapubic cystostomy is placed under sonographic guidance. Reconstruction of anastomosis is a difficult surgery and it is best to perform a cystostomy and attempt antegrade passage of a catheter. In presence of severe hematuria, open suprapubic cystostomy may be done.
3. Erectile dysfunction: It is defined as inability to maintain erection for penetration with/without help of phosphodiesterase type 5 (PDE5) inhibitors. Several factors influence the return of erectile function, e.g., age, preoperative potency, extent of nerve sparing done unilaterally or bilaterally, diabetes, hypertension and medications. Technical factors include avoiding local cauterization, recognition of nerve bundles and preservation of surrounding tissues, avoiding placement of deep sutures for control of bleeding, traction injury and freeing nerves completely before division of the urethra. Erections return within 3-6 months postoperatively and patients can be encouraged to use various erectile aids such as intracavernosal injection (ICI) therapy, PDE5 inhibitors to hasten the return of erections.

RADICAL CYSTECTOMY

Midline incision, from umbilicus to symphysis pubis. Space of Retzius is entered. Blunt dissection is performed to release the bladder from the pelvic sidewall attachments bilaterally. This is carried in a cephalad direction to the level of the vas deferens in men and the round ligament in women. Next, the urachus is controlled and divided as high as possible and peritoneum between the two median umbilical ligaments is included in dissection. On either side, mobilization is done to adequately expose the great vessels and the ureters.

Bilateral ureters are dissected free and divided close to the bladder. Superior vesical artery can be ligated and divided for ureteral dissection. Distal margin of ureter maybe sent for frozen section for presence of urothelial carcinoma, depending upon surgeons' preference. In the males, after completely ligating vascular pedicles, peritoneum is incised over seminal vesicles. Rectum is dissected from midline and dissection carried at level of prostate. It is preferable to do sharp dissection to avoid rectal injury. Dissection is carried laterally and the posterior vesical pedicles are identified. After dissection, surgeon should be able to reach prostate and palpate the urethra. Anterior dissection is similar to radical prostatectomy. After ligation of dorsal venous complex, anterior urethra is identified and dissection is completed. Nerve sparing radical cystectomy and subtotal resection are described techniques for prevention of erectile dysfunction. In the females, it included total pelvic exenteration inclusive of the bladder, urethra, anterior vagina, uterus, and cervix. Most of the steps are similar to radical cystectomy in males. However, knowing the steps of hysterectomy and identification of posterior fornix, gaining entry into vaginal canal, dissection of uterus, cervix, anterior vaginal cuff and bladder is essential. Urethral meatus can be excised from the pelvis or the vagina. Closure of vaginal defect is necessary. At times, vaginal sparing surgery is done in absence of bladder neck involvement.

COMPLICATIONS

1. Hemorrhage is the most common complication as the all organs—bladder, prostate, urethra, uterus and vagina, are vascular and require careful and secure vascular control. The anterior trunk of internal iliac artery maybe individually ligated and clipped. The posterior trunk is preserved to avoid gluteal claudication. The other source of bleeding is DVC which would be described under radical prostatectomy.
2. Rectal injury: It is a grave complication if not identified intraoperatively. Its incidence is 0.3-9%. Predisposing factors include:
   a. Prior pelvic surgery
   b. Colonic inflammatory disease
   c. Prior TURP
   d. Extension of the mass posteriorly
   e. Pelvic irradiation

   Intraoperative recognition, appropriate repair, adequate decompensation, adequate pelvic drainage, antibiotics and nutrition support are necessary in treatment. Plane between rectum and Denonvilliers fascia should be made with sharp dissection. Insufflation of the rectum by air when the pelvis is filled with fluid and per rectal examination maybe used to detect suspected injury. Two layer closure with greater omental interposition or if need be, sigmoid loop colostomy maybe done when injury is large or impaired healing is likely due to pelvic irradiation or colonic inflammatory disease.

3. **Venous thromboembolism:** Reported in 1-4% of cystectomy and leads to further complications such as fatal and nonfatal pulmonary embolism. Routine prophylaxis with low dose unfractionated heparin or intermittent pneumatic compression, compression stockings is recommended especially in patients with multiple risk factors such as obesity, smoking, advanced age, immobility, cardiovascular catheterization, oral contraceptives, acute medical illness and thromboembolic disease.
4. **Ileus:** Postoperative ileus is most common complication and cause of morbidity with an incidence of 7-23%. It is defined as delayed return of bowel function beyond 4th postoperative day. Ileus fails to resolve beyond 10th postoperative day after correction of hypokalemia and other electrolyte imbalances will warrant investigations to find out additional causes—intestinal or urinary leak. Bowel decompression and routine fluid management are advocated for treatment.
5. **Bowel leak:** Finding of fever, wound infection, sepsis, delay of return of bowel function should raise suspicion of intraperitoneal abscess from bowel leak or unrecognized trauma. Findings of enteric contents in drain confirm the diagnosis. CT scan is necessary to rule out a leak and distal intestinal obstruction. Conservative management can be done in the absence of peritonitis and controlled fistula along with proximal decompression, hyperalimentation, parenteral nutrition, use of somatostatin analogs. If displaying signs of sepsis or peritonitis, patient will require emergency laparotomy to cleanse the abdominal cavity and proper drainage of pelvis and peritoneum and creation of proximal enterostomy.

Complications After Radiation Therapy

Complications with preoperative radiation vary from 30 to 70% and are commonly wound or pelvic complications, gastrointestinal or genitourinary fistula, and small bowel obstruction. Late complications include stenosis and fistula of both urinary and gastrointestinal system.

ADRENALECTOMY

PREOPERATIVE PREPARATION FOR ADRENALECTOMY

Endocrine Society Clinical Practice Guideline (ESCPG) recommends that all patients with a hormonally functional pheochromocytomas and paragangliomas should undergo preoperative blockade to prevent perioperative cardiovascular complications. They recommend preoperative medical treatment for 7-14 days to allow adequate time to normalize blood pressure and heart rate. Preoperative cardiac evaluation is important, because patients with pheochromocytoma are at risk for cardiomyopathy.

Alpha-adrenergic receptor blockers are the first choice of drugs.

Alpha-1-selective adrenergic receptor blockers are associated with lower preoperative diastolic pressure, a lower intraoperative heart rate, better postoperative hemodynamic recovery and fewer adverse effects such as reactive tachycardia and sustained postoperative hypotension than nonselective adrenergic blockers.

Phenoxybenzamine irreversibly blocks α receptor. Therefore, intraoperative catecholamine surges typically do not override its actions. Oral administration of 10 mg twice daily is initiated and titrated by increase of 10–20 mg to a blood pressure of 120 to 130/80 mm Hg in a seated position. It causes presynaptic inhibition of adrenergic control thus leading to increase in beta adrenergic outflow.

Selective reversible α1-blockers, such as terazosin, doxazosin, or prazosin, are used at some centers. These agents may have fewer side effects than phenoxybenzamine. Prazosin is a selective alpha-1 blocker. No beta-blockade is required. It causes incomplete alpha blockade. Dose is 1–5 mg BD.

Roizen Criteria

To assess the efficacy of preoperative alpha blockade:
- No recording of BP > 160/90 mm Hg for 24 hours before the operation
- No orthostatic hypotension or BP < 80/45 mm Hg
- No ST/T wave changes for 1 week before the operation
- Not more than 5 premature ventricular contractions/minute.

Preoperative coadministration of β-blockers is indicated to control tachycardia only after administration of α-adrenergic receptor blockers. Use of β-blockers in the absence of an α-blocker is not recommended because of the potential for hypertensive crisis due to unopposed stimulation of alpha-adrenergic receptors. Treatment with α-blockers alone has shown to reverse blood volume contraction in only about 60% of patients.

In the absence of α-blockade, β antagonists cause a potentiation of the action of epinephrine on the α1 receptors owing to blockade of the arteriolar dilation at the β2 receptor. Beta blocker may precipitate bronchospasm and CHF.

Esmolol (250 µg/kg/min) can be used intraoperatively to control BP.

Calcium Channel Blockers

Calcium channel blockade lowers blood pressure by generating smooth muscle relaxation. Calcium channel blockers are the most often used add-on drug class to further improve blood pressure control in patients already treated with α-adrenergic receptor blockers. Monotherapy with calcium channel blockers is not recommended unless patient has very mild preoperative hypertension or has severe orthostatic hypotension with α blockers (**Table 1**).

TABLE 1: Drugs used in pre-operative preparation for patients of pheochromocytoma.

Drug	Starting time	Starting dose	Final dose
Preparation 1 Phenoxybenzamine	10–14 days before surgery	10 mg BID	1 mg/kg/day
or Doxazosine		2 mg/day	32 mg/day
Preparation 2 Nifedipine	As add-on to preparation 1 when needed	30 mg/day	60 mg/day
or Amlodipine		5 mg/day	10 mg/day
Preparation 3 Propanolol	After at least 3–4 days of preparation 1	20 mg TID	40 mg TID
Atenolol		25 mg/day	50 mg/day

Catecholamine Synthesis Blockade (α-Metyrosine)

It prevents the conversion of tyrosine to L-dihydroxyphenylalanine (L-DOPA) by inhibiting the tyrosine hydroxylase enzyme. Metyrosine may be used in combination with α blockers for a short period before surgery to further stabilize blood pressure to reduce blood loss and volume depletion during surgery. Blockade of catecholamine synthesis is incomplete if used alone, therefore must be used in combination. Dose: 250 mg QID to 1 g QID. Side effects include sedation, mood depression, extrapyramidal symptoms and galactorrhea.

Volume Replacement

Treatment should also include a high-sodium diet and fluid intake to reverse catecholamine-induced blood volume contraction preoperatively to prevent severe hypotension after tumor removal. Initiation of a high-sodium diet a few days after the start of alpha-adrenergic receptor blockade reverses blood volume contraction, prevents orthostatic hypotension before surgery, and reduces the risk of significant hypotension after surgery. Continuous administration of saline (1–2 L) is also helpful if started in the evening before surgery. Caution is required for volume loading in patients with heart or renal failure.

OPEN ADRENALECTOMY

Laparoscopic adrenalectomy is replacing open adrenalectomy. However, there are few absolute contraindications of laparoscopic approach:
1. Locally recurrent adrenal mass
2. Locally advanced adrenocortical carcinoma
3. Severe cardiopulmonary disease
4. Pregnancy
5. Very large adrenal tumors

Principles: Minimal handling of tumor and en-bloc resection of adrenocortical carcinoma.

Incision:
- Flank incision
- 11th rib or higher up approach
- Lumbodorsal approach
- Anterior transabdominal approach

Steps

The dissection should expose adrenal gland, renal vein, and IVC. Plane between adrenal gland and lateral wall of IVC is developed to expose the adrenal vein. Care must be taken to avoid avulsion of the vein. Adrenal gland is dissected superiorly. Many a times, arterial branches are not identified but whatever vessels are encountered should be ligated and cut. Lastly, anterior and medial margins are taken care of and gland is removed. On the left side, the adrenal gland is approached by mobilizing the descending colon and splenic flexure. Superior retraction of spleen will expose the left adrenal vein as it opens into left renal vein. The medial attachments to the aorta need to be taken either with monopolar diathermy or safely ligated. Inferior dissection is relatively easy. However, left renal artery is to be protected.

Thoracoabdominal approach is used for large tumors and incision is along the 8th or 9th rib and extended into the abdomen. Diaphragm is divided and rest of the dissection is same as any other adrenal surgery.

Intraoperative Management

Preoperative fluid loading is necessary to avoid precipitous fall in blood pressure after adrenalectomy. If there are significant hemodyanamic changes, expected arterial line and other general management is warranted. Correction of hypokalemia and glycemic control should be strictly done. Patients with Cushing syndrome should receive glucocorticoids in perioperative period. Induction of pneumoperitoneum may be associated with significant catecholamine release.

COMPLICATIONS

Intraoperative

Vascular injury is the most common injury especially to the IVC and adrenal vein. Avulsion of vein causes significant bleeding especially on the right side. Vascular injury can be managed with the help of clamps, intracorporeal suturing, exposure of the IVC and suturing. Use of staples and metal clips should be avoided as it may cause adjacent organ injury. Multiple adrenal vessels and accessory vessels occur in 10% of patients. Identification and ligation of branch of inferior phrenic artery may be difficult. Adrenal sparing surgery is considered in patients with MEN syndrome but patient requires close monitoring of adrenal insufficiency.

Postoperative

1. Close blood pressure monitoring is necessary in postoperative period. Any concerns for bleeding should be kept in mind. Patients with pheochromocytomas may develop hypotension due to alpha adrenergic blockers and carry postoperative risk of hyperglycemia. Volume replacement and judicious use of catecholamines is warranted.
2. Primary hyperaldosteronism: Hypokalemia may be present due to continuous potassium loss. Hyperkalemia is also present secondary to failure of contralateral adrenal gland. Daily monitoring of potassium levels should be done and patient should be regularly monitored for salt wasting.
3. Cushing syndrome: Patients undergoing bilateral adrenalectomy are at risk of Nelson disease and recurrent episodes of Addisonian crisis. Short-term mineralocorticoids and long-term corticosteroids are necessary. Acute adrenal insufficiency manifests with fever, nausea, lethargy and hypotension and can be treated with dexamethasone. Patients with Cushing syndrome are prone to hyperglycemia, poor wound healing, infection and fractures secondary to osteoporosis.

PENILE MASS

PARTIAL PENECTOMY

Steps (Figs. 5A to D)

1. The lesion and urine should be cultured preoperatively and appropriate antibiotics started prior to the surgical procedure.
2. The penis is prepared with a povidone-iodine solution, and the tumor isolated using a sterile glove to avoid spillage of cells during penile manipulation.
3. Outline the planned incision with a marking pen, providing an adequate minimum 1-cm margin.
4. A tourniquet is placed around the base of the penis to minimize blood loss.
5. The incision is circumferentially carried through the skin, dartos (superficial fascia), and Buck fascia (deep fascia) to the tunica albuginea.
6. On the dorsum of the penis, the dorsal neurovascular bundle is individually ligated and cut with absorbable sutures.
7. Ventrally, a 1-cm stump of the urethra is created
8. The corpora cavernosa are divided upto the urethra
9. Frozen section can be sent at this point if any doubt exists regarding the surgical margins.

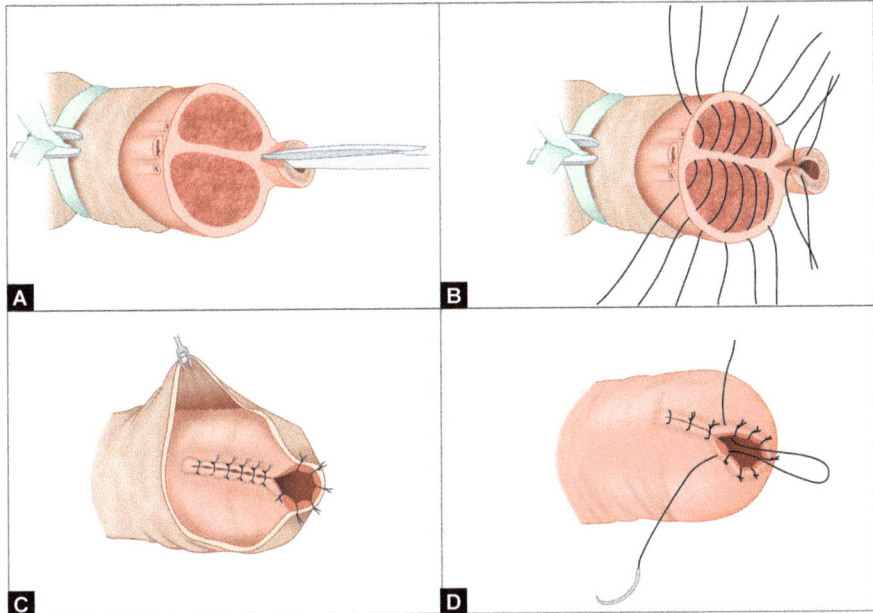

Figures 5A to D: Steps in partial penectomy.

10. The corporal ends are closed with 2-0 absorbable sutures, including the Buck's fascia and tunica albuginea.
11. The penile base tourniquet is then released, and all minor vessels are fulgurated or ligated until adequate hemostasis is achieved.
12. The urethra is spatulated to prevent stenosis of the neomeatus and sutured to the ventral penile skin.
13. A Foley catheter is left indwelling for 48 hours.

TOTAL PENECTOMY

- The patient is placed in low lithotomy position.
- The lesion is prepared and covered with sterile glove and antibiotics are given according to preoperative urine and penile tumor culture.
- Incision is placed circumferentially at the base of the penis with extension into the median raphe of the scrotum.
- The suspensory ligament of the penis is identified and divided at the base of the penis.
- The dorsal vein and penile arteries are identified, ligated and divided.
- The penis is then reflected superiorly, the Buck's fascia is opened ventrally, and the urethra is dissected away from the corpora cavernosa.
- The urethra and corpus spongiosum are mobilized away from the corpora between clamps and divided at the distal bulbar region with adequate length for construction of a perineal urethrostomy.

- The corpora cavernosa are dissected up to the ischiopubic rami, clamped, sectioned, and sutured.
- The perineal urethrostomy is constructed by removing a 1-cm ellipse of skin and subcutaneous tissues from the midperineum, midpoint from the anus and scrotum.
- Midline perineal urethrostomy is performed.
- The urethra is spatulated dorsally, and a V-inlay of skin is created and sutured to the urethra using 3-0 absorbable sutures.
- An 18 Fr Foley catheter is inserted, and drains are kept
- The scrotal incision is closed transversally for elevation of the scrotum away from the perineal urethrostomy using absorbable sutures.
- The Foley catheter is kept for at least 5 days.

Complications

1. Meatal stenosis
2. Bleeding
3. Wound infection
4. Urethral necrosis

RADICAL ORCHIECTOMY

- *Indication*: Carcinoma of testis or its appendages
- *Incision*: Over the inguinal canal, 2 cm superior to inguinal ligament following the lines of Langer (**Fig. 6**).

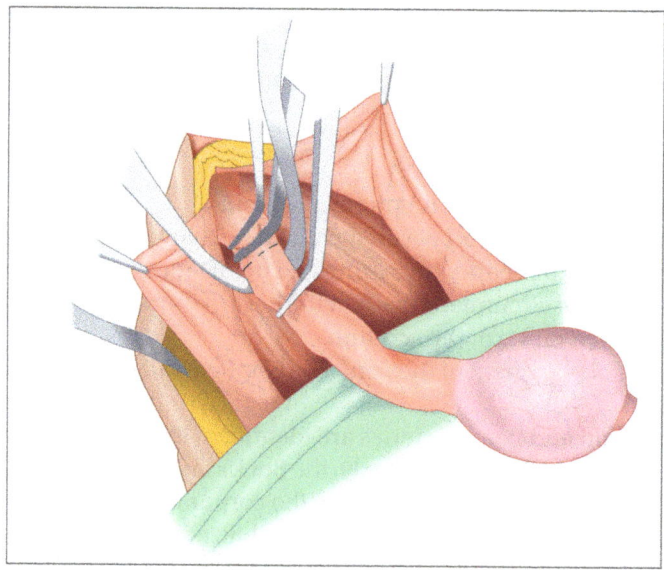

Figure 6: Radical inguinal orchiectomy.

- After incision of skin, subcutaneous tissue and external oblique aponeurosis, the ilioinguinal nerve in the spermatic cord should be encircled and isolated, if possible.
- Mobilize the testis from the scrotum through the external inguinal ring
- Delivery of testicle is done after incising gubernaculum.
- Spermatic cord is ligated anterior at the internal inguinal ring. Vas deferens and gonadal vessels are ligated separately, vas deferens with non-absorbable dark suture so that stump can be retrieved during subsequent retroperitoneal lymph node dissection (RPLND).
- Vas deferens is not taken as a part of specimen.
- Repositioning of ilioinguinal nerve is done followed by closure.

PARTIAL ORCHIECTOMY

- **Indication**: 1. Polar tumors < 2 cm.
- 2. When contralateral testis is subnormal or absent.
- Intraoperative sonography can be used to facilitate localization of mass.
- The testis is delivered from inguinal incision (**Figs. 7A to E**).

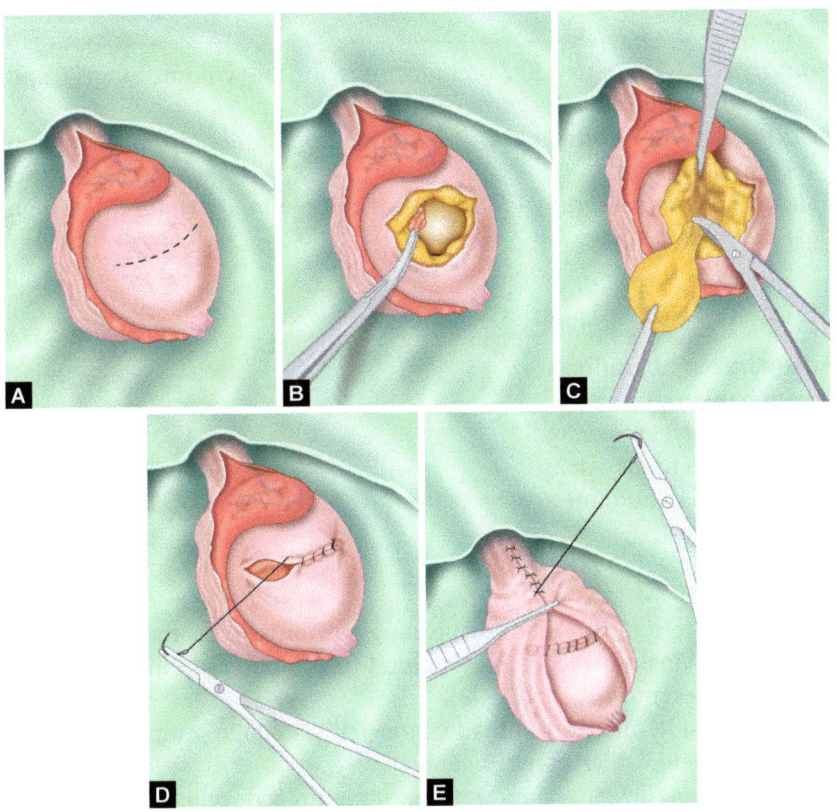

Figures 7A to E: Partial orchiectomy procedure.

- The cord can be clamped and the testis can be kept over crushed ice for cold ischemia.
- Tunica vaginalis and albuginea are opened and the tumor is enucleated with rim of surrounding tissue.
- Additional biopsies can be taken for frozen section.
- After hemostasis, the testis is placed back into the dependent portion of scrotal compartment and secured at three points of internal fixation to the gubernaculum.

COMPLICATIONS

1. Testicular pain/chronic orchialgia
2. Bleeding due to slippage of ligature
3. Tumor spillage, especially during partial orchiectomy
4. Scrotal or inguinal hematoma
5. Retroperitoneal hemorrhage from spermatic cord

RETROPERITONEAL LYMPH NODE DISSECTION

TYPES

1. *Primary RPLND*: Done after orchidectomy for low volume stage 1 and stage 2 nonseminomatous germ cell tumors.
2. *PC-RPLND*: After completion of systemic chemotherapy or remission after chemotherapy.
3. *Salvage postchemotherapy RPLND*: After completion of standard or high dose chemotherapy.

PREOPERATIVE PLANNING

- Adequate blood products
- Sperm banking
- Assess bleomycin toxicity
- Prevention of lung toxicity
- Recent CT scan abdomen, pelvis, chest—within 6 weeks of surgery

STEPS

1. Exposure of retroperitoneum by incising peritoneum on right side from foramen of Winslow to cecum and then from cecum upto medial aspect of inferior mesenteric vein (**Fig. 8**).
2. On the left side, incision is made from left paracolic gutter to inferior mesenteric vein, which can be ligated.
3. Plane between mesentery and retroperitoneum is developed at the level of gonadal vein and extended along its anterior surface.

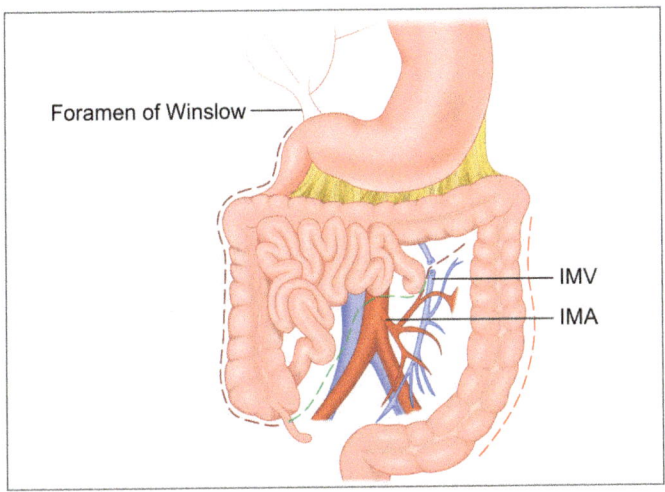

Figure 8: Marking of peritoneal incisions.

4. Falciform ligament maybe divided.
5. Superior mesenteric artery needs to be identified.
6. Split and roll technique started over anterior surface of aorta, rather than IVC.
7. If possible, fibers of superior hypogastric plexus need to be identified.
8. The split is started at the 12 o'clock position of the aorta, immediately inferior to the left renal vein and continued caudally upto inferior mesenteric artery (IMA).
9. If possible, preserve postganglionic sympathetic fibers.
10. Lower extent of dissection is upto left ureteric crossing of common iliac artery.
11. If necessary, lumbar artery and veins need to be doubly ligated and divided.
12. Left gonadal vein also needs to be ligated.
13. Entire packet dissected over lower pole of kidney and left genitofemoral nerve and sympathetic trunk preserved.
14. The lumbar veins and lumbar arteries should be identified and controlled.
15. Superiorly, the packet is rolled up to the crus of the diaphragm.
16. Lymphatics should be ligated as they course through the crus and into the retrocrural region.

Interaortocaval Packet

- Split and roll technique can be commenced on medial side of aorta, extending to IVC and from the renal hilum to the crossover of the right common iliac artery (at the point where it is crossed by right ureter) (**Fig. 9**).

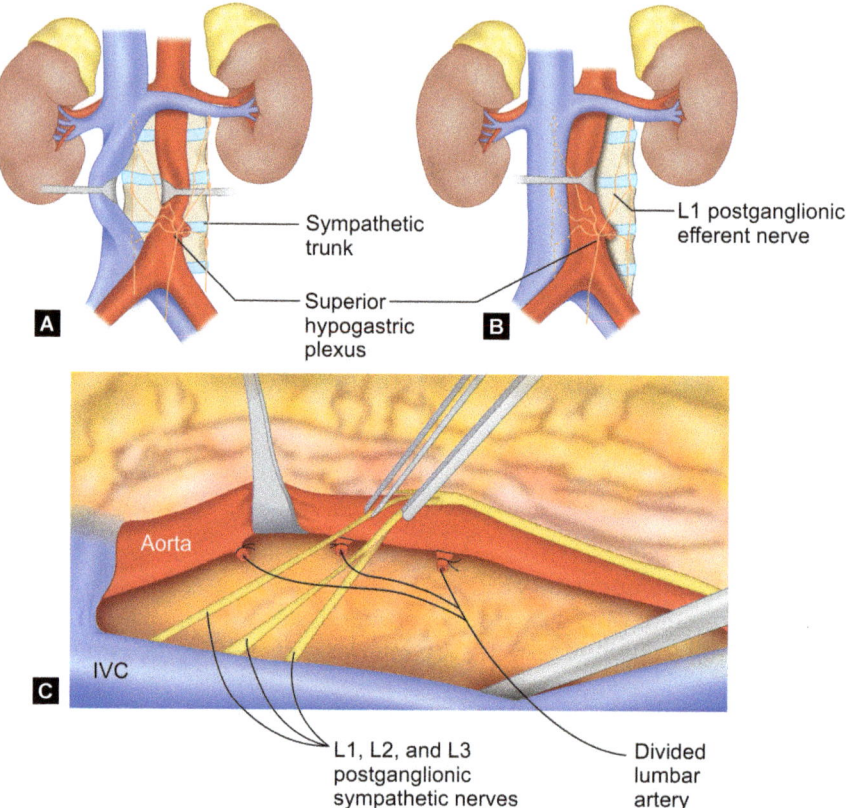

Figures 9A to C: Surgical technique of retroperitoneal lymph node dissection.

- Right gonadal vein is also ligated and divided at the IVC.
- The packet is rolled laterally off of the IVC and any lumbar veins encountered between renal hilum and common iliac veins are ligated and divided.
- Lumbar arteries must be ligated and divided.
- The lymphatic tissue is dissected upto anterior spinous ligament.
- The right sympathetic trunk is encountered at the right lateral border of the interaortocaval packet and should be preserved when possible.
- The superior aspect of the packet is rolled inferiorly off of the renal vessels exposing the crus of the diaphragm and lymphatics coursing into the retrocrural region must be ligated.

Right Paracaval Packet

- Lymphatic tissue is removed from right common iliac artery upto renal hilum, taking care to preserve the right sympathetic trunk and the genitofemoral nerve.

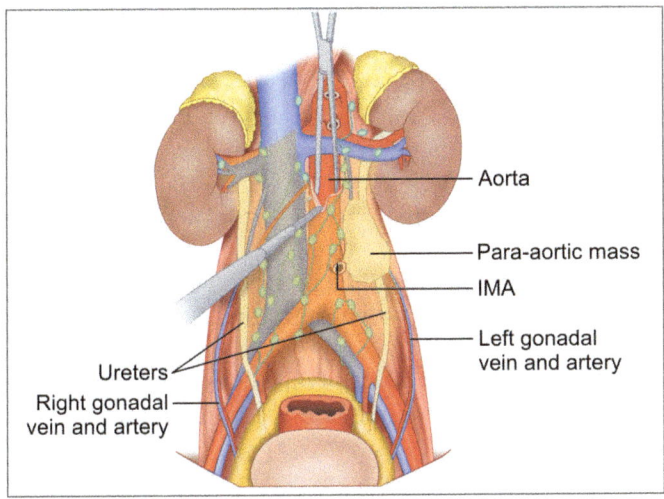

Figure 10: Template boundaries for retroperitoneal lymph node dissection (RPLND).

- Superiorly, lymphatics upto crus of diaphragm are removed. Gonadal vein needs to be removed right upto the internal ring and care needs to be taken on left side to prevent injury to sigmoid colon mesentery (**Fig. 10**).

Preservation of Nerves

- Left postganglionic sympathetic nerves are seen along the lateral border of the aorta and left common iliac artery and onto the anterior surface of these vessels immediately caudal to the IMA.
- They are dissected upto their origin at the sympathetic trunk.
- The right-sided postganglionic nerve fibers are best identified on the anterior surface of the IVC and interaortocaval space and seen going into superior hypogastric plexus.
- When the nerve fibers have been dissected free for the entirety of their courses through the RPLND template, the lymphatic packets around the fibers should be dissected.

Complications

1. Arterial:
   a. Postchemotherapy, there is substantial fibrosis which renders major retroperitoneal blood vessels to injury.
   b. Preoperative signs such as lower limb edema, collateral veins, visualization of IVC on CT scan, need to be kept in mind for need of IVC dissection or reconstruction.
   c. Vascular anomalies of renal vessels need to be noticed.

d. Superior mesenteric artery should be identified early as its injury can lead to major catastrophe.
e. Lymphatic trunks at the base of SMA need to be properly ligated to prevent chylous ascites.
f. Though IMA can be ligated in young patients, ischemic colitis may develop in older patients.
g. Approximately 1% of patients require resection of aorta and aortic replacement.
h. Peeling of tumor in subadventitial plane can leave the aorta devoid of support and may require graft substitution.

2. Venous:
   a. Inferior mesenteric veins (IMV), gonadal vein and lumbar vein can be easily divided. Injury to left side is common because of multiple tributaries.
   b. Injury to left renal vein can be managed by simple sutures, saphenous vein graft or gortex graft.
   c. It may require clamping of renal artery and cooling of kidney.
   d. Extensive injury can mandate nephrectomy.
   e. Injury to IVC is due to laceration and avulsion of lumbar vein.
   f. They enter IVC at its posterolateral aspect and are a common source of bleeding.
   g. Persistent bleeding from lumbar veins may be controlled by oversewing of perivertebral soft tissue along with use of hemostatic agent.
   h. Resection of IVC may be required if tumor is invading the IVC wall or if IVC has desmoplastic reaction.
   i. The incidence of IVC reconstruction is about 8.6% and it is important to resect IVC rather than doing incomplete resection of tumor.
   j. IVC resection leads to venous congestion of lower extremities and accumulation of lymph in them, leading to Budd–Chiari syndrome and chylous ascites.
   k. Contralateral testicular, lower lumbar and pelvic veins can be preserved if possible to allow venous drainage.

3. Lymphocele and chylous ascites:
   a. Unrecognized injury to cysterna chyli, thoracic duct or their tributaries leads to retroperitoneal lymphocele.
   b. Some lymphoceles may lead to retroperitoneal abscess and require percutaneous drainage.
   c. Persistent active lymphatic leakage may require ligation of lymphatic channel and shunting.
   d. Treatment of chylous ascites is repeated paracentesis, hyperalimentation, somatostatin analogs.

4. Ejaculatory dysfunction:
   a. It can occur due to injury to postganglionic sympathetic fibers, which on left side are just below IMA and on right side merge with the IVC.

INFERIOR VENA CAVA THROMBECTOMY

Surgical approach depends upon level of IVC thrombus:
- Early ligation of renal artery
- Mobilization of kidney and necessary vascular structures

Thrombi level I
With Satinsky clamp applied to IVC

Thrombi level II
- Control of caudal IVC, contralateral renal vein, cephalad IVC.
- Ligation of lumbar veins in segment of IVC with thrombus.
- Distal bland emboli can be left in situ and IVC ligated cephalad to this.
- IVC grafting/reconstitution is required only in some cases as collateral supply is usually established.

Thrombi level III/IV
- Exposure of liver, suprahepatic IVC, portal vein, control porta hepatis, cardiopulmonary bypass and venovenous bypass are associated with increased risk of CVA, myocardial infarction, thromboembolic phenomenon and disseminated intravascular coagulation (DIC)
- Measures to decrease possibility of bypass should be considered. Possibility of postoperative Budd–Chiari syndrome should be kept in mind.
- Advocating this surgery in a patient with metastasis with severe intractable edema, ascites may not have any benefit due to perioperative morbidity and low life expectancy.

POLITANO-LEADBETTER TECHNIQUE

- Suprahiatal tunnel medial and superior to the original tunnel in direction of trigone and medial to the orifice is made.
- It is necessary to prevent hooking of ureter at entry into neohiatus.
- The tunnel maybe created with use of right angle clamps or submucosal infiltration.
- The tunnel should be capacious enough and ratio of 5:1 needs to be maintained (**Fig. 11**).
- Before suture anastomosis, it is important to confirm patency and absence of kinks.
- The mucosa of neohiatus should be handled with care.

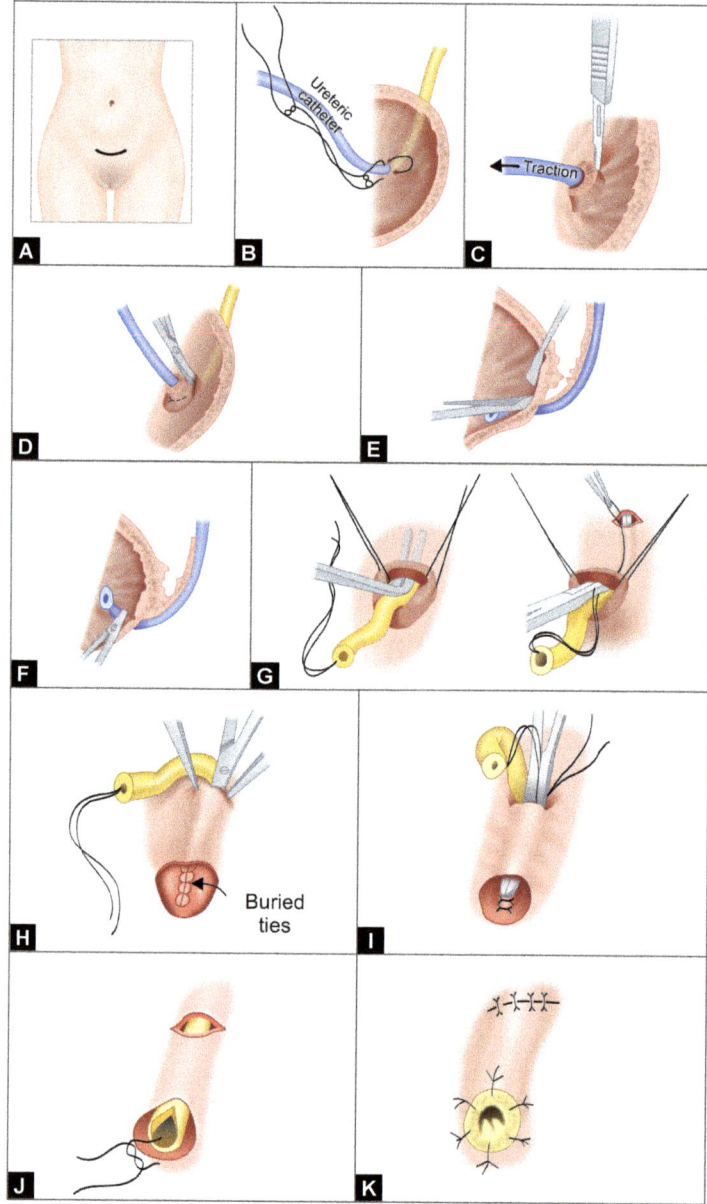

Figure 11A to K: Politano-leadbetter technique.

GLENN ANDERSON TECHNIQUE

- Infrahiatal tunnel is created toward the bladder neck using the same hiatus (**Fig. 12**).
- The detrusor are then reapproximated.
- So, in short it is an advancement of ureter in the bladder neck.

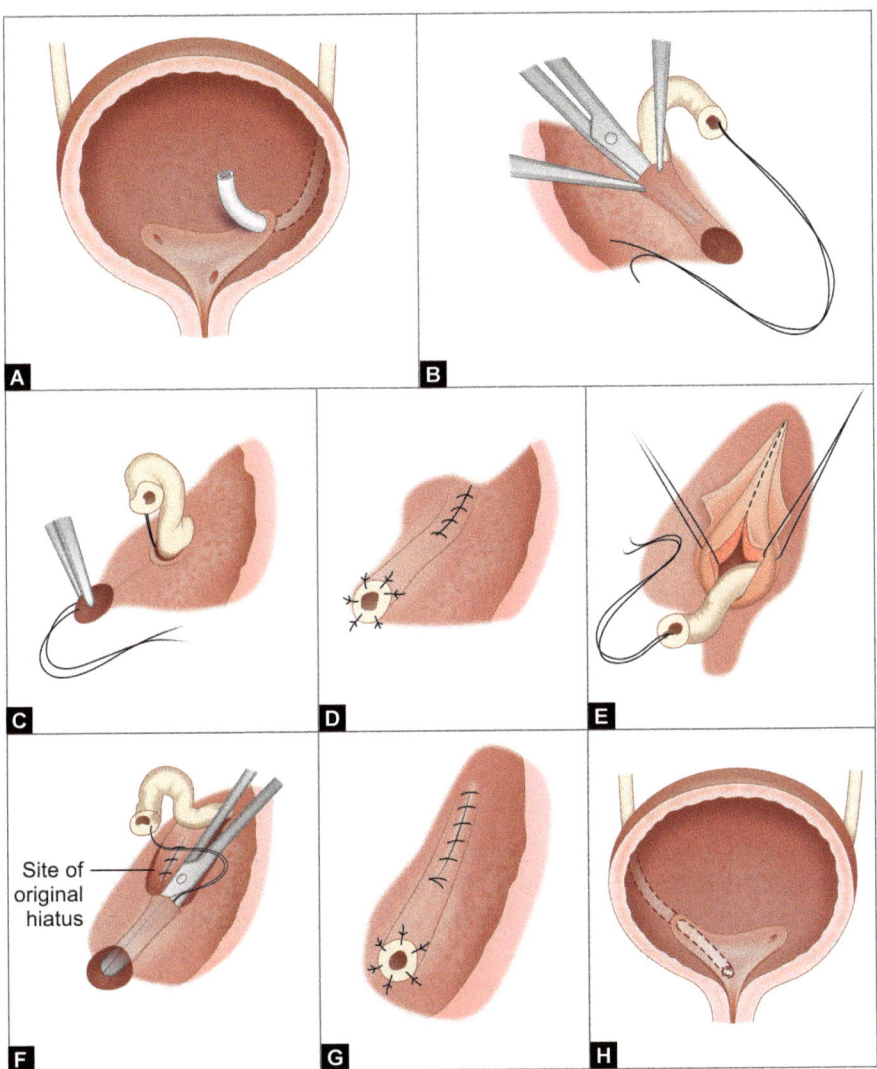

Figure 12: Glenn-Anderson technique.

COHEN'S CROSS TRIGONAL TECHNIQUE

- The tunnel is dissected across the trigone toward the contralateral bladder wall and cross trigonal reimplantation is done (**Fig. 13**).
- Superior displacement of ureter allows bladder neck reconstruction, if necessary.
- Retrograde access to the ureteric orifice postoperatively maybe challenging.
- It is useful when bladder wall is thickened and hiatus is excessively spatulated.

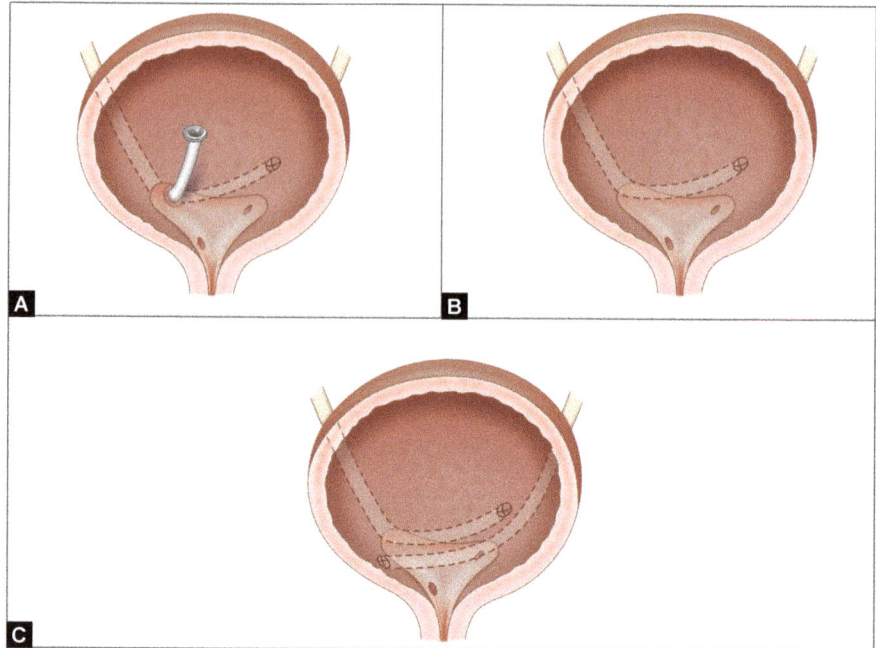

Figure 13: Cohen's Cross-trigonal technique.

LEICH-GREGOIR EXTRAVESICAL APPROACH

- It allows the advancement of ureter without opening the bladder.
- Transient voiding inefficiency has been reported due to excessive stretching of detrusor along medial aspect of ureter just outside the Waldeyer's sheath.
- The ureter is approached extravesically and obliterated umbilical artery maybe divided if necessary.
- To prevent nerve injury, it is necessary to limit dissection to ureteric surface.
- The bladder is made full and a new submucosal tunnel is created by dissecting detrusor flaps (**Fig. 14**).
- The detrusor is dissected off the mucosa along the entire length of tunnel.
- The distal end of ureteric orifice can be advanced by using two vertical sutures as described by Zaontz.
- The ureter is approximated mucosa to mucosa and detrusor closed over it.
- Absence of any constriction or contracture of ureter needs to be checked for.

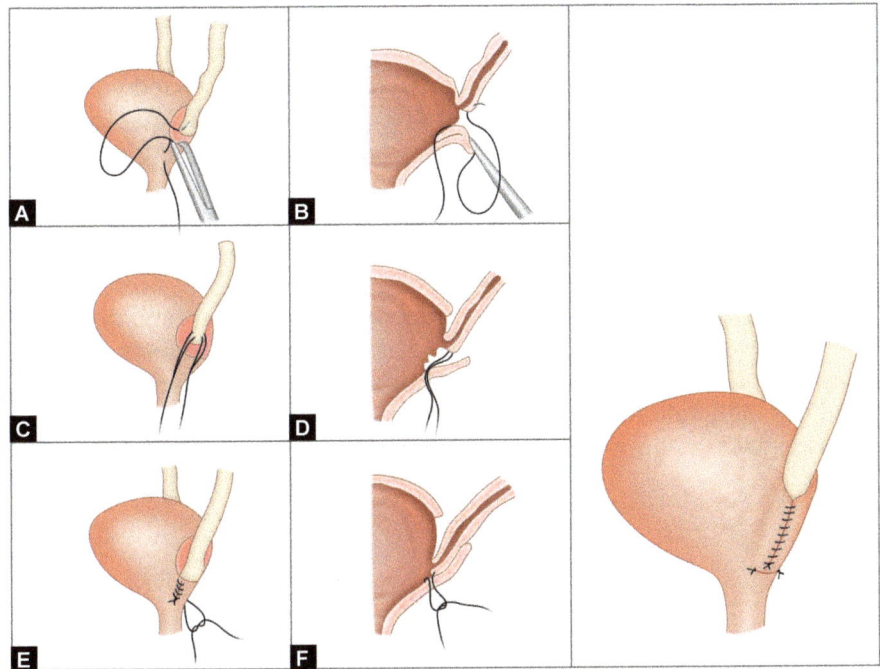

Figure 14: Lich-Gregoir technique.

COMPLICATIONS

Early

1. Decreased urine output maybe secondary to transient edema of VUJ and postoperative dehydration. It can also be due to bladder spasm and obstruction of the neo-orifice by balloon of Foley's catheter.
2. Postoperative urine extravasation is uncommon and related to improper closure of the detrusor.
3. Voiding dysfunction is common after reimplant is done in patients of urge incontinence and it is related to bladder inflammation and can be treated with anticholinergics. Urinary retention due to neuropraxia has been reported in 2–5%.

Late

1. Ureteral obstruction: It maybe asymptomatic or associated with pain and repeated UTI. It is usually due to mechanical obstruction of distal ureter. There maybe ureteric obstruction in few cases and maybe associated with significant renal loss if not recognized early. Devascularization of distal

ureter maybe due to electrocautery, torsion of ureter in new submucosal tunnel, too lateral placement of the neohiatus leading to J-hooking and obstruction of ureter as the bladder fills. There could also be redundancy of ureter medially with relation to posterior detrusor wall. The original hiatal defect, if not closed properly, can interfere with morbidity of neohiatus. Development of postoperative diverticulum can cause reflux. It can be due to adhesions in transperitoneal course of ureter in relation to bowel segment and broad ligament of females. In males, care should be taken to avoid injury to vas deferens.
2. Reflux: Ipsilateral reflux is due to persistent inflammation of submucosal tunnel, inadequate tunnel length, devascularization of ureter in the tunnel and ureterovaginal fistula. Contralateral reflux is common in patients with voiding dysfunction and patients with abnormal ureters. It also maybe a pop-off mechanism or undilated abnormal contralateral ureter.

CHAPTER 32

Biostatistics

STATISTICS

The practice or science of collecting and analyzing numerical data in large quantities, especially for the purpose of inferring proportions in a whole from those in a representative sample.

BIOSTATISTICS

It is the branch of statistics that deals with data relating to living organisms.

The purpose of this chapter is to not make one expert in biostatistics or biostatistician. It just to acquaint one to biostatistics, so that one can collect, interpret, and describe data scientifically well.

The first step is to understand the types of study design (**Flowchart 1**).
- *Descriptive*: The researcher just reports variables as they are happening, no one has control over the variables. For example, case report and case series. For example, population survey of serum prostate-specific antigen (PSA) in village of healthy men between 60 and 70 years.
- *Analytical*: The researcher uses information that is already available and analyses them to make critical evaluation of the material.

For example, cohort study—10-year follow-up of serum creatinine after donor nephrectomy.
- Case-control study—evaluation of smoking as risk factor for cancer bladder
- Randomized control study—a randomized controlled trial of retrograde intrarenal surgery (RIRS) versus mini-percutaneous nephrolithotomy (PCNL).
- Cross-sectional study—prevalence of urolithiasis at a tertiary center or prevalence of cancer prostate in a camp organized.

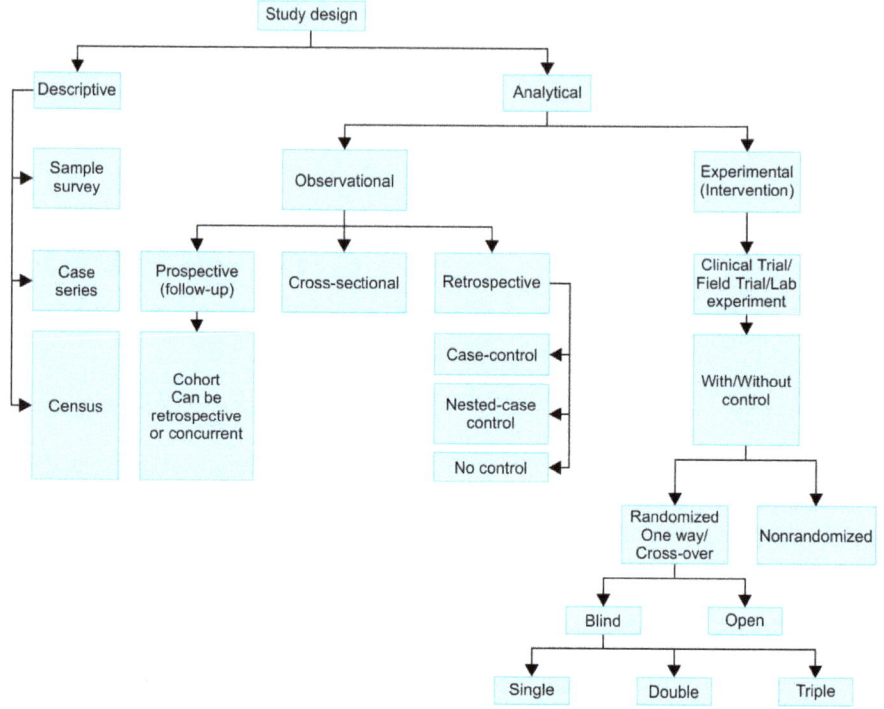

Flowchart 1: Types of study design

The next step is to know the types of variables:
- Quantitative:
  - *Continuous*: This variable lies on continuity on continuity, any value between two ends, e.g., PSA value can be 1.2 or 4.3, creatinine can also be in decimals
  - *Discrete*: Can take only discrete value, it does not have any decimal, e.g., previous number of surgeries, we cannot have 1.5 as surgery count or number of punctures/tracts in PCNL.
- Qualitative (categorical):
  - *Ordinal*: Ordered categories, e.g., Likert Scale or pain—mild, moderate, and severe

    Degree of hydronephrosis—mild, moderate, or severe, but if degree of hydronephrosis is quantified as 10 mm, 12 mm, and 15 mm, then it is quantitative data.
  - *Nominal*: Nonordered categories, e.g., requirement of ureteric dilatation before RIRS, use of double-J (DJ) stent

The quantitative data collected has to be described as **"measure"** of central tendency and **"measures"** dispersion values. The measures for central tendency (**averages**) are:

For example, duration of surgery in mini-PCNL in seven patients
The readings were 17, 20, 22, 31, 15, 10, and 22.

- **Mean:** It is average of all data, mean = sum of all values/number of values

    Mean = Sum of all values/Number of observations = 137/7 = 19.6
- **The value which divides whole data into two equal parts when data is put in to ascending order is known as median. Median is also known as positional average.** It also defined as It is the middle value, when the data is arranged in the ascending order.

    For example, if we arrange the above, 10, 15, 17, 20, 22, 22, and 31

    Thus, then median is 20.
- *Mode*: It is the observation that occurs the most frequently.

    For example, 22 is most commonly occurring value.

The measures for the dispersion of data are as follows:
- *Range*: It is the range from the lowest to largest observation.

    For example, the range for the above example is 10–31.
- *Inter Quartile Range (IQR)*: It is measure of dispersion which includes 50% observations of dataset,

    Interquartile range = $Q_3 - Q_1$

    For example, values are 10, 15, 17, 21, 25, 30, 35, and 40

    The above underlined values are interquartile range.
- *Mean deviation:* It is the average of all the absolute deviations **taken** from central value.
- *Standard deviation (SD) (degree of variability)*: Variability of the observation about the mean (scatter of population)

    Square root of mean squared deviations taken from mean.

$$SD = \sqrt{Variance} = SD = \sqrt{\frac{\sum(x-\bar{x})^2}{\eta}}$$

For example, the SD in the above-mentioned example would be 6.6.

Which implies that mean ± SD, i.e., 19.6 ± 6.6 would contain 68% of values 19.6 ± 13.2 would contain 95% of values.

The other way of describing quantitative is by partition values:
- *Quartile (**Positional Averages**)*: For an ungrouped data arranged in ascending order, the three numbers which divide them into four equal parts known as quartiles.

    They are denoted as Q_1, Q_2, and Q_3. Q_1 has 25% observations to its left and 75% to its right. For example, values are **10, 15,** 17, 21, 25, 30, 35, and 40. The bold values are Q_1 and the underlined values are after Q_3.
- *Percentiles*: Total frequencies are divided into hundred equal parts.

    $Q_1 = P_{25}$, $Q_2 = P_{50}$ = Median, $Q_3 = P_{75}$

The first and most important step in analyzing data is to check whether the data is normal or non-normal.
- *Normal/Gaussian data*:
    - Introduced in 1733 by Abraham de Moivre
    - It is a bell-shaped curve, smooth, and perfectly symmetrical curve

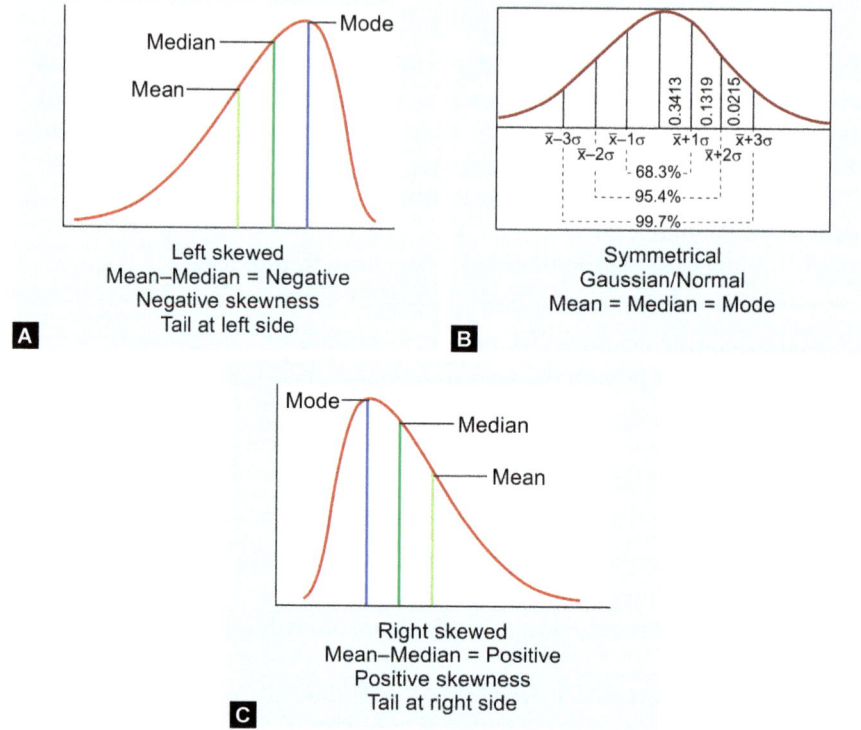

Figure 1: Distribution depicting symmetrical and non-symmetrical data. (a) showing non-normal data with skewed towards left, (b) showing normal/Gaussian data, (c) showing non-normal data with skewed towards right.

- The two tails of curve extend up to infinity.
- AUC (area under the curve) = 1, skewness = 0, kurtosis = 3
- The frequency graph is symmetrical, with mean = median = mode
- This data is analyzed by parametric tests.

- *Non-normal:* The frequency graph is not symmetrical and is skewed to one side (**Fig. 1**).

The various tests to detect the normality of the data to be interpreted are as follows:
- D'Agostino-Pearson normality test
- Anderson-Darling test
- Shapiro-Wilk normality test (n <50), but can be used for large samples
- Kolmogorov-Smirnov test (n ≥50)

The normality of data can be checked online or any computer software. The shape of frequency graph also helps to know the distribution (**Fig. 2**). One of the easy ways to check normality of data prior to starting statistical analysis is as follows https://www.gigacalculator.com/calculators/normality-test-calculator.php (**Fig. 3**).

If the *p* value is >0.05, then the data is normally distributed.

Tests of normality

	Kolmogorov–Smirnov[a]			Shapiro–Wilk		
	Statistic	df	Sig.	Statistic	df	Sig.
Prostate size	0.184	15	0.184	0.889	15	0.064

a. Lilliefors significance correction

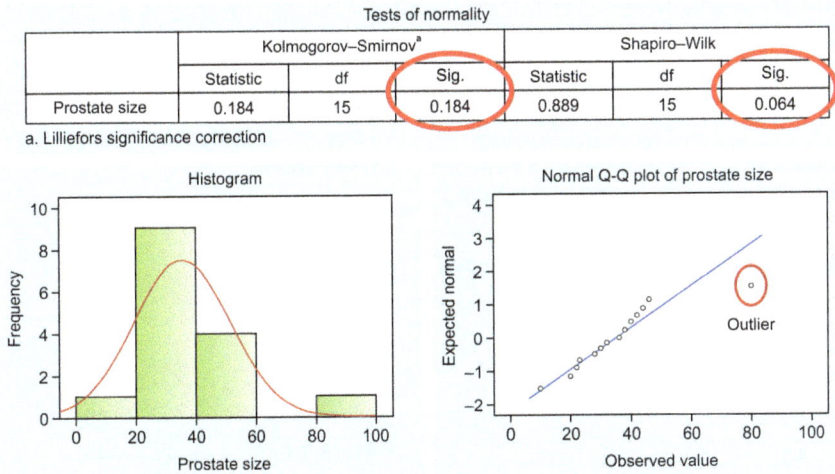

Figure 2: Shows various ways of detecting normalcy of data.

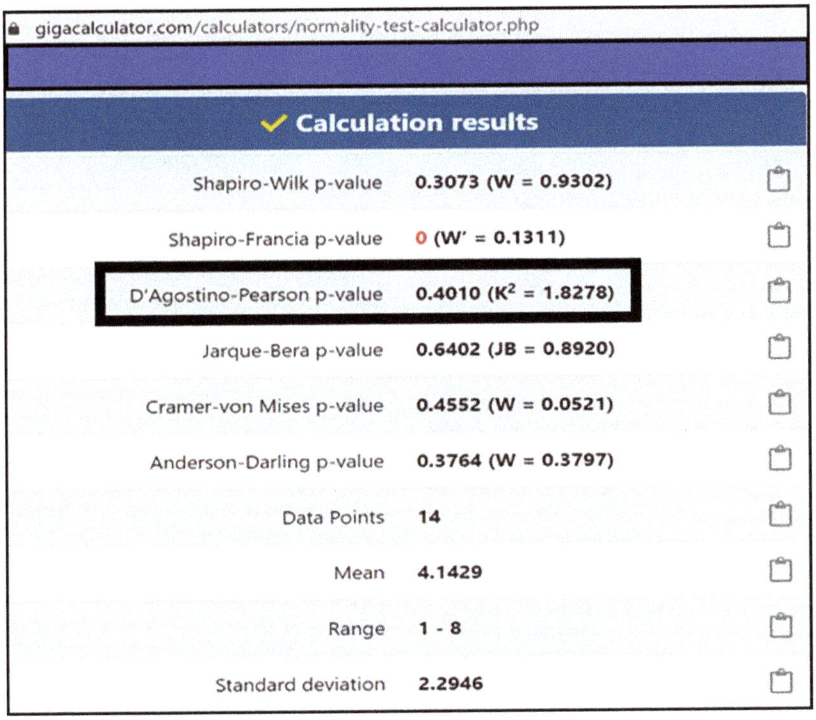

Figure 3: Online calculator showing various tests for normalcy of data.

For example, we have a data of prostate size of 15 patients as described (**Table 1A**), which has been arranged in ascending order (**Table 1B**) and its descriptive analysis is in **Table 1C**.

The correct way of describing data according to variable is as follows (**Flowchart 2**):

TABLE 1A: Prostate size data of 15 patients.	TABLE 1B: Prostate size data of 15 patients arranged in ascending order.	TABLE 1C: Descriptive statistics of these patients.		
Prostate size	Prostate size (arranged)	Mean		35.3
10	10	Median		36
20	20	Mode		38
23	22	Standard deviation		15.96
40	23	Range		70
36	28	Minimum		10
22	30	Maximum		80
80	32	Percentiles	25	23
44	36		50	36
38	38		75	42
28	38			
32	40			
46	42			
30	44			
42	46			
38	80			

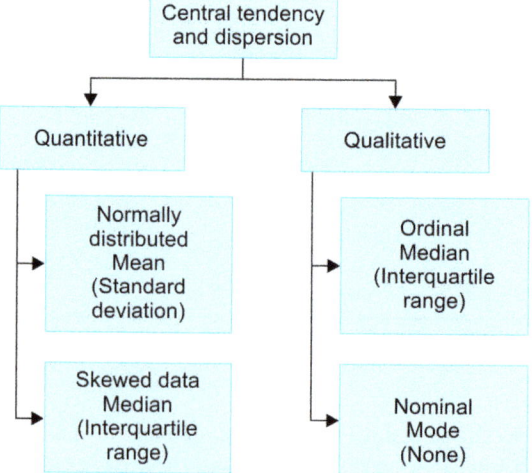

Whisker and box plot representing the data with the outliers (explained later)

Flowchart 2: Showing the correct way of describing data according to variable.

Central tendency and dispersion
- Quantitative
  - Normally distributed: Mean (Standard deviation)
  - Skewed data: Median (Interquartile range)
- Qualitative
  - Ordinal: Median (Interquartile range)
  - Nominal: Mode (None)

KURTOSIS

Skewness is representative of tail of the distribution. Negative value of skewness represents negatively skewed data (tail on left side). Positive value of skewness represents the positively skewed data (tail on right side).

Kurtosis is representative of peak of the data distribution. Leptokurtic (Thin curve): Kurtosis value is greater than 3. Mesokurtik: Kurtosis value is equal to 3. Platykurtik (Flat curve): Kurtosis value is less than 3.

Standard Deviation (SD) and Standard Error of Mean

In statistics, we study some sample from entire population. In this case, we need to how far is sample mean (M) from the population mean (M1), if repeated samples of size "n" are taken (**Fig. 4**). The measure of such variability is standard error of mean (SEM). What SD is to sample, the SEM is to the population mean. Standard error shows the sampling stability of the estimator (generally known as mean).

$$SEM = SD/\sqrt{n}$$

Example: *In a village of population of 20,000 people, the mean population uroflow (M1) was 13 mL/s and if we select 100 sample from the population and their sample mean (M) is 12 mL/s with SD of 5 mL/s.*

Then,

$$SEM = 5/\sqrt{100} = 0.5$$

Probability and p Value

Probability

It is the measure of the likelihood that an event will occur (where 0 indicates impossibility and 1 indicates certainty). In inferential statistics, in "*null*

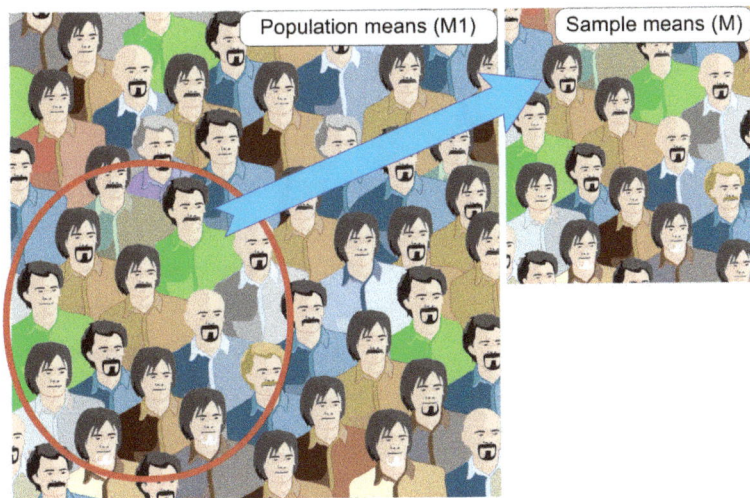

Figure 4: Showing the pictorial depiction of population and sample mean.

hypothesis" (H_0 "H-naught," "H-null"), there is no relationship (difference) between the population variables in question. *Alternative hypothesis (H1)* states that there is a difference between the variables in question. The *p value* is the probability of occurrence of the difference by chance. If *p* value <0.05, then result is statistically significant and thus rejects the null hypothesis (H_0).

If *p* value for null hypothesis is <0.05, then null hypothesis is true only in 5% cases, it means null hypothesis is rejected and alternate hypothesis is accepted and the difference is statistically significant (**Fig. 5**). *p* values alone do not permit any direct statement about the direction or size of a difference or of a relative risk (RR) between different groups. However, this would be particularly useful when the results are not significant. For this purpose, confidence limits contain more information.

Confidence Interval

Confidence interval (CI) is the range of values which contains the desired parameter [e.g., mean and odds ratio (OR)] with a probability defined in advance. A 95% CI means that the CI covers the true value in 95 of 100 studies. In other words, we have 95% confidence that the true value in the population from which the sample was taken lies within the 95% CI. A *wide CI suggests an imprecise* result and indicates that the results should be interpreted with caution regardless of statistical significance. Also, wide CI represents SE (mean) is greater. Thus, *p value is of statistical significance* and *CI is of clinical significance*.

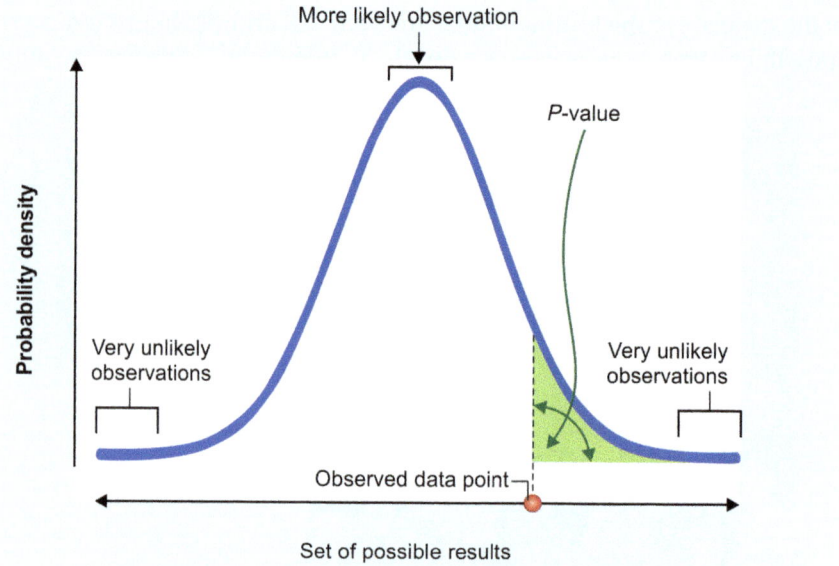

Figure 5: A *p*-value (shaded in green) is the probability of an observed (or more extreme) result assuming that the null hypothesis is true.

The CI size depends upon the sample size and dispersion of data. If sample size is small and the data is widely dispersed, then the CI is wide. *p* value tells about statistical significance, but CI tells about the direction of effect. If the CI does not include the value of zero effect, it can be assumed that there is a statistically significant result.

Although point estimates, such as the arithmetic mean, the difference between two means or the OR, provide the best approximation to the true value, they do not provide any information about how exact they are. This is achieved by CIs. We obviously cannot estimate the difference between the studied sample mean and the true population mean, as the true population mean is not known. We have 95% confidence that the true value in the population from which the sample was taken lies within the 95% CI. CIs can be used to describe the probability that the true value is within a given range.

Suppose we select many samples from population. We calculate the mean of these sample means and SD.

$$\text{Standard error of sample mean SE (mean)} = SD/\sqrt{n}$$

95% CI for a mean = mean − 1.96 SE (mean) to mean + 1.96 SE (mean). The various multiplying factors for different confidence intervals are as shown in **Table 2**.

Odds ratio and RR should always be presented with CI (it gives estimate of statistical significance as well as precision of the ratio).

- CI depends upon:
  - Dispersion of data (SD)
  - Sample size

Thus, if data is less dispersed or sample size is large, then SEM is small and thus *CI is narrow*.

- If the CI does not include the value of *zero effect (0 for mean, 1 for OR)*, it can be assumed that there is a statistically significant result.

For example, we are evaluating the prostate cancer risk reduction by finasteride. The null hypothesis would be reduction of 0%. In the Prostate Cancer Prevention Trial, they randomly assigned 18,882 men 55 years of age or older with a normal digital rectal examination and a PSA level of 3.0 ng/mL or lower to treatment with finasteride (5 mg/day) or placebo for 7 years. The study found 24.8% reduction in prevalence of cancer over the 7-year period (95% CI 18.6–30.6%; *p* <0.001). The null hypothesis of no risk reduction with finasteride does not fall within the 95% CI, and the result is

TABLE 2: Tabulated standard normal values.	
Confidence interval (CI)	Multiplying factor
90%	1.64
95%	1.96
99%	2.58

therefore statistically significant. The CI is narrow. The reasonably large RR reduction with narrow CI suggests that the result is not only statistically meaningful, but also clinically meaningful.

Numbers Needed to Treat

Numbers needed to treat (NNT) is straightforward measure that conveys an estimate of a treatment's clinical effect. For a study of treatment effect, the NNT is defined as the number of patients that must be treated in order to prevent one additional adverse outcome. In general, a large treatment effect is associated with a small NNT, while a small treatment effect is associated with a large NNT. This concept is needed as the absolute or relative risk reduction provides discrete statistical significance, but the magnitude of treatment's clinical effect is often difficult to determine.

Hazard Ratio

Hazard ratio (HR) is a measure of association used in prospective studies. The HR is the ratio of (chance of an event occurring in the treatment arm)/(chance of an event occurring in the control arm). The HR has also been defined as the ratio of (risk of outcome in one group)/(risk of outcome in another group), occurring at a given interval of time. The term "hazard" refers to the probability that an individual, under observation in a clinical trial at time t, has an event at that time. The HR is a measure of the magnitude of the difference between the two curves in the Kaplan–Meier plot, while the p value measures the statistical significance of this difference. A HR of exactly 1.0 means that the study drug provides zero risk reduction, compared to the control treatment. A HR of 0.75 means that the study drug provides 25% risk reduction compared to control treatment.

Hazard ratios differ from RRs and ORs in that RRs and ORs are cumulative over an entire study, using a defined endpoint, while HRs represents instantaneous risk over the study time period.

Outliers: During analysis of data, sometimes some values are extreme from others, which skew the data. They are known as outliers. If they are due to typographical errors, then they have to be removed from the final analysis.

One-tailed and two-tailed test: When comparing groups of two continuous data, the null hypothesis says that there is no real difference (A and B). If we are sure that the difference is only one-sided, e.g., A > B, then one-tailed test can be used. If we consider both possibilities or not absolutely sure about direction of difference, then two-tailed test is used. Generally, two-tailed p value is considered norm.

TYPES OF ERROR IN ANALYSIS

There are two main errors in statistics (**Tables 3 and 4**):

TABLE 3: Showing true or false positives and negatives.

	Disease present	Disease absent
Test positive	True positive	False positive
Test negative	False negative	True negative

TABLE 4: When our decision is to reject null hypothesis (H_0), while the actual situation is that H_0 is true, then it is Type I error. Similarly, when our decision is to accept null hypothesis, while the actual situation is that alternate hypothesis is true (i.e null hypothesis is rejected), then we introduce the Type II error.

	Actual situation	
Decision	H_0 true	H_1 true
Accept H_0	1-α	Type II error (β)
Reject H_0	Type I error (α)	Power (1-β)

- *Type I error (α error) (level of significance):* It occurs if the null hypothesis is rejected when it is true. A value of 0.05 is most commonly used. It is generally less serious.
- *Type II error (β error):* It is the chance of a false-negative result. It is set at a level of 0.20, which translates into <20% chance of a false-negative conclusion. It is more serious error.

Power is the complement of beta, i.e., *(1-beta).* A power is 0.80 or 80% when beta is set at 0.20. It represents chance of avoiding a false-negative conclusion, or the chance of detecting an effect if it really exists.

α—*level of significance* is the maximum probability of making type I error. Commonly used 0.05 or 0.01. For example, if 5% level of significance, then is a chance that we will reject a null hypothesis when it is true in 5 decisions out of 100 decisions.

Steps in Doing Statistical Analysis

The sequential steps in doing statistical analysis are:
1. Specify the hypothesis of interest as a null and alternative hypothesis
2. Calculate sample size
3. Check normality of data
4. Decide what statistical test is appropriate
5. Use the test to calculate the *p* value
6. Weigh the evidence from the *p* value in favor of the null or alternative hypothesis

One of the most important steps in any study to have appropriate statistical significance and correct outcomes, is to have proper sample size (n).

Sample Size

- Has to be predetermined
- Analytically approached
- Sufficiently large to represent the population.
- *Larger sample*: Wastage of resources, time consuming, true treatment effect may be missed due to heterogeneity of large population, very small clinically insignificant differences are detected.
- *Smaller size*: Not provide the suitable answer to research question, not possible to detect significant difference even if it exists, false results.

The determinants of sample size are as follows:
- *p* value (depends on α)
- Power (related with β)
- Effect size (clinically relevant assumption): It refers to the smallest difference that would be of clinical importance. Ideally, the basis of effect size selection should be on clinical judgment. The researcher has to determine this effect size with scientific knowledge and wisdom. Available previous publications on related topic might be helpful in this regard.

The factors affecting sample size are:
- Feasibility—whatever maximum is feasible according to the resources available
- Dropouts/Nonresponders—some would not respond even after getting selected for the studies

The sample size can be calculated online or by any software. One of the way to calculate sample size (simplified way) is as given below: **Figures 6 and 7**.

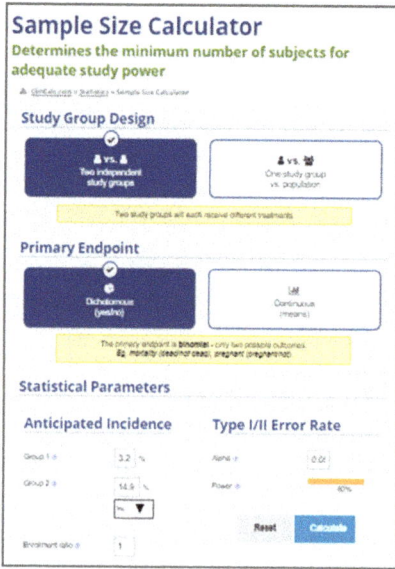

Figure 6: Online sample size calculator.

- Visit website—https://clincalc.com/stats/samplesize.aspx
- For example, incidence of dizziness in silodosin versus tamsulosin

Just answer simple questions and find anticipated incidence of events from previous studies or pilot study and calculate sample size generally by keeping α as 0.05 and power as 80%.

There are three questions to be answered to choice the appropriate statistical test[1] (**Flowcharts 3 to 5**):

Question 1: Are the variables unpaired?
Question 2: Are the variable paired?

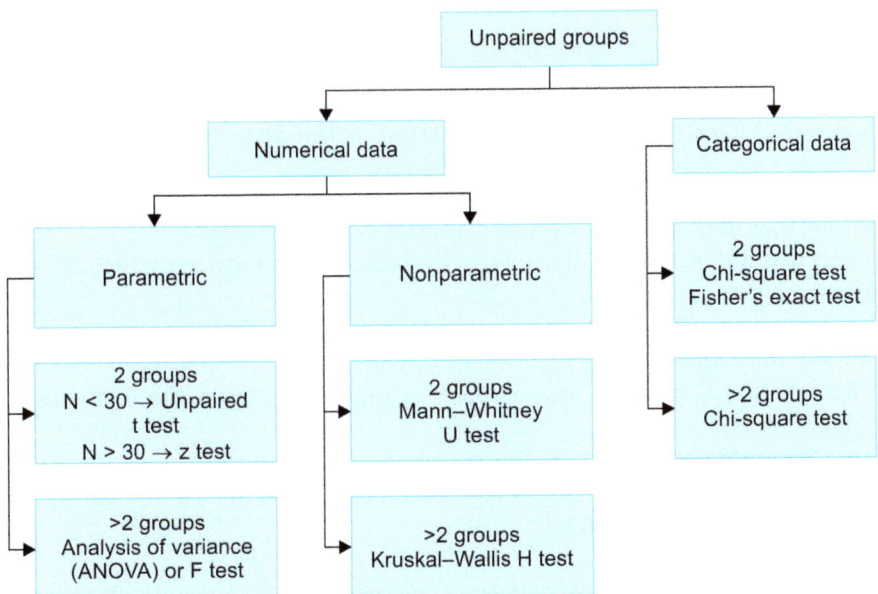

Figure 7: Online sample size calculator.

Flowchart 3: Choice of appropriate statistical test-unpaired data.

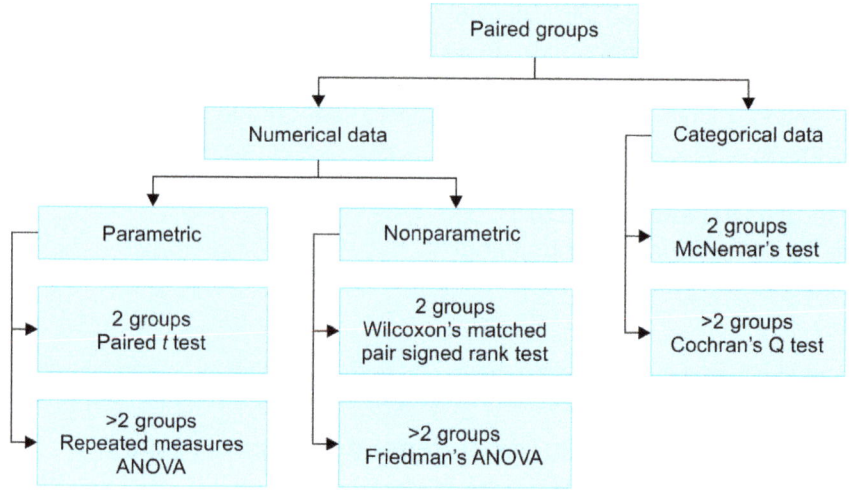

Flowchart 4: Choice of appropriate statistical test-paired data.

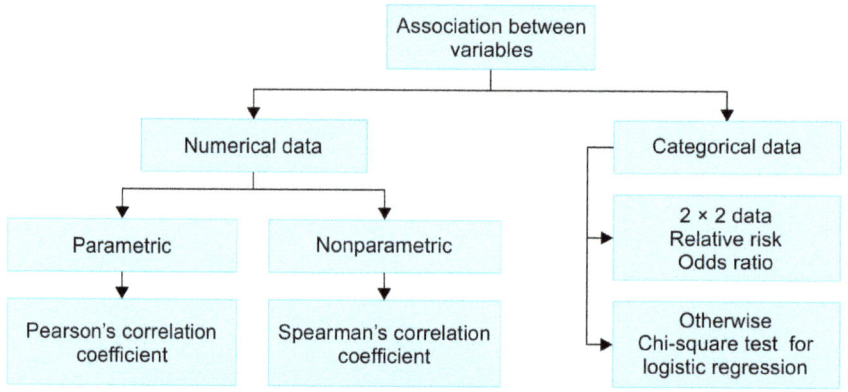

Flowchart 5: Choice of appropriate statistical test - if there association between the variables.

Question 3: Is there need to test association between variables?
Now let us understand the above facts by analyzing an example which is as follows:
We are analyzing IPSS outcomes of tamsulosin versus placebo
Questions to be answered:
- Sample size (Calculate the sample size depending upon the following parameters):
  ○ Standard deviation (previous studies or pilot studies)
  ○ Effect size (minimum expected difference—decided by investigator)
  ○ $\alpha - 0.05$ and β: 80%/0.80
- Which statistical test:
  ○ Check if data follows *normal distribution* (D'Agostino–Pearson normality test).

- Depends on *hypothesis question*
  - IPSS at 0 and 12 weeks—*unpaired "t" test with two-tailed test as directions of result is non-specific*
  - IPSS before and after taking tamsulosin—*paired "t" test*
  - IPSS in both groups at 0.6.12 weeks—*repeated measure analysis of variance (ANOVA)*
  - if retrograde ejaculation to be evaluated (Yes/No)—*Chi-square test*
- Any correlation between variables to find association between age and IPSS—*Pearson correlation coefficient test*

SCREENING AND DIAGNOSTICS TESTS

A screening test is performed on healthy, asymptomatic individuals to identify who is at sufficiently high risk of a specific disorder to justify a further diagnostic test, or direct preventive management.

A diagnostic test is utilized to determine a diagnosis.

Validity of diagnostic tests: Validity of a diagnostic test is the ability of the test under study to provide accurate measurements in comparison to a reference test (i.e., gold standard). Accurate measurement refers to the ability of the test to identify which people have the disease and which do not, i.e., Is the test accurately measuring what it is supposed to measure?

Sensitivity = $TP/(TP + FN) = A/(A + C) \times 100$ (defined as the proportion of true positives among patients with the disease). A sensitive test is a good screening test because it identifies most of the patients with disease and only few who do not. Thus, it is the ability to correctly identify patients who have the disease.

Specificity = $TN/(FP + TN) = D/(B + D) \times 100$ (is defined as the proportion of true negatives among patients without the disease). A specific test is a good diagnostic test because it identifies most of the patients who do not have disease. Thus, it is the ability to correctly identify patients who do not have the disease.

Positive predictive value (PPV) = $TP/(TP + FP) = A/A + B \times 100$ (is defined as the number of diseased patients with a true-positive test divided by the number of patients diagnosed with positive tests). PPV refers to the likelihood that a patient with a positive outcome for a disease actually will have the disease.

TABLE 5: Cross-table showing relation between the disease and the test.

	Disease present	Disease absent	Total
Test positive	A (True positive)	B (False positive)	A + B
Test negative	C (False negative)	D (True negative)	C + D

Negative predictive value (NPV) = TN/(TN + FN) = D/C + D × *100* (is defined as the number of nondiseased patients with true-negative tests divided by the number of patients diagnosed with negative tests). NPV refers to the likelihood that a patient with a negative outcome for a disease will actually not have the disease.

Positive likelihood ratio: Sensitivity/1 – specificity

(This gives a ratio of the test being positive for patients with disease compared with those without disease. Aim to be much greater than 1 for a good test).

Negative likelihood ratio = 1 – sensitivity/specificity

(This gives a ratio of the test being negative for patients with disease compared with those without disease. Aim to be considerably <1 for a good test).

Diagnostic accuracy (efficiency): It is the proportion of correct results of the diagnostic tool. It is calculated by adding those actually found to be positive (TP) and those who actually are negative (TN) = (TP + TN)/(TP + FP + FN + TN)

General rule: *A screening test needs high sensitivity, a diagnostic test needs high specificity.*

Criteria for screening test:
- Disease:
    - Asymptomatic long enough period to allow detection
    - Prevalence of the disease enough to justify screening
    - Sufficient effect on quality/length of life
- Test:
    - Sensitive
    - Reliable and valid
    - Simple and inexpensive
    - Cost-effective
    - Safe
- Population tested:
    - High disease prevalence
    - Acceptable
    - Good compliance

The description of the important statistical tests is as follows:
- *Student's "t" test*: Mr. William S Gosset (Student—pen name), a civil service statistician, a head brewer at Guinness brewery, introduced "t" distribution of small samples and published his work under the pseudonym "Student." It is applicable only when the data is normally distributed.

    There are two types of "t" test:
    1. *Unpaired "t" test*: Used to test statistical significance of difference between two independent sample means or sample mean and population mean.

2. *Paired "t" test*: It is used to measure statistical difference between paired measurements (Dependent sample) or observations, taken before and after application of an intervention.

Procedure:
- Define null and alternate hypothesis
- Calculate *t* score by using formula
- Calculate degree of freedom, $Df = (n-1)$
- See "t" value table for the degree of freedom
- If $t_{calculated} > t_{table}$, then null hypothesis rejected
- If $t_{calculated} < t_{table}$, then null hypothesis accepted
- ANOVA test:
    ○ One-way ANOVA
        - *Unmatched data*: Measures three or more unmatched groups when data is categorized in one way
            For example, IPSS comparison in tamsulosin, silodosin, and alfuzosin
        - *Matched data*: For example, IPSS comparison before, during, and after tamsulosin
            Here, use repeated measures ANOVA test
            The term repeated measures applies strictly when you give treatments repeatedly to one subjects.
    ○ Two-way ANOVA/Two factors ANOVA:
        - How a response is affected by two independent factors
        - For example, IPSS comparison in tamsulosin, silodosin, and alfuzosin from urban, semi-urban, and rural population
        - Generally complicated
    ○ *Post-hoc tests*: ANOVA test only tells whether there is a difference, but does not tell us at what point the difference between various groups subsist. Post-hoc test is capable to pinpoint the exact difference between the different groups of comparison.

How to select a post hoc-test?
- *Dunnett's post-hoc test*: If one column represents control group and we wish to compare all other columns to that control column but not to each other
- *Test for linear trend*: If the columns are arranged in a natural order (i.e., dose or time) and we want to test whether there is a trend so that values increases (or decreases) as you move from left to right across the columns. For example, dose responses of 0.2 mg, 0.4 mg, and 0.8 mg tamsulosin
- *Bonferroni, Turkey's, or Newman's test*: If we want to compare all pairs of columns

3. Chi-square test:
    ○ This test was developed by Karl Pearson.
    ○ *Basis*: The test is based on the chi-squared distribution with n degrees of freedom where n is given by (no. of rows - 1) × (no. of columns - 1).

- Rationale:
  - It calculates the frequencies that would be expected if there were no association (i.e., null hypothesis is true).
  - It compares the observed frequencies with these expected values.
  - If the observed frequencies are very different to the expected values, this provides evidence that there is an association.
  - The test uses a formula based on the chi-squared distribution to give a p value.
- Assumption (**Table 6**):
  - Large sample size
  - All expected values should be >5
  - It gives p value, but does not give estimate of CIs

4. Wilcoxon-matched-pairs signed-ranks test:
   - It is the analog of the t test for two independent means (paired groups)
   - It is based on the ranks of the data in each group
   - So, it is used if data has non-normal distribution.
   - It gives a p value but no estimate of the difference between the groups
5. Mann–Whitney test
   - It is a Student's "t" test performed on ranks.
   - For large numbers, it is almost as sensitive as Student's "t" test.
   - For small numbers with unknown distribution, this test is more sensitive than Student's "t" test.
   - This test is generally used when two unpaired groups are to be compared and the scale is ordinal (i.e., ranks and scores), which are not normally distributed.

- Pearson's correlation:
  - It is used to estimate the strength of linear relationship between two continuous variables.
  - Correlation coefficient—denoted as "r" (−1 to +1)
  - R = 0, no linear relationship, if r is negative then variables have negative linear relationship and so (**Table 7**).

TABLE 6: Statistical tests for categorical/qualitative data.		
Chi-square test	**Fisher's exact test**	**McNemar's test**
Unpaired data	Unpaired data	Paired data
Sample size: Large	Sample size: Small and large	Any sample size
Expected counts in a cell should be >5	Expected counts in a cell is <5	
Relies on approximation	Gives exact values	
Yate's continuity correction for chi-square is used when the sample size is sample		

TABLE 7: The difference between Pearsons correlation and simple linear regression.	
Pearson correlation	**Simple linear regression**
Strength of linear relationship	Nature of linear relationship
Used when neither of the variable predicts the other	Used when the predictor variable affects the outcome variable
Gives correlation coefficient, *p* value, and confidence interval	Gives equation of best fitting straight line through data in the form of intercept and slope of line, with confidence intervals
Example: Age and prostate volume	Example: Age and PSA trends

(PSA: prostate-specific antigen)

RECEIVER OPERATING CHARACTERISTIC CURVES

It is a graphical method to compare the sensitivity and specificity for all possible cut-offs. This allows the most appropriate cut-off to be chosen for the particular context.

The plot of true positive (sensitivity) on y-axis versus false positive (1−specificity) on x-axis across varying cut-offs generates a curve in the unit square called a receiver operating characteristic (ROC) curve. ROC curve corresponding to progressively greater discriminate capacity of diagnostic tests is located progressively closer to the upper left-hand corner in "ROC space." A horizontal line is shown at 45° and the "curve" joins the points. Sensitivity and specificity are inversely related. If the diagnostic test performs well then the curve will be distinctly above the 45° line. If the curve rises steeply and is close to the y-axis and then flattens out, the "best" possible cut-off will give high sensitivity and specificity (**Fig. 8**).

The AUC can be interpreted as the probability that a randomly chosen diseased subject is rated or ranked as more likely to be diseased than a randomly chosen nondiseased subject. This interpretation is based on nonparametric Mann–Whitney U statistics that is used in calculating AUC.

AUC → 1: The diagnostic test is perfect in the differentiation between the diseased and nondiseased. This happens when the distribution of test results for the diseased and nondiseased do not overlap.

AUC → 0.5: Curve located on diagonal line

AUC → 0: Test incorrectly classify all subjects with diseased as negative and all subjects with nondiseased as positive that is extremely unlikely to happen in clinical practice.

Advantages of Receiver Operating Characteristic

- It is independent of prevalence of disease as it is dependent on sensitivity and specificity.

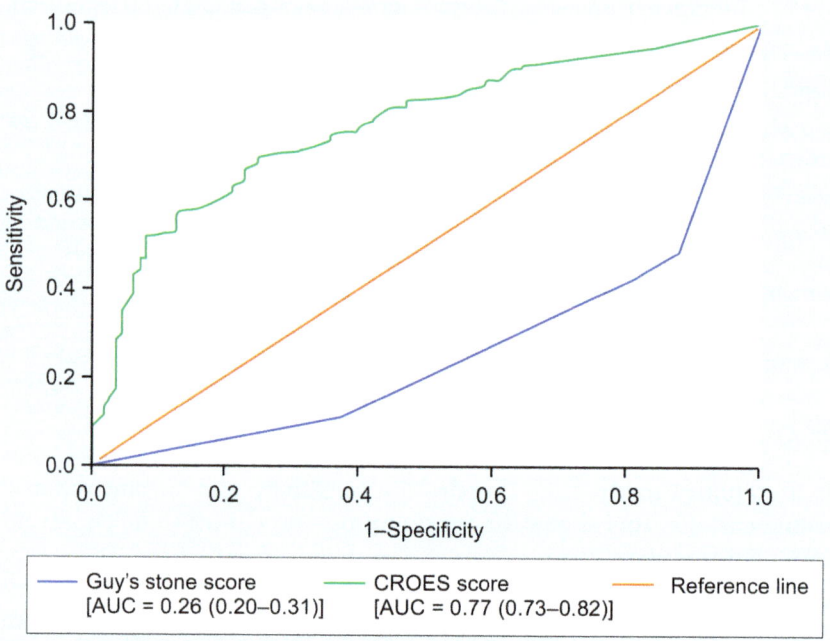

(AUC: area under the curve)

Figure 8: Receiver operating characteristic curve shows that the CROES nephrolithometry scoring system is above the reference line, that means the scoring system is performing well than the other score.

Source: Yarimoglu S, Polat S, Bozkurt IH, Yonguc T, Aydogdu O, Aydın E, et al. Comparison of STONE and CROES nephrolithometry scoring systems for predicting stone-free status and complication rates after percutaneous nephrolithotomy: a single center study with 262 cases. Urolithiasis. 2017;45(5):489-94.

- Several diagnostic tests on the same subjects can be simultaneously compared.
- The optimal sensitivity and specificity can be determined by using ROC curve analysis.
  The various ratios in statistics are given in **Table 8**.
- *Risk difference, attributable risk* = Risk of exposure group − Risk of unexposed group = $a/(a + c) - b/(b + d)$
- *Risk ratio (RR)*, relative risk = Incidence of exposed/Incidence of unexposed =
  $$[a/(a + c)]/[b/(b + d)]$$
  - Measure of incidence of an outcome
  - Used in prospective studies (cohort), where the population is known
  - "Risk of developing the outcome"
- *Odds ratio (OR)* = Odd of exposed/Odds of unexposed group = $[a/c]/[b/d]$

TABLE 8: Cross table showing relationship between exposure of a risk factor and the occurrence of disease.

	Exposure	No exposure	Total
Disease	a	b	a + b
No disease	c	d	c + d
Total	a + c	b + d	
Incidence	a/(a + c)	b/(b + d)	

- Odds of an event happening is defined as the likelihood that an event will occur, expressed as a proportion of the likelihood that the event will not occur.
- OR is a measure of association between exposure and an outcome. The OR represents the odds that an outcome will occur given a particular exposure, compared to the odds of the outcome occurring in the absence of that exposure.
- OR of 1 = no difference, OR >1 indicates increased occurrence of event
- OR <1 indicates decreased occurrence of event (protective exposure)
- Look at CI and *p* value for statistical significance of value
- Looks at prevalence
- Used in case control studies, when the outcome is unknown
- "Odds of developing the outcome"

There is difference between the probability and odds:

Probability: The extent to which an event is likely to occur, measured by the ratio of the favorable cases to the whole number of cases possible (0–1), e.g., probability of 50 times heads among 100 trials is 50/100 = 0.5.

Odds: Probability of favorable event occurring versus not occurring, e.g., odds of having heads in above example = (probability of heads/1 – probability of heads) = 0.5/1 – 0.5 = 1.

REGRESSION ANALYSIS[2]

Definition

Regression analysis is a technique used to find out the relationship between different variables. Regression looks closely into how a dependent variable is affected upon varying an independent variable while keeping the other independent variables constant. The various types of regression analysis are given in **Table 9**.

Linear Regression Analysis

The first step for possible relationship between the two variables can be made on the basis of scatter plot (scatter graph). This plot can be linear/non-linear. Linear regression is to be done only if the scatter graph is linear.

TABLE 9: Various types of regression analysis.

Type of regression	Application	Dependent variables	Independent variables
Linear regression	Description of a linear relationship between dependent variable and independent variable	Continuous (blood pressure)	Continuous/Categorical (age, weight, and sex)
Logistic regression	Prediction of the probability of belonging to groups (outcome: Yes/No)	Dichotomous (success of treatment: Yes/No)	
Proportional hazard regression (Cox regression)	Modeling of survival data	Survival time (time from diagnosis to event)	

- *Univariable linear regression*: It studies linear relationship between dependent variable (outcome) Y and single independent variable (predictor) X. It is explained by the formula

$$y = a + bx$$

where y is the outcome, 'a' is the intercept, 'b' is the slope of the line, and 'x' is the predictor variable

The regression line enables one to predict the value of the dependent variable Y from that of the independent variable X. For example, one can estimate person's blood pressure (BP) (dependent variable) from height (independent variable). The slope b of regression line → regression coefficient. It helps us to understand the change in dependent variable as per unit change in independent variable.

- *Multivariable regression analysis*: It is used when multiple independent variables affect a single dependent variable.

$$Y = a + b_1 \times X_1 + b_2 \times X_2 +...+ b_n \times X_n$$

The model permits the computation of a regression coefficient b_i for each independent variable X_i. Each of the coefficients b_i reflects the effect of the corresponding individual independent variable X_i on Y, where the potential influences of the remaining independent variables on X_i have been taken into account, i.e., eliminated by an additional computation. Thus, in a multiple regression analysis with age and sex as independent variables and weight as the dependent variable, the adjusted regression coefficient for sex represents the amount of variation in weight that is due to sex alone, after age has been taken into account. This is done by a computation that adjusts for age, so that the effect of sex is not confounded by a simultaneously operative age effect.

Thus, multivariable analysis describes a statistical relationship and helps individual prognostication. Many times large number of factors (independent variables) affects dependent variable. The goal of statistical analysis is to find out which of these factors truly have an effect on the dependent variable. In general, the number of observations should be at least 20 times greater than the number of variables under study. If too many irrelevant variables are included in the model, over adjustment is likely to be the result: that is, some of the irrelevant independent variables will be found to have an apparent effect, purely by chance.

Sometimes, multiple independent variables may be interdependent. An independent variable that would be found to have a strong effect in a univariable regression model might not turn out to have any appreciable effect in a multivariable regression with variable selection. This will happen if this particular variable itself depends so strongly on the other independent variables that it makes no additional contribution toward explaining the dependent variable. So, if independent variables are mutually dependent, then finally other independent variables will end up being included in the final model.

Multivariate analysis refers to statistical models that have two or more dependent or outcome variables and multivariable analysis refers to statistical models in which there are multiple independent or response variables.

Correlation[3]

Concept

Denote association between two quantitative variables. We also assume that the association is linear, that one variable increases or decreases a fixed amount for a unit increase or decrease in the other.

The degree of association is measured by a correlation coefficient (Pearson's correlation coefficient after its originator), denoted by r (−1 to +1).

When one variable increases as the other increases, the correlation is positive; when one decreases as the other increases, it is negative. Complete absence of correlation is represented by 0 (**Fig. 9**).

Statistical significant association can be calculated from "t" test after assuming that both variables are plausibly normally distributed, there is a linear relationship between them and the null hypothesis is that there is no association between them.

Spearman rank correlation is used to assess association if the data is not normally distributed, such as outlying points well away from the main body of the data could unduly influence the calculation of the correlation coefficient. For n >10, the Spearman rank correlation coefficient can be tested for significance using the *t* test. The difference between correlation and regression is highlighted in **Table 10**.

There are different ways of summarizing data (**Table 11**).

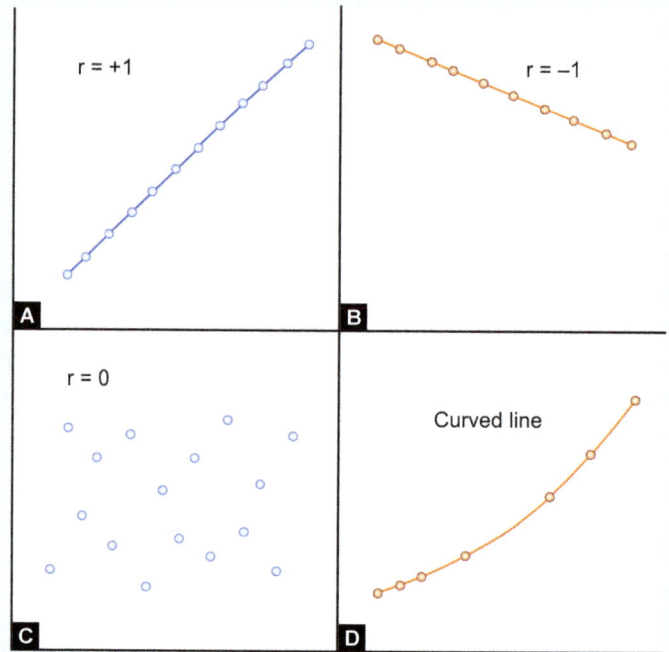

Figure 9: Correlation coefficient.

TABLE 10: Difference between correlation and regression.

	Correlation	Regression
Main purpose	Know association or absence of relationship between two variables under study; if variables are correlated, it allows measuring the strength of their association	Helps determine a functional relationship between two variables so as to estimate the unknown variable with the help of known variable and make future projections
Meaning	Statistical measure to determine co-relationship or association of two variables	How an independent variable (x) is numerically related to dependent variable
Use	Linear relationship between variables	Estimate random variable on the basis of value of fixed variable
Nature of variables	They are not designated as dependent or independent. Both the variables need to be quantitative	One variable is dependent and another is independent. Dependent variable needs to be quantitative, while the independent variable can be even categorical
Range	−1.0 to +1.0	
Association	Extent and direction of linear association between two variables	Describe one variable as a linear function of another variable

TABLE 11: Different ways of summarizing data.

Chart	Variable type	Purpose	Statistics
Bar/Pie chart (**Fig. 10 and 11**)	One categorical	Shows frequencies/ Proportions/ Percentages	Individual percentages
Stacked bar chart (**Fig. 12**)	Two categorical	Compares proportions within groups	Percentages within groups
Histogram (**Fig. 13**)	One scale	Shows distribution of results	Mean and SD
Scatter graph (**Fig. 14**)	Two scale	Relationship between two variables and detects outliers	Correlation coefficient
Box and whisker plot (**Figs. 15 and 16**)	One scale/One categorical	Compares spread of values	Median and IQR

(IQR: interquartile range; SD: standard deviation)

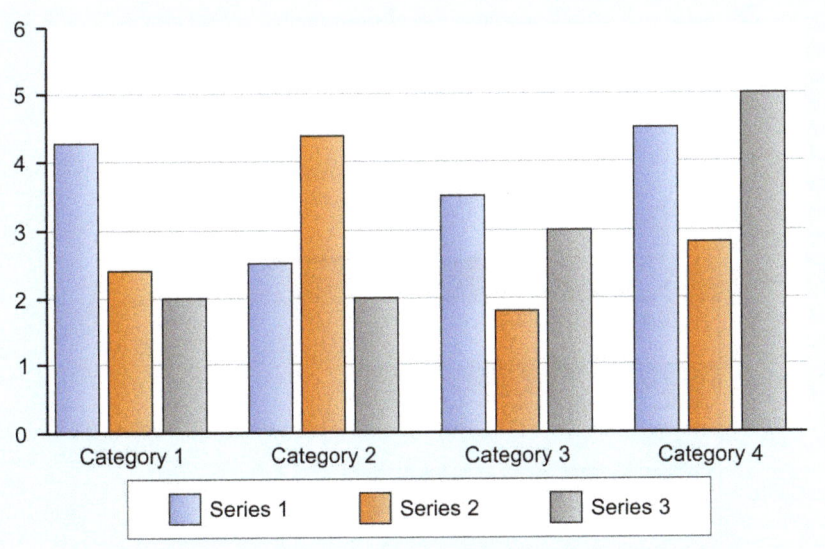

Figure 10: Bar chart.

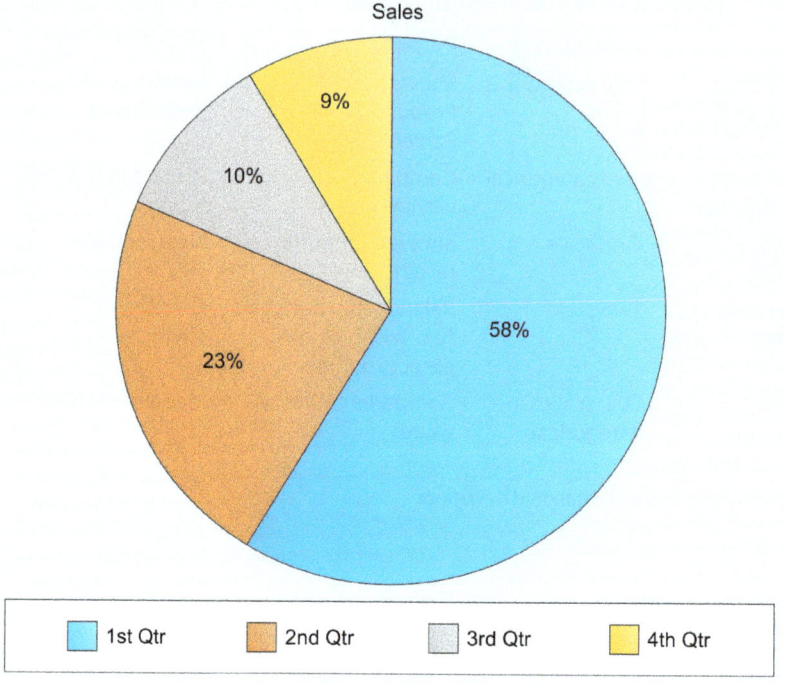

Figure 11: Pie chart.

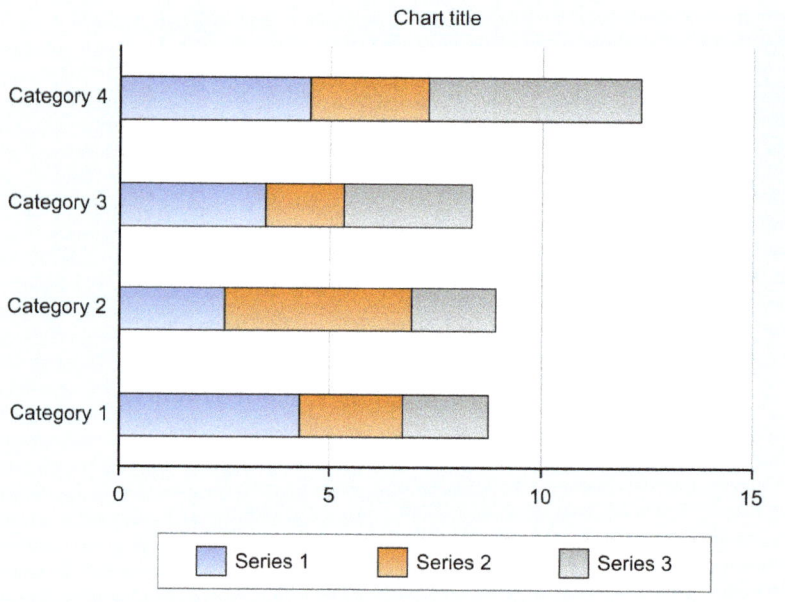

Figure 12: Stacked bar chart.

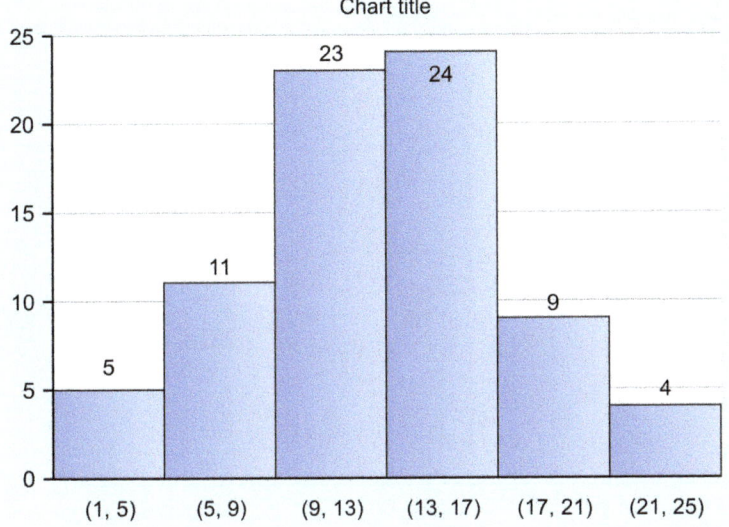

Figure 13: Histogram.

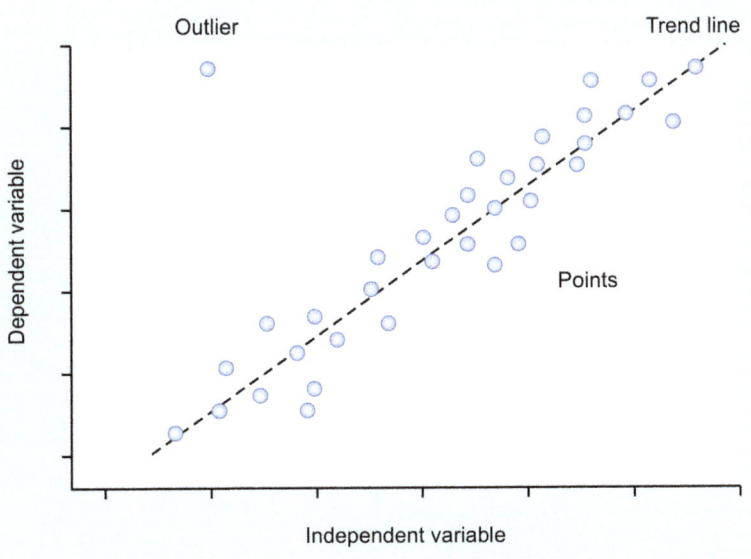

Figure 14: Scatter graph.

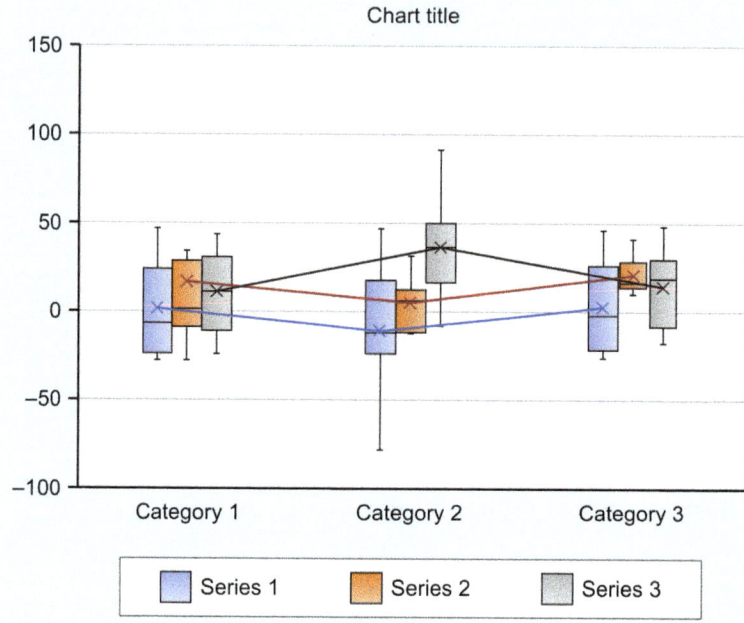

Figure 15: Box and whisker plot.

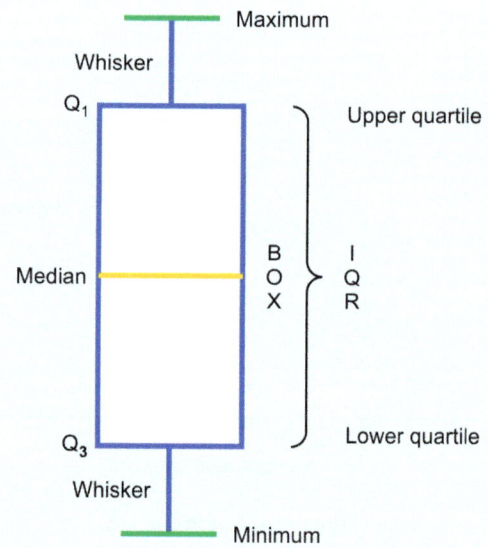

Figure 16: An enlarged box and whisker.

SURVIVAL ANALYSIS KAPLAN–MEIER CURVES

Survival analysis is concerned with studying the time between entry to a study and a subsequent event. Initially, it was concerned with only mortality, but it can be applicable for any other events. The x-axis depicts the length of survival time and the y-axis depicts the cumulative survival probability. This only changes when there is a death (or any event occurs) and so the graph is not smooth but is stepped. Median survival is the time when half of the subjects survive is useful summary for medical research (**Fig. 17**).

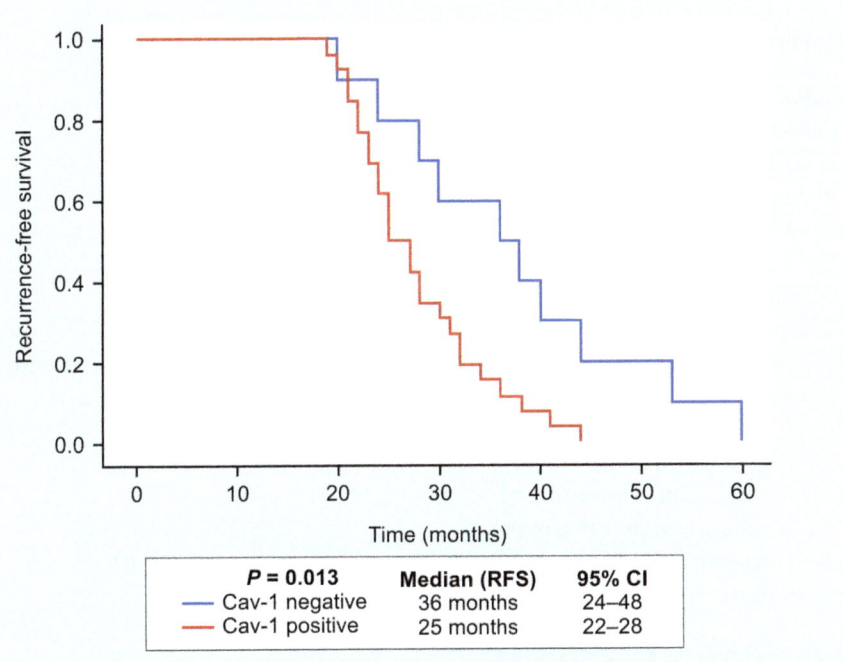

Figure 17: Survival analysis kaplan–meier curves.
Source: Gao Y, Li L, Li T, Ma L, Yuan M, Sun W, et al. Simvastatin delays castration-resistant prostate cancer metastasis and androgen receptor antagonist resistance by regulating the expression of caveolin-1. Int J Oncol. 2019;54(6):2054-68.

REFERENCES

1. Nayak BK, Hazra A. How to choose the right statistical test? Indian J Ophthalmol. 2011;59(2):85.
2. Schneider A, Hommel G, Blettner M. Lineare Regressionsanalyse–Teil 14 der Serie zur Bewertung wissenschaftlicher Publikationen; 2011.
3. BMJ. Correlation and regression. [online] Available from: https://www.bmj.com/about-bmj/resources-readers/publications/statistics-square-one/11-correlation-and-regression. [Last Accessed March, 2021].

CHAPTER 33

Research Methodology

STUDY DESIGNS

Broadly, there are three types of study designs.[1]
1. *Observational*: The subjects are merely observed.
    a. Case-reports/Case series
    b. Case–control (retrospective) studies
    c. Cohort (prospective)
    d. Historical cohort studies
    e. Cross-sectional/Prevalence studies
2. *Experimental*: Studies in which some intervention is done.
    a. Controlled (where cases with intervention done are compared with controls)
        i. Parallel/Concurrent
            a. Randomized controlled trials (RCTs)
            b. Non-randomized
        ii. Sequential (crossover)
    b. Non-controlled (only cases with intervention are evaluated)
3. Systematic reviews/Meta-analysis

OBSERVATIONAL STUDIES

Observational studies have population as subject of interest, while analytical studies have individual as subject of interest. The individuals are evaluated and the inference is extrapolated to the entire population from which the sample is drawn.

Case–Control Study

It is also known as retrospective studies to test casual hypothesis. The question that is generally answered is—"What happened?" The design of case–control study is described in **Figure 1**.

The steps involved in case-control study are as follows:
1. *Selection of cases*: The cases should be well-defined before study. Source—generally hospital based

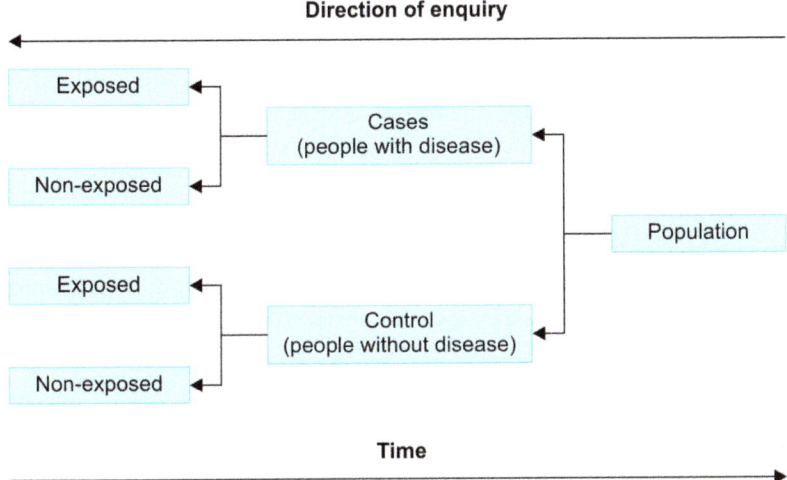

Figure 1: Design of case–control study.

2. *Selection of controls*: Controls are without disease, but should be comparable with the cases to all aspects except the disease under study. Bias and confounding factors should be taken into consideration.
3. *Matching*: Matching is defined as the process by which we select controls in such a way that they are similar to cases with regard to certain pertinent selected variables (e.g., age) which are known to influence the outcome of disease and which, if not adequately matched for comparability, could distort or confound the results. A "confounding factor" is defined as one which is associated both with exposure and disease, and is distributed unequally in study and control groups. More specifically a "confounding factor" is one that, although associated with "exposure" under investigation, is itself, independently of any such association, a "risk factor" for the disease.
4. *Measurements of exposure*: The variables and the outcomes should be exactly specified.
5. *Analysis and interpretation*: The final step is analysis of the data by odds ratio (OR) which is a measure of the strength of the association between risk factor and outcome.

Advantages
- Relatively easy to carry out
- Rapid and inexpensive
- Require comparatively few subjects and rare diseases
- No risk to subjects

- Risk factors can be identified. Rational prevention and control programs can be established
- No attrition problems, because case–control studies do not require follow-up of individuals into the future
- Ethical problems are minimal

Disadvantages

- Retrospective nature and thus recall bias and accuracy of data uncertain.
- Incidence cannot be calculated and thus relative risk cannot be calculated.
- Natural history of the disease cannot be established

Cross-sectional Studies/Prevalence Studies

The data of the specified population is analyzed at one point of time, rather than over period of time. They generally answer the question, "What is happening now?" They help to know about the prevalence of disease in question. Surveys and polls are also cross-sectional studies.

Cohort Study

It is also known as prospective/longitudinal or incidence study. Case–control study is "effect to cause", while cohort study is "cause to effect". A cohort is a group of people who have something in common and who remain part of a group over an extended time. They generally answer the question, "What will happen?"

The design of cohort study is described in **Figure 2**.

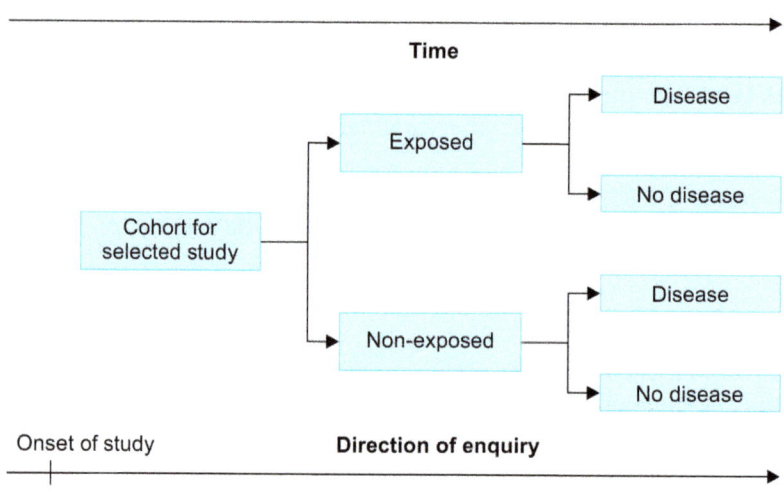

Figure 2: Design of cohort study.

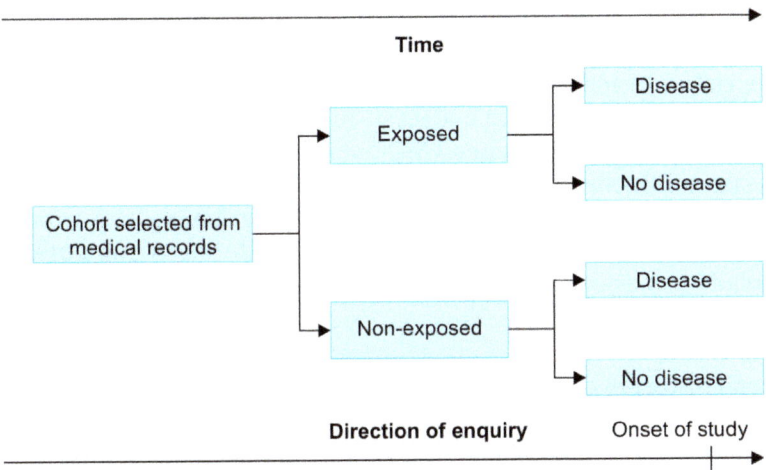

Figure 3: Design of retrospective cohort study.

There are two different types of cohort studies:
1. *Prospective cohort studies/Current cohort study*: The outcome (disease) has not occurred at the time investigation begins. For example, effect of type of diet (vegetarian/non-vegetarian), risk of developing urolithiasis.
2. *Retrospective cohort studies/Historical cohort study, prospective study in retrospect and non-concurrent prospective study*: In this study, the investigators go back in time to evaluate medical records. They form study groups and trace them forward through the time generally upto present (**Fig. 3**).

The components of this study are:
1. *Selection of study subjects*: It can be from general population or special groups (professional population)
2. *Obtaining data on exposure*: Data about the exposure can be obtained from the cohorts via interview, review of medical records, medical examination/test
3. *Selection of comparison groups*: It could be internal comparisons (some subjects in the cohort acts control for a specific outcome) or external comparisons (the study and control cohorts should have comparable demographic data)
4. *Follow-up*: It could be regular examination or review of medical records/questionnaire
5. *Analysis*:

	Developed cancer bladder	Not developed cancer bladder	Total
Cigarette smoking (Yes)	70 (a)	30 (b)	100 (a + b)
Cigarette smoking (No)	6 (c)	94 (d)	100 (c + d)

Incidence rate of cancer bladder (among smoker) = 70/100 = 7 per 10
(among non-smokers) = 6/100 = 0.6 per 10
Relative risk = Incidence of disease among exposed/incidence of disease among non-exposed = 7/0.6 = 11.66
Attributable risk/Risk difference: (Attributable risk indicates to what extent the disease under study can be attributed to the exposure) = Incidence of disease among exposed – incidence of disease among non-exposed/incidence of disease among exposed × 100 = 7 – 0.6/7 = 0.91 × 100 = 91%, i.e., 91% of bladder cancer can be eliminated if smoking factor is removed.

Advantages

- Natural history of disease can be studied
- One exposure to multiple outcomes can be studied
- Incidence rate and therefore relative risk and attributable risk can be calculated
- There is no recall bias

Disadvantages

- Large number of people involved
- Therefore, more time required and more expensive
- Rare diseases cannot be assessed
- Attrition problem—patient lost to follow-up

EXPERIMENTAL STUDIES

They are almost similar to analytical studies except that the conditions in which study is carried out are under the direct control of the investigator. The aim of this study is: (1) Provide scientific proof of etiological factors; and (2) Measuring the effectiveness and efficiency of health services for prevention and control of the disease.

Randomized Controlled Trials

Randomized controlled trials are quantitative, comparative, controlled experiments in which investigators study two or more interventions in a series of individuals who receive them in random order. The RCT is one of the simplest and most powerful tools in clinical research. Ethics committee approval is must before the study. Written informed consent in the language spoken and understood by patient is also very important and mandatory before the study. The clinical trials should be registered with "Clinical Trials Registry-India (CTRI)" by Indian Council of Medical Research (ICMR) (http://ctri.nic.in/). Nowadays, editors of major journals have made it mandatory for CTRI registration for publication of the study in journals.

The basic steps in conducting a RCT include the following:
1. *Drawing up a protocol*: The protocol specifies the aims and objectives of the study, questions to be answered, criteria for the selection of study and control groups, size of the sample, the procedures for allocation of subjects into study and control groups, treatments to be applied when and where and how to what kind of patients, standardization of working procedures and schedules as well as responsibilities of the parties involved in the trial, upto the stage of evaluation of outcome of the study.
2. *Selecting reference and experimental populations*
3. *Randomization*
4. *Intervention*: This is done if required by the investigator.
5. *Follow-up*: This implies examination of the experimental and control group subjects at defined intervals of time, in a standard manner, with equal intensity, under the same given circumstances, in the same time frame till final assessment of outcome.
6. *Assessment of outcome*: The final step is to applying statistical test and inferring the results (**Flowchart 1**).

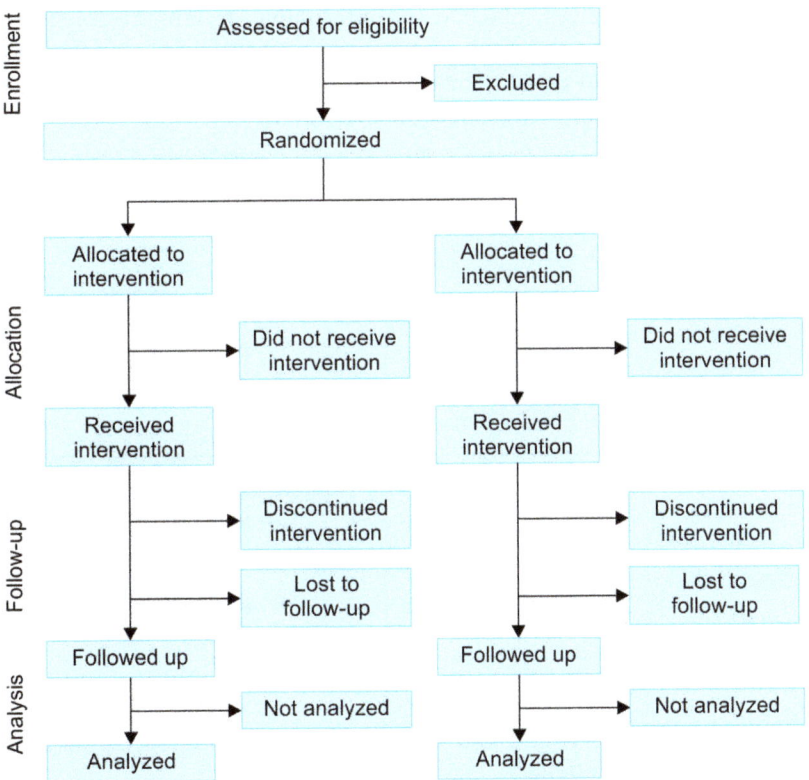

Flowchart 1: Randomized Controlled Trials.

Advantages of RCT
- Randomization ensures removal of bias and confounding factors
- Strongest evidence among all study designs
- It can be tailored to answer any specific question

Disadvantages
- It is labor intensive and expensive
- Lost to follow-up or attrition can happen
- Ethical issues regarding new drug or treatment as some study population might drop.

Types of RCT
There are two types of RCT (**Figs. 4A and B**):
1. *Concurrent parallel study designs*: The patients randomized to treatment exposure or unexposed, remain in the same group for the entire duration of the study.
2. *Crossover study designs*: The study group receives treatment and the control group receives placebo or alternative treatment for some specified duration in the study, following which they are observed for some time (wash-out period) for elimination of the drug effect. Both the groups then crossover with respect to each other.

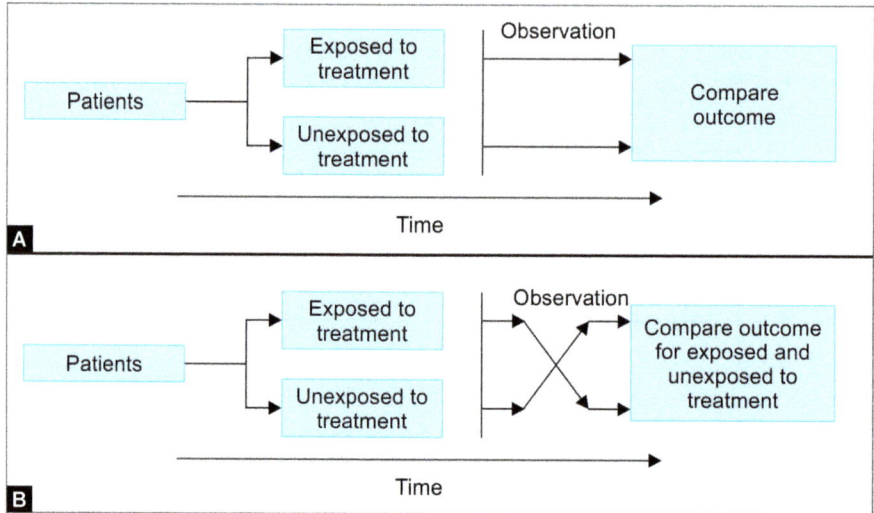

Figures 4A and B: Types of randomized controlled trials: (A) Concurrent parallel study designs; (B) Crossover study designs.

Bias in Clinical Trials

Definition: Bias is defined as any tendency which prevents unprejudiced consideration of a question. In research, bias occurs when "systematic error is introduced into sampling or testing by selecting or encouraging one outcome or answer over others" (**Table 1**).[1]

TABLE 1: Different types of bias in clinical trials.	
Type	Description
Selection bias	This occurs when the subjects included in the study are not truly representative of the target population. This can happen if the sample size is too small or nonrandom sampling or serious cases die of and thus are not available for comparison with the mild cases
Channeling bias	Channeling bias occurs when patient prognostic factors or degree of illness dictates the study cohort into which patients are placed. For example, bias of younger population in operative intervention arm while older population in conservative treatment arm
Definition bias	The study subjects should be sharply defined to avoid ambiguity. For example, effect of drug on erectile dysfunction. The definition of erectile dysfunction should be clearly defined
Evaluator/ Investigator bias	The investigator taking end-point variable measurement intentionally or unintentionally favors one group over other. It is more common with subjective or quality of life end-points
Chronology bias	This occurs when historic cohorts are used as comparison group for patients. Preoperative computed tomography (CT) urography helps kidney puncture planning and decreases puncture time. When historic cohorts are used when CT was not available, the conclusion would be puncture time decrease as surgeon experience increases, but CT urography currently available introduces chronology bias. This can be minimized by prospective studies or RCT
Recall bias	Recall bias refers to the phenomenon in which the outcomes of treatment (good or bad) may color subjects' recollections of events prior to or during the treatment process
Performance bias	It occurs when participant knows of exposure to intervention or its response, be it inactive or active
Misclassification of exposure or outcome	This occurs when the exposure is poorly defines or the outcome is poorly defined as nonobjective measures
Instruction bias	If no discrete instructions are made then investigators can use their own discretion

Contd...

Contd...

Type	Description
Length bias	A case–control study is generally based on prevalent cases rather than incident cases. Prevalence is dominated by those who survive for a longer duration. And these patients are qualitatively different from those who die early. Thus the sample may include disproportionately more of those who are healthier and survive longer. The conclusions cannot be generalized to those who have less survival time
Lead time bias	All cases are not detected at the same stage of the disease. In cancers some may be detected at the time of screening and some may be detected after clinical manifestation. The follow-up is generally from time of detection. This difference in "lead time" can lead to errors. For example, false impression of improved survival in a screened population without affecting mortality, because the cancer is diagnosed earlier in the natural history of the disease but the patient still dies of the cancer
Ascertainment or information bias	It occurs due to measurement error or misclassification of patient. For example, diagnostic bias (more diagnostic procedures performed in cases as compared with controls), recall bias (error of categorization, investigator aggressively search for exposure variables in cases)
Allocation bias	Allocation bias occurs when the measured treatment effect differs from the true treatment effect
Detection bias	It occurs when observations in one group are not as vigilantly sought as in the other
Attrition bias/ Loss-to-follow-up bias	It occurs when patient is lost to follow-up preferentially in a particular group
Citation bias	It refers to the fact that some researchers or trial sponsors may publish only positive findings it their study, to prevent negative impact on their personal abilities
Berkson's bias/ Admission bias	It is due to different rates of admission to hospital for people with different disease
Neyman bias (Prevalence-incidence)	It is a selection bias where the very sick or very well or both are erroneously excluded from a study. The bias ("error") in your results can be skewed in two directions: • Excluding patients who have died will make conditions look less severe • Excluding patients who have recovered will make conditions look more severe
Hawthorne effect/ Observer effect bias	Here the individuals modify an aspect of their behavior in response to their awareness of being observed. This can affect the integrity of research by affecting the relationship between the variables

Randomization

Randomization ensures that each patient has an equal chance of receiving any of the treatments under study, generate comparable intervention groups, which are alike in all the important aspects except for the intervention each groups receives.

Importance
- Method to allocate individuals in an arm
- Minimize selection and allocation bias
- Maximize statistical power
- Leads to all characteristics to be distributed equally in both groups
  The different types of randomization are described in **Table 2**.
  The key differences between stratified sampling and cluster sampling are given in **Table 3** and **Figure 5**.

TABLE 2: Different types of randomization.			
Method	Definition	Used when	Example
Simple/ Unrestricted	Each individual of the population has the same chance of being included in the sample	Population is small and homogeneous	Lottery method, table of random numbers, computer generated
Stratified	When specific variables are known to influence the outcome, stratification of the sample is required to keep the variables (e.g., age, gender, weight, prognostic status, etc.) as similar as possible in between the treatment groups. This method achieves a balance between baseline characteristics	Population in non-homogeneous	• Variable identified → Strata created → Simple randomization applied • In case of assessing results of immunotherapy for viral warts, stratification can be done with respect to the types of warts viz. verruca vulgaris, verruca plana, plantar warts, condyloma acuminata
Cluster	Population is divided into a finite numbers of distinct and identifiable units (sampling units/ element). A group of such elements is a cluster and sampling of these clusters is done	Large geographical area	

TABLE 3: Key differences between stratified sampling and cluster sampling.		
Key	Stratified sampling	Cluster sampling
Meaning	Stratified sampling is one, in which the population is divided into homogeneous segments, and then the sample is randomly taken from the segments	Cluster sampling refers to a sampling method wherein the members of the population are selected at random, from naturally occurring groups called 'cluster'
Sample	Randomly selected individuals are taken from all the strata	All the individuals are taken from randomly selected clusters
Selection of population elements	Individually	Collectively
Homogeneity	Within group	Between groups
Heterogeneity	Between groups	Within group
Bifurcation	Imposed by the researcher	Naturally occurring groups
Objective	To increase precision and representation	To reduce cost and improve efficiency

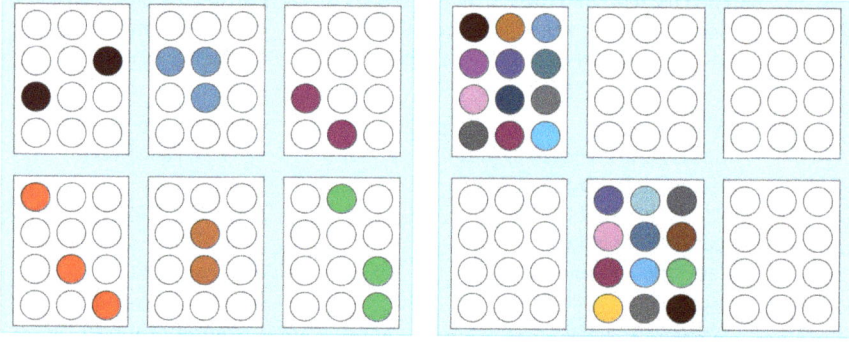

Figure 5: Diagrammatic differences between stratified sampling and cluster sampling.

Blinding

Blinding refers to the concealment of group allocation from one or more individuals involved in a clinical research study, most commonly a RCT. The optimal strategy to minimize the likelihood of differential treatment or assessments of outcomes is to blind as many individuals as possible in a trial. It is generally difficult to blind in surgical trials than in medical trials.

The types of blinding are described in **Table 4**.

If blinding is not possible:
- Standardize the treatment of the groups (apart from the intervention)
- Consider an expertise-based trial design

TABLE 4: Types of blinding.		
Type	Description	Purpose
Open labeled/ Unblinded	All parties are aware of treatment	
Single blinded	Participant (generally) or investigator	Knowledge about the intervention in group assignment may affect their behavior
Double blind	Participant + Investigator	Avoids clinicians having differential attitude toward a group with an intervention
Triple blind	Participant + Investigator + Data analyst	This leads to unbiased data collection and analysis and prevents biased results toward an intervention

- Use objective, reliable outcomes if possible
- Consider duplicate assessment
- Acknowledge the limitations

Allocation Concealment

Allocation concealment refers to the process ensuring the person who generates the random assignment remains blind to what arm the person will be allotted. For example, less sicker patients allotted to a particular group in which the investigator is interested. The allocation should be concealed from investigator till the initiation of intervention. The different ways of allocation concealment are:

- *Central randomization*: Some centrally independent authority performs randomization and informs the investigators via telephone, e-mail or fax
- *Pharmacy controlled*: Pharmacy provides coded drugs for use
- *Sequentially numbered containers*: Identical containers equal in weight, similar in appearance and tamper-proof are used
- *Sequentially numbered, opaque, sealed envelopes*: The randomized numbers are concealed in opaque envelope to be opened just before intervention and are *the most common and easy to perform method.*

The needs for allocation concealment are:
- The investigator may allocate favorable subjects to the group of his interest
- If subject knows about allocation to placebo group, then the subject might opt out of study.

There differences between blinding and allocation concealment are descried in **Table 5**.

TABLE 5: Differences between blinding and allocation concealment.		
	Blinding	**Allocation concealment**
Purpose	Makes participant or investigator or both unaware of treatment received	Conceals randomization sequence
Bias prevented	Subjective bias	Selection bias
Time in trial	Done when patient enters the trial (during recruitment)	Occurs after patient has entered trial (after recruitment)

Formulating a Research Question

The most important aspect of any study is the research hypothesis. The importance of good research question is:

A clearly defined question enhances the chances of developing:
- The appropriate protocol
- Preparation of optimal study design
- Helps in guiding analysis and decision making
- Ensures better chances of publication
- Getting a good question increases the likelihood of finding a correct solution to problem

The questions that need to be answered while formulating a good research question are described by three criteria:

1. **PICOT**[2]

Component	Related questions
Population	• What is the target population? • Is the target population narrow or broad? • Is the target population vulnerable? • What are the eligibility criteria? • What is the most appropriate recruitment strategy?
Intervention	• What is the intervention? (treatment, diagnostic test, procedure) • Is there any standard of care for the intervention? • Is the intervention the most appropriate for the study design? • Is there a need for standardizing the intervention? • What are the potential side effects of the intervention? • Will potential side effects be recorded? • If there is no intervention, what is the exposure?
Comparator	• How has control intervention been chosen? • Are there any ethical concerns related to the use of placebo? • Has a sham intervention been considered? • Will statistical analyses be adjusted for multiple comparisons?

Outcome	• What is the primary outcome? • What are the secondary outcomes? • Are the outcomes exploratory, explanatory or confirmatory? • Have surrogate and clinical outcomes been considered? • Are the outcomes validated? • Have safety outcomes been considered? • How are the outcomes going to be measured? • Will the dependent and independent variables be numerical, categorical or ordinal? • Will be enough statistical power to measure secondary outcomes?
Time frame	• Is the study designed to be cross-sectional or longitudinal? • How long will the recruitment phase take? • What is the time frame for data collection? • Have frequency and duration of the intervention been specified? • How often will outcomes be measured? • Which strategy will be used to prevent/decrease dropouts?

2. **FINER**[2]

Component	Criteria
Feasible	• Ensures adequacy of research design • Guarantees adequate funding • Recruits target population strategically • Aims an achievable sample size • Prioritizes measurable outcomes • Optimizes human and technical resources • Accounts for clinicians commitment • Procures high adherence to the treatment and low rate of dropouts • Opts for appropriate and affordable frame time
Interesting	• Engages the interest of principal investigators • Attracts the attention of readers • Presents a different perspective of the problem
Novel	• Provides different findings • Generates new hypotheses • Improves methodological flaws of existing studies • Resolves a gap in the existing literature
Ethical	• Complies with local ethical committees • Safeguards the main principles of ethical research • Guarantees safety and reversibility of side effects
Relevant	• Generates new knowledge • Contributes to improve clinical practice • Stimulates further research • Provides an accurate answer to a specific research question

3. **FINERMAPS**[3]
- FINER (As described previously)
- M (Manageable)—can be managed by the researcher
- A (Appropriate)—appropriate logically and scientifically for the community and institution
- P (Potential value and publishability)—must address a topic that has clear implications for resolving important dilemmas in health and healthcare decisions made by one or more stakeholder groups.
- S (Systematic)—structured with specified steps to be taken in a specified sequence in accordance with the well-defined set of rules though it does not rule out creative thinking.

SYSTEMATIC REVIEWS AND META-ANALYSIS[4]

A systematic review collects all possible studies related to a given topic and design, and reviews and analyzes their results. A systematic review is an objective, reproducible method to find answers to a certain research question, by collecting all available studies related to that question and reviewing and analyzing their results. A meta-analysis is a valid, objective, and scientific method of analyzing and combining different results. Usually, in order to obtain more reliable results, a meta-analysis is mainly conducted on RCTs, which have a high level of evidence.

The steps involved in the process are given in **Flowchart 2**.

Quality of evidence: If the Grading of Recommendations, Assessment, Development and Evaluation (GRADE) system (http://www.gradeworkinggroup.org/) is used, the quality of evidence is evaluated on the basis of the study limitations, inaccuracies, incompleteness of outcome data, indirectness of evidence, and risk of publication bias, and this is used to determine the strength of recommendation.

Data extraction: It is done by two different investigators and they resolve the differences by consensus.

Data analysis: The final aim is to increase power and accuracy. If it is determined that the different research outcomes cannot be combined, all the results and characteristics of the individual studies are displayed in a table or in a descriptive form; this is referred to as a qualitative review (**Table 6**).

The quantitative review of meta-analysis is evaluated by calculating the weighted pooled estimate. The pooled estimate is the outcome of the meta-analysis, and is typically explained using a forest plot. The black squares in the forest plot are the ORs and 95% confidence intervals in each study. The area of the squares represents the weight reflected in the meta-analysis. The black diamond represents the OR and 95% confidence interval calculated across all the included studies. The bold vertical line represents a lack of therapeutic effect (OR = 1); if the confidence interval includes OR = 1, it

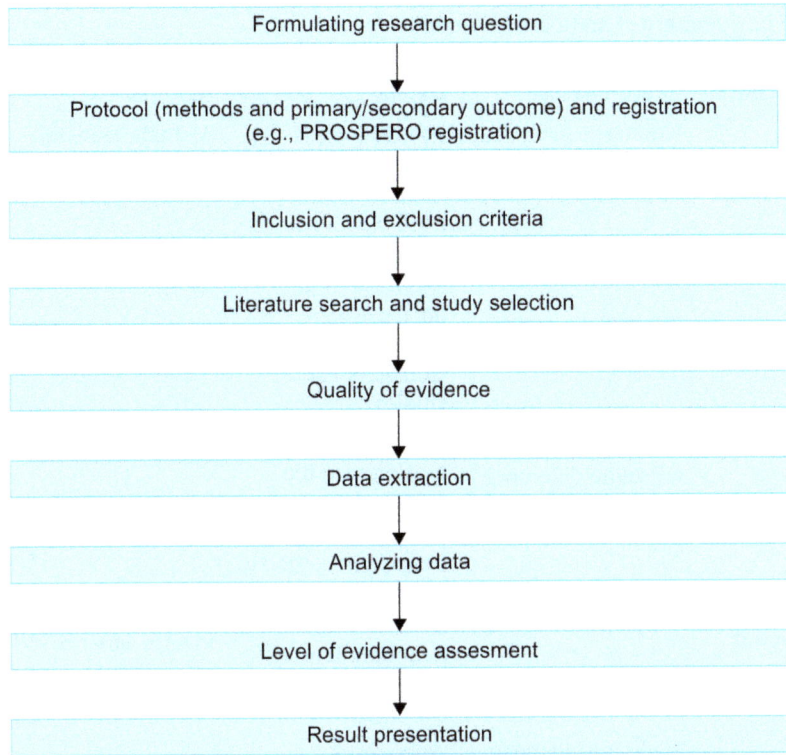

Flowchart 2: A systematic review.

means no significant difference was found between the treatment and control groups.

Homogeneity of data: Homogeneity test is a method whether the degree of heterogeneity is greater than would be expected to occur naturally when the effect size calculated from several studies is higher than the sampling error. Tests for homogeneity are:
- *Forest plot*: Greater overlap between confidence intervals → Homogeneity
- *Chi-square test calculated from forest plot*: <0.1 then statistical heterogeneity
- *Higgins I^2 statistics*: <23% → Strong homogeneity, 50% → Average, >75% → Strong heterogeneity.

Results presentation:
- Flowchart with literature search and selection process
- Table of characteristics of included studies
- Table of quality of evidence such as GRADE
- *Data analysis*: Forest plot and funnel plot
- Data analysis with Review Manager software (The Cochrane Collaboration, UK):
  ○ P value from z test → Tests the null hypothesis that the intervention has no effect

Type of data	Effect measure	Details	Meta-analysis method
Dichotomous	Odds ratio (OR)	Used for other case–control studies or cross-sectional studies	Mantel–Haenszel (M-H)
	Risk ratio (RR)	Used for randomized controlled trials (RCTs), quasi-experimental studies, or cohort studies	Mantel–Haenszel (M-H)
	Risk difference (RD)		Inverse variance (IV)
Continuous	Mean difference (absolute difference in means of two groups)	When results are presented in the same units (MD < 0 → new treatment method is less effective MD > 0 → new treatment is more effective than existing method)	Inverse variance (IV)
	Standardized mean difference (mean difference/standard deviation)	When results are presented in different units	

TABLE 6: Summary of meta-analysis methods.

- P value from chi-square test → Tests the null hypothesis for a lack of heterogeneity.

Funnel Plot[5]

A funnel plot is a scatter plot of the effect estimates from individual studies against some measure of each study's size or precision. The standard error of the effect estimate is often chosen as the measure of study size and plotted on the vertical axis with a reversed scale that places the larger, most powerful studies toward the top. The effect estimates from smaller studies should scatter more widely at the bottom, with the spread narrowing among larger studies. In the absence of bias and between study heterogeneity, the scatter will be due to sampling variation alone and the plot will resemble a symmetrical inverted funnel (**Fig. 6**). A triangle centered on a fixed effect summary estimate and extending 1.96 standard errors either side will include about 95% of studies if no bias is present and the fixed effect assumption (that the true treatment effect is the same in each study) is valid.

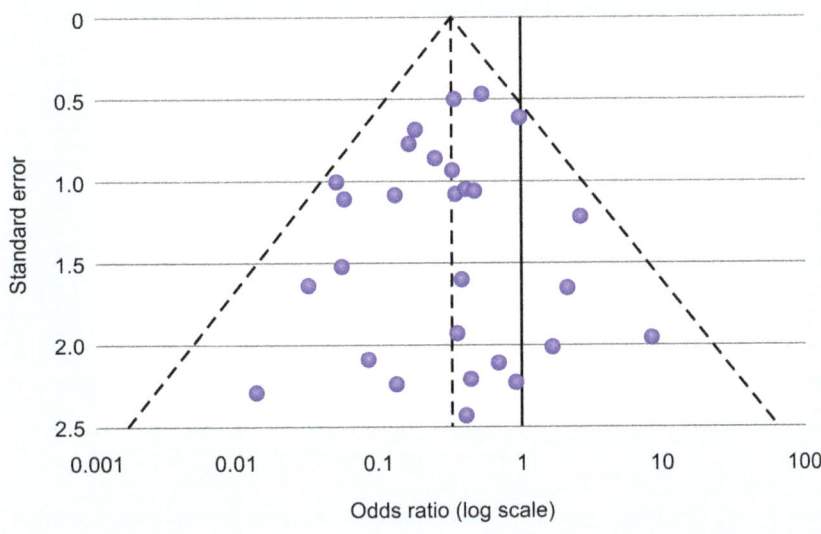

Figure 6: Example of symmetrical funnel plot.

Possible sources of asymmetry in funnel plots:
- Reporting biases
- Publication bias
  - Selective outcome reporting
  - Selective analysis reporting
- Poor methodological quality leading to spuriously inflated effects in smaller studies
- True heterogeneity
- Chance

Symmetrical funnel plot: The outer dashed lines indicate the triangular region within which 95% of studies are expected to lie in the absence of both biases and heterogeneity (fixed effect summary log odds ratio ± 1.96 × standard error of summary log odds ratio). The solid vertical line corresponds to no intervention effect.

Forest Plot/Blobbogram
- It is used for displaying data analyzed in systematic reviews and meta-analysis.
- X axis—null effect, Y axis—odds ratio or relative risk
- Box—point estimate of a study with its size displaying sample size
- Horizontal lines—95% confidence intervals

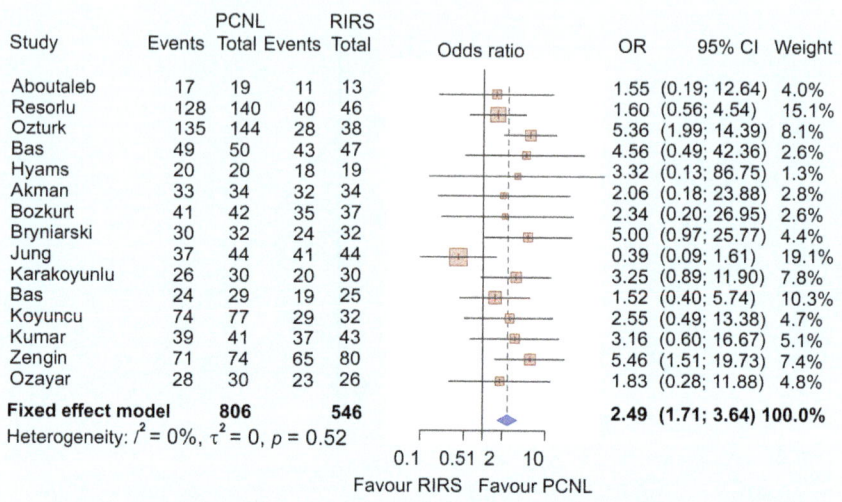

Figure 7: Pairwise meta-analysis of success rate in percutaneous nephrolithotomy (PCNL) and retrograde intrarenal surgery (RIRS).

Source: Chung DY, Kang DH, Cho KS, Jeong WS, Jung HD, Kwon JK, et al. Comparison of stone-free rates following shock wave lithotripsy, percutaneous nephrolithotomy, and retrograde intrarenal surgery for treatment of renal stones: A systematic review and network meta-analysis. PLoS One. 2019;14(2):e0211316.

- The diamond represents the point estimate and confidence intervals when you combine and average all the individual studies together
- Powerful studies (those with more participants) have narrower (shorter) confidence intervals. A study with an odds ratio of one and a very narrow confidence interval would indicate no significant effect.

The **Figure 7** explains the example of forest plot/blobbogram.

Institutional Ethics Committee

Every trial or thesis requires approval from Institutional Ethics Committee (IEC) before proceeding. It constitutes of:
1. Chairperson (outside the institution)
2. Member secretary (belongs to the institution and conducts the business of the committee)
3. 1–2 Persons from basic medical science area
4. 1–2 Clinicians
5. 1 Legal expert
6. 1 Social scientist
7. 1 Philosopher/Ethicist/Theologian
8. 1 Lay person from the community

Institutional Animal Ethics Committee

This committee takes care of all aspects of animal research and care. This committee is formed as per the guidelines of the Committee for the Purpose of Control and Supervision of Experiments on Animals (CPCSEA).

The committee[6] of Institutional Animal Ethics Committee (IAEC) consists of 5 members (all from science background including one Veterinarian).
- A Biological Scientist
- Two Scientists from different biological disciplines
- A Veterinarian involved in the care of Animals
- Scientist In-charge of Animal House Facility
  The Chairman of the IAEC (preferably Head of the Institution/Department) and Member Secretary need to be nominated by the establishment from the above five members
  The validity of this committee is 3 years and needs to be renewed thereafter.

The functions of the IAEC are as follows:
- To review, modify and approve research proposals involving lab animals
- To conduct periodic supervision of Institute's animal facility and correct research activity if it is not conducted as per CPCSEA guidelines
- To see that all those persons involved in animal care and research are adequately trained to handle the animals
- To ascertain ethical use of animals and protection of wellbeing of animals during and after research

References

Referencing is a scientific approach to delineate a data source by providing a standard set of information, allowing its easy identification, searchability, and retrieval.

References: Only the source of information referred in the research paper.

Bibliography: List of relevant sources for reading even if they are cited in paper.

In-text citations: Validate authors' statements and establish relation between several studies.

The references format may be classified as:
1. **Name-year (or author-date):** Which is a parenthetical citation including the author(s)' last name(s) and publication year (in this style, the reference list is ordered alphabetically) **(APA and Harvard)**;
2. **Citation-sequence:** With the numbers presented sequentially in the text, either superscripted, in brackets, or in parentheses, and the reference list formatted in numerical order **(Vancouver)**; and
3. **Citation-name:** Wherein the number in a citation (superscript, brackets, parentheses) refers to an item on the reference list. The reference list is

ordered alphabetically, and as a result, the citation numbers in the text will not be sequential.

The other way of classifying referencing formats is:
1. Publication Manual of the American Psychological Association **(APA)** uses a name-year format (APA, 2009).
2. American Medical Association **(AMA)** uses a citation-sequence format (AMA, 2007).
3. National Library of Medicine **(NLM)** style, which is used for references in MEDLINE/PubMed (US NLM, 2014). [Recommended by the International Committee of Medical Journal Editors (ICMJE)]
4. **Vancouver style**: Citation-sequence style ~ AMA style
5. **Harvard style**: Name-year format ~ APA
6. **Chicago style** (The Chicago Manual of Style): Generally used in Social Sciences
7. **MLA** (Modern Language Association): Generally used by theater related literature.

The differences between Vancouver and Harvard style of referencing are given in **Table 7**.

References are generally to be styled according to the ICMJE recommendations of National Library of Medicine's (NLM) citation style. The journal article format is:

Author AB, Writer, CD. Article Title. Journal Title. Year Month Day of Publication; Volume (Issue):Page Range.

TABLE 7: Differences between Vancouver and Harvard style of referencing.

Vancouver style	Harvard style
References are listed **numerically** in the same order that they were cited in the body of the paper	References are listed **alphabetically** by the surname of the author or title of the book or journal article
In the in-text, a cited text is indicated by a **number**, e.g., In BPH, alpha blockers are useful[6]	In the in-text, a cited text is indicated by the **author's surname and the date** In BPH, alpha blockers are useful (Xyz, 2017)
Maximum number of authors that must be mentioned → **6**	Maximum number of authors that must be mentioned → **8**
If > 6 authors, then write "et al." OR "and others"	If > 8 authors, then write "et al." OR "and others"
Journal titles are abbreviated and are **not in italics**	Journal titles are written in full and are in **italics**
Date of publication is normally given at the **end of the reference**	Date of publication is normally given **immediately after the author**. Hence the style is also known as **Author-date Style**

The format for referencing a book chapter is—
Authors. Title. Edition. Secondary Authors. Place of Publication: Publisher; Date of Publication. Page Range.

Level of Evidence (Table 8 and Fig. 8)

TABLE 8: Depicting Level of evidence and grade of recommendation.

Grade of recommendation	Level of evidence	Interventions
A	1a	Systematic review (SR)/randomized controlled trials (RCT)
	1b	Individual RCT
B	2a	SR of cohort studies
	2b	Individual cohort study
	2c	"Outcomes" research; Ecological studies
	3a	SR of case-control studies
	3b	Individual case-control study
C	4	Case series
D	5	Expert opinion

Source: Home - 2020 - The Centre for Evidence-Based Medicine (cebm.net)

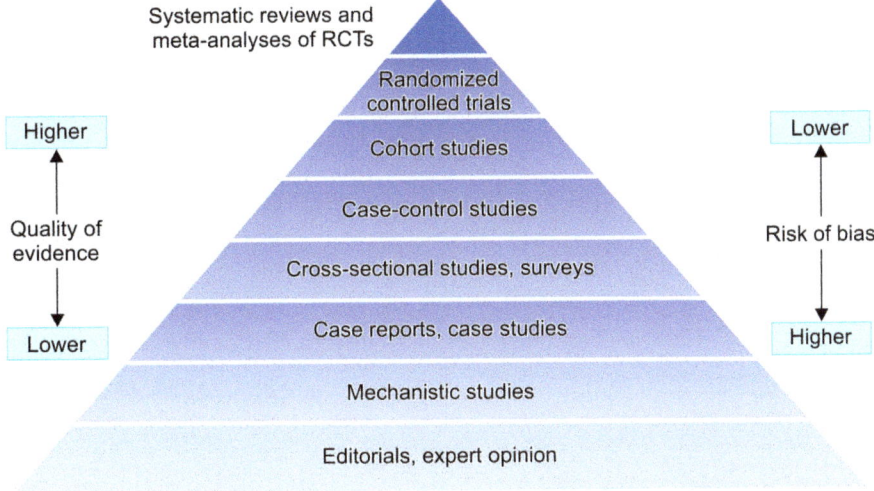

Figure 8: Pyramid depicting level of evidence in medical literature.

REFERENCES

1. Pannucci CJ, Wilkins EG. Identifying and avoiding bias in research. Plast Reconstr Surg. 2010;126(2):619-25.
2. Fandino W. Formulating a good research question: Pearls and pitfalls. Indian J Anaesth. 2019;63(8):611-6.
3. Ratan SK, Anand T, Ratan J. Formulation of research question–stepwise approach. J Indian Assoc Pediatr Surg. 2019;24(1):15-20.
4. Ahn E, Kang H. Introduction to systematic review and meta-analysis. Korean J Anesthesiol. 2018;71(2):103-12.
5. Sterne JA, Sutton AJ, Ioannidis JP, Terrin N, Jones DR, Lau J, et al. Recommendations for examining and interpreting funnel plot asymmetry in meta-analyses of randomised controlled trials. BMJ. 2011;343:d4002.
6. Committee for the Purpose of Control and Supervision of Experiments on Animals. Reconstitution of IAEC. [online] Available from: http://cpcsea.nic.in/content/109_1_ReconstitutionofIAEC.aspx. [Last Accessed March, 2021].

Index

Page numbers followed by *f* refer to figure, *fc* refer to flowchart, and *t* refer to table.

A

Abdomen 269*f*
Absolute neutrophil count 335
Access devices 96
Access needles 48, 48*f*
Access sheath 153, 156*t*
Accessories 79, 87, 137
 channel 9
 sterilization of 171
Acucise endopyelotomy 80, 80*f*
Adapters 14*f*
Adenomas 269
Adequate lymph node dissection 306
Adrenal adenoma, percentage of 319
Adrenal gland 318*f*
Adrenal mass 268, 318
Adrenal oncocytoma 319
Adrenal tumor 318, 318*f*
Adrenalectomy 374
 complications 377
 laparoscopic 376
 preoperative preparation for 374
Adrenocortical carcinoma 271
 chemotherapy for 346
 diagnosis of 319
Advance bipolar systems 126
Air
 drying 169*f*
 well termination 205
Airseal 103*f*
Alanine aminotransferase 334
Albarran lever 7, 8*f*
Alcohol 164
Aldehyde 165
Alken dilators 50
 over alken rod 53*f*
Alken needle 158*f*
Alken telescopic metal dilator 53*f*
Allergic reactions 330
Allport clips 112*f*
Alpha-adrenergic receptor blockers 374

Ambu® ascope™ 16*f*
Amino acid 164
Amlodipine 376
Amplatz dilator 50, 52*f*
 entering calyx 53*f*
Amplatz fixed core guidewire 141
Amplatz renal dilator set 51
Amplatz sheath 46, 58*f*
Anderson-Darling test 396
Anesthesia, general 220
Angioedema 345
Angioembolization, indications for 256
Angiomyolipoma 254
 medical management for 256
Angle tipped ureteric catheter 138, 138*f*, 139*f*
Antireflux surgery, principles of 369
Antiseptics 160
Argon
 beam coagulator 132, 132*f*
 properties of 132
Armamentarium 91
Aspartate aminotransferase 334
Atenolol 376
Atraumatic graspers 92
Autosuture and ethicon veress needles 97*f*
Axitinib 336, 338, 340

B

Bacillus Calmette-Guérin 328
 contraindications 329
 dose and schedule 329
 indications 329
 mechanism of action 328
 toxicity 329
Balanitis xerotica obliterans 216, 355
Balfour retractor 174
Ball electrode 17
Ball tip fiber 206
Balloon dilator 50, 54
 parts of 55*f*

Balloon ureteric catheter 138
Bar chart 417f
Baskets devices 150
Baumrucker system 30
Benign prostatic hyperplasia 199
   management of 199, 210
Bias 429
   allocation 430
   ascertainment 430
   attrition 430
   Berkson's 430
   channeling 429
   chronology 429
   citation 430
   Hawthorne effect 430
   in clinical trials, types of 429t
   information 430
   instruction 429
   lead time 430
   length 430
   Neyman 430
   observer effect 430
   performance 429
   recall 429
   selection 429
Bioabsorbable stent 144
Biopsy 260, 263, 267, 309, 312
   forceps 17
   sample 313
Biostatistics 393
Bipolar
   button electrode 41
   circuit 126f
   electrode 38
   technology, limitations of 39
Bisected radical nephrectomy 300
Bisected radical nephroureterectomy 304f, 308
Bladder 262, 304, 307
   cancer
      chemotherapy for 327
      immunotherapy for 333
      palliative chemotherapy for 332
   capacity 217, 235
   carcinoma, types of 305
   diseases, benign 225
   diverticulum 225
   evacuator, modification of 36f, 37
   mass 265, 266
   mucosa 361
   neck
      absence of 373
      involvement 323
      tumor, treatment for 304
Bland thrombus 259
Bleeding 354
Bleomycin 342, 343
Blinding 432, 434t
   types of 433t
Blobbogram 439
Blue-light flexible cystoscopy 17
Blunt dissection 372
Blunt tipped obturator 104
Bonferroni test 409
Bookwalter retractor 174, 174f
Bowel leak 374
Box and whisker plot 420f
Bridge 3, 8
   parts of 8f, 9
   types of 9
Broken loop 32
Bugbee electrode 20, 20f, 190f
Bugiogram, disadvantages of 221
Bulbar urethra 216, 223
Bulldog clamp 177, 177f
Bulldog clip applier 114
Burst laser therapy 207

C

Cabazitaxel 335
Cabozantinib 337
Calcium channel blockers 375
Calyceal stone, lower 237f
Camera control unit 91, 93
Cannula 92, 100
Capacitative coupling 134, 135f
Carbon dioxide
   cylinder 92
   pressure regulator valve 92
Carboplatin single agent adjuvant 341
Carcinoma
   penis
      conditions of 312
      types of 312
   prostate, chemotherapy for 334
   testis, incidence of 316
Case-control study 422
   advantages 423
   design of 423f
   disadvantages 424

Catecholamine synthesis blockade 376
Catheter, loss of 372
Centers for Disease Control and
 Prevention Guidelines 161
C-flex 143
Charge-coupled device 15, 16, 86, 93
Chemical
 agents 164
 disinfectants, aldehyde group of 164
Chemotherapy 347
 adjuvant 332
Chip-on-the-tip principle 86
Chi-square test 409
Choriocarcinoma 316
Chylous ascite 386
Circle nephrostomy tubes 150
Cisplatin 340, 343, 345, 346
Clip applicator and staplers 91, 108
Close-end catheter 137
Clutton metallic bougie 182
Coaxial cable laparoscopes 115
Cohen's cross trigonal technique 389, 390f
Cohort study 424
 design of 424f
Color code disk 4, 7
Compact operating fiber
 ureterorenoscope 78
Complementary metal oxide
 semiconductor 16
 image sensors 15, 86
Cone tipped ureteric catheter 137, 138f
Continuous flow resectoscope 27f
Continuous irrigation sheath 23, 26, 57
Continuous laser 199
Contralateral testicular biopsy, role of 316
Conventional fiberoptic flexible
 ureteroscope, parts of 82
Conventional rod-lens system 13, 13t
Cook flexor access sheath 155f
Cooley vascular clamp 178, 178f
Councilman catheter 149
Creatinine 232, 233
Cryotherapy 133
Culp-DeWeerd spiral flap 368
Cystectomy 304-306
Cystogram 220, 226f
Cystolithotomy, laparoscopic 46
Cystolithotripsy
 adapter 46f
 percutaneous 46

Cystolithotrity instruments 43
Cystoprostatectomy 304, 304f, 307f
Cystoscope 3
 beak 6
  types of 6f
 color coding for 11f
 obturator 3
 parts of 4f, 13f
 sheath 3-5, 5f
 urethroscope sheath 189, 189f
Cystoscopies, sterilization of 172
Cystourethroscope 186, 186f
 adolescent 188f
 types of 10

D

D'Agostino-Pearson normality test 406
Dangler stents 144
Data
 analysis 436
 continuous 438
 detecting normalcy of 397f
 dichotomous 438
 extraction 436
 Gaussian 396f
 homogeneity of 437
 non-normal 396f
 non-symmetrical 396f
 normal 396f
 normalcy of 397f
 symmetrical 396f
 type of 438
De Pezzer catheters 150
Debakey vascular
 clamps 178, 179f
 forceps 179, 180f
Deflux 195
 injection, instruments for 194
 needles, cystoscope for use with 189
Denis brown abdominal retractor 175, 175f
Desiccation 125
Desjardins forceps 179, 180f
Dextérité surgical system DEX® 116, 116f
Diagnostic tests 407
 validity of 407
Digital cystourethroscopes 15
Digital flexible ureteroscope 86
 advantages of 87
 disadvantages of 87
 parts of 84
Dilators 182

Diode laser 200, 211
Direct coupling 134, 134f
Disengageable ratchet 106
Disinfection 160, 161
Dissection
  hook 92
  template of 300f
Distal bulbar stricture 217
Distal hypospadias 350
Distal tubularized incised plate repair 350
Distal ureteric tumor 308, 309
Distal urethra
  dissection of 358
  incision of 358
Diverticulum 226
  acquired 227
  cause of 226
  congenital 227
Docetaxel 335
Double J stents 142, 144f, 153
Double lumen ureteric catheter 138
Doxazosine 376
Doxorubicin 346
Drug-eluting stents 144
Dual-operating channel ureteroscope 78
Dunnett's post-hoc test 409

E

Echo-tipped ureteral catheter 139f
Ectopic kidney, calculus in 246
Ejaculatory dysfunction 387
Electrocautery 122
Electrodes 193
Electrosurgery 122
Electrosurgical
  cutting 125
  generator 123
  tissue effect 125, 125f
Ellik evacuator 36, 36f
Embolization, preoperative 364
Endocameleon 115
Endoclip™ multiclip applier 112
Endocrine Society Clinical Practice Guideline 374
Endopyelotomy stent 144, 144f
Endoscopic management 46, 216
EndoTIP port 103f
Energy

  sources 66, 122
  transmission 205
Enseal 128f
Enucleation, techniques of 211
Epididymoorchitis 222
Erectile dysfunction 372
  prevention of 373
Ergonomic body support 117, 117f
Ethicon endosurgery generator 128
ETHOS™ platform 117, 118f
Ethyl alcohol 164
Ethylene oxide 89, 164, 173
  gas 163
  sterilization 163
Ethylene tetrafluoroethylene 206
Etoposide 342, 343, 345, 346
Everolimus 338
Excision 355
Exophytic component 254f
Exophytic mass 260f
Extended length cystoscope-urethroscope 10
Extension cord 92
Extracapsular extension 322
Extracorporeal shock wave lithotripsy 248
Extragonadal germ cell tumor, chemotherapy for 345
Extrarenal pelvis 254
Eyepiece 76, 82
  lateral 194
  types of 79f

F

Fairhurst formula 217
Fan retractor 106
Fascial dilator 50, 51f
Fever, persistent high-grade 330
Fiber 206
  cystourethroscope 187f
  hub 204
  size 206
Fiberoptic
  cystourethroscopes 13
  flexible ureteroscope 81
  telescope 62f
  ureteroscope 86
Fistula, urethrocutaneous 354
Flaps

epilation of 355
vascularity of 355
Flexible biopsy forceps 17, 18f
Flexible cystourethroscopes 13, 14f, 16t
   advancements in 15
   advantages of 15
   indications of 15
Flexible fiberoptic ureteroscope, basic design of 82
Flexible ureteroscopes 81, 82f, 84, 172
   evolution of 81
   tip of 83f
   types of 81
Fluorouracil 340
Foley adapter 217
Foley catheter 23, 145, 146, 148f, 149, 216, 217, 361, 368
   color coding for 147t
   simple 146
   types of 146
Forceps, types of 157
Formaldehyde 164, 166
Frequency spectrum 123, 123f
Fulguration 125
   anticipate after 233
Funnel plot 438

G

Gapometry index 221
Gelpi retractor 175
Gemcitabine 328
   contraindications 328
   indications 328
Genitourinary system 345
Germ cell tumor 315, 316
Germicide 160
Gibbons catheter 145
Gil vernet hilar retractor 176, 177f
Glans wings, adequate mobilization of 353f
Gleason's grade 322
Glenn–Anderson technique 388, 389f
Glutaraldehyde 164, 165
Gonadal tumor, chemotherapy for 345
Gorget 183, 185f
Grasping forceps 17
Green light laser 200, 211
Guidewire 140
   parts of 141f
   types of 141f
Guy's STONE score 242f

Gyrus loop 40f
Gyrus PK tissue management system 127

H

Harrington retractor 175
Hassan trocar 104
Haygrove sound 183, 184f
Hematological reasons, dose modification for 335t, 346t
Hematoma 273, 354, 365
Hematopoietic tumor 315
Hematuria catheters 146
Hem-O-lok clip applicator 109, 110, 110f, 111
Hemorrhage 300f, 373
Hemostasis 363
Hemostat style ratchet 106
Hendrickson's classical lithotrite 45f
Heparin 144
Hepatic dysfunction, dose modification to 334t
Hexaminolevulinate 17
High frequency cable 33, 35f
High pressure reflux 235
High watt holmium laser 204, 207
Histogram 419f
Holmdahl formula 217
Holmium laser 200, 210
   lithotripsy
      pulse frequency in 207
      pulse variation in 208
Holmium:yttrium aluminum garnet laser 200, 202, 202f
Hook electrode 189f
Hopkins rod-lens system 12, 13, 13t
Hormone refractory prostate cancer 335
Hounsfield unit 240
Human prostate tissue 322f
Hutch diverticulum 196
Hydrogen peroxide gas plasma sterilization 162
Hydronephrosis 263
   bilateral 246
   classify 252
Hydrophilic coating 156
Hyperoxaluria, types of 244
Hyperplasia, prostatic 322f
Hypersensitivity reaction 344
Hypospadias 350
Hypotension 345

Hypothyroidism 337
Hysterectomy, steps of 373

I

Ifosfamide 343, 345
　dose modification for 344t
Iglesias outer sheath with nephroscope 46
Ileus 374
Incidentaloma 270
Indoscope 89f
Inguinal orchiectomy 314
Initial puncture needle 49, 50
Inlet and outlet vent 4, 7
Inlet channel 23
Inner preputial skin graft 353f
Instruments 1, 48
　insert of 105
　laparoscopic 91
Insufflators 92, 96
　types of 96
Insulation failure 134, 135f
Integrated ultrasound and advanced bipolar generators 131
Interlacing video 95
Interlocking clips, types of 111
Intracavernosal injection therapy 372
Intraductal carcinoma 322
Intrarenal holmium laser lithotripsy 208f
Intravenous pyelogram 142, 229, 240f
Intravenous urogram 252f
Iodophors 167
Ipilimumab 339
Isopropyl alcohol 164
Isotope renogram 253

K

Karl Storz
　bipolar resectoscope loop 40
　cystoscopes sheaths 3t
　endoscopes, specifications of 77f
　semirigid ureteroscope 76
Kaye's tamponade balloon 149
Kelly retractor 175
Keyhole sign 232
Kidney 246, 273, 307
　mass 254f
　nonfunctional 196, 266
Kilian septum speculum 183, 184f

Kink resistant sheath 156
Koff's formula 217
Kolmogorov-Smirnov test 396
Koraitim's Golden triad 358
Kurtosis 399

L

Lambert-Kay vascular inferior vena cava clamp 179, 180f
Laparoscopes 115, 115f, 116f
Laparoscopic camera 92, 93f
Laparoscopic dissecting instruments 91
Laparoscopic instruments 91
　sterilization of 171
Laparoscopic needle holder 92
Laparoscopic scissors 92, 107, 108
　parts of 101f
　types of 108f
Laparoscopic video monitor 94
Laparoscopy 370
　instruments 91
　new platforms for 117
Laser 199
　beam production in holmium laser, mechanism of 201
　fiber
　　anatomy of 204, 205f
　　configuration of 206
　　freshen tip of 212
　lithotripsy 212
　　settings 207
　　techniques of 210
　properties and mechanism of action 200
　system 204
Latzko repair 361
Leich-Gregoir extravesical approach 390
Lesion, differential diagnoses of 312
Leusch obturator 28
Lich-Gregoir technique 391f
Li-Fraumeni syndrome 272
Ligasure 126, 127f
　devices 126
Light
　amplification by stimulated emission of radiation 132, 199
　cable 3
　pillar 13
　source 91
　transmission fiberoptic cable 91
Linear regression analysis 413

Linear trend, test for 409
Lister's dilators 182*f*
Lister's metallic bougie 183
Lithoclast master 69*f*
Lithoclast
  mechanism of action of 67*f*
  with suction 68, 68*f*
Lithotripsy 198
Lithotripter 67
Lithovue 88*f*
Logic type flexible ureteroscope 82*f*
Loops
  classification of 31
  control mechanism 29
  types of 33, 34*f*
Low power suction with drainage 65*f*
Lower polar exophytic large mass 259
Lower ureter, filling defect in 262*f*
L-size clip color code 110*f*
Ludwik's straight knife waveform 22
Lymph node 306, 311
  status 311
Lymphadenectomy, regional 366
Lymphocele ascite 386
Lymphoid tumor 315

M

Malecot catheter 145, 149, 149*f*
Malleable retractor 174
Manhes style ratchet 106
Mann–Whitney test 410
Manual ventilation bags 164
Marberger compact operating fiber
   ureterorenoscope 78
Mauermayer stone punch 44, 45*f*
Meatal
  retrusion 355
  stenosis 354
Meatotomy scissor 17, 18*f*
Medial lobe resection 211
Medium-flow rates 97
Megaureter, etiology of 231
Memokath deployment, steps of 143
Mesenteric artery, inferior 278
Meta-analysis 436
  methods 438*t*
Metal cannula 104*f*
Metallic bougie 182
  use of 183
Metallic serial telescopic dilators 53
Metallic stent 143

Metastatic disease 257
Michel ureteroscope 78
Microperc 60, 62*f*, 66
Microwave ablation 133
Micturating cystourethrogram 216,
   219*f*, 222*f*, 223, 223*f*, 224*f*, 232*f*, 234*f*
  anteroposterior plate 228*f*
Mid ureteric stone stent 247
Millin's self-retaining bladder retractor
   175, 176*f*
Miniaturized percutaneous
   nephrolithotomies 63
Minimally invasive percutaneous
   nephrolithotomy 60, 63*f*
Minimally invasive surgery 134
Miniperc 58
  accessories 61*f*
Mitomycin C 327
  contraindications 327
  indications 327
Mitotane 346
Monopolar circuit 124, 124*f*
Moses technology 207
Multiload applicator 112*f*
Muscle
  invasive bladder
    cancer, chemotherapy for 330
    tumor 304
  invasive disease, high-grade 267

N

Narrow band imaging 16
Necrosis with cystic changes 300*f*
Needle
  driver, parts of 107
  holder 107
    parts of 107*f*
  types of 49, 49*f*
Needloscopes 115
Negative predictive value 408
Nelaton catheter 145, 149, 150*f*
Neoadjuvant chemotherapy 330
  advantage of 331
Neobladder, contraindications of 306
Neodymium:yttrium aluminum 200
  garnet 199
    laser 199, 202
Nephrectomy 362
  preoperative evaluation 362
  segmental 364
  simple 362

Nephrocalcinosis 243
 types of 244
Nephrometry score 260
Nephroscopes 46, 55, 56f, 58
 grips of 57f
 types of 55
Nephrostomy 245
 tubes 148
Nephroureterectomy 306, 309
 specimen of 307f
Nerves, preservation of 385
Nesbit system 29
Neuroblastoma 319
Neuroendocrine tumors, chemotherapy for 345
Neurogenic bladder 227, 228
 type of 228
Newman's test 409
Nickel 143
Nifedipine 376
Nitinol core hydrophilic guidewire 141
Nivolumab 339
Non-functional adrenal incidentaloma 320
Non-germ cell tumors 315
Noninterlocking titanium 109
Nottingham urethral dilator 154f

O

Obstructive megaureter, bilateral primary 229
Obturator 9, 22, 101
 specifications of 9
 types of 10f, 10t
Ocular lens 82
Olympus
 electrode 40f
 Turis system 39
 ureteroscopes 79
One-tailed test 402
Onlay island flap technique 351f
Online sample size calculator 404f, 405f
Open abdominal surgery 370
Open adrenalectomy 376
Open cystolithotomy 46
Open end catheter 137, 145
Open surgery 122, 123
 retractors 174
Open urology instruments 174
Optical system 82

Optiview 102, 102f
Orthophthalaldehyde 166
Orthotopic kidney 247
Otis maurmyers urethrotome 21, 23, 24f

P

P value 399
Paclitaxel 343
 dose modification for 344t
Pan anterior urethral stricture 215
Pancreatic injuries 365
Paragangliomas, assessment of 271
Paraureteric diverticula 235
Parenchyma 239
Partial nephrectomy 261, 363
 complications of 364, 365
 indications 363
 procedures 363
 relative contraindications 363
Partial orchiectomy 381
 procedure 381f
Partial penectomy 311, 313, 378
 specimen 312f
 steps in 379f
Passive dilators 153
Passive element, advantages of 31
Pazopanib 337
Pearson's correlation 410, 415
 and simple linear regression, difference between 411t
Pearson's normality test 396
Pediatric
 cystoscope-urethro-fiberscope 189f, 190f, 196f, 197
 cystourethroscope 188f
 endourology instruments 186
 instruments 47
 operating cystourethroscope 189
 optical urethrotome 190, 190f
 resectoscope 191, 191f, 192f
 uretero-reno-fiberscope 196, 197f
 ureterorenoscope 193, 193f, 197t
 urology 186, 229
Pelvic
 stone, right 237f
 ureteric junction obstruction 250
Pelvicalyceal system 240f, 258
Pelvis 269f
Pelviureteric junction 142, 308
 obstruction, diagnose secondary 235

Pembrolizumab 333, 336, 340
  exclude 333
  indication 333
Penile length, stretch of 310
Penile
  mass 310, 378
  tumor 310
  urethra 216, 223
    abnormal 353*f*
    stricture 356
Penis 340
  carcinoma 311, 312
Penoscrotal junction 223
Per acetic acid 167
Percuflex 143
Percutaneous nephrolithotomy 48, 157, 173, 440*f*
  accessories 157
  forceps 171
  instruments 48
  tract dilators 50
Percutaneous universal nephroscope 56
Perineal urethroplasty, progressive 357
Perineal urethrostomy 379
Peritoneal incision, marking of 383*f*
Peritoneum 373
Phaeochromocytoma, assessment of 271
Phenoxybenzamine 375, 376
Pheochromocytoma 376*t*
  diagnose 269
  metastatic 319
  tumors 269, 319
Pie chart 418*f*
Pig tail ureteric catheter 138, 145, 149*f*
Pirads scoring 323
PK system 127*f*
Plasma
  aldosterone concentration 271
  kinetic resection loop 40
  renin activity 271
  sterilization 162
Politano–Leadbetter technique 387, 388*f*
Polymer 143
  clips 109
Polytetrafluoroethylene 50
Polyurethane 143
  stents 143
Polyvinylchloride 145

Positive predictive value 407
Posterior urethra 220*f*, 222, 223
Post-hoc tests 409
Post-traumatic posterior urethral injuries 218
Potassium titanyl phosphate 199, 200
  laser 202
Prednisolone 335
Primary pelviureteric junction obstruction 254
Propanolol 376
Prostate
  bipolar transurethral resection of 38, 39
  carcinoma 323
  chips 36
  enlarged 227
  instruments, transurethral resection of 25
  removal of 370
  sparing radical cystectomy 305
  syndrome, transurethral resection of 35
  transurethral enucleation of 42*f*
  transurethral resection of 10, 25, 34, 38, 38*f*, 173
  transurethral vaporization of 41
Prostatic urethral length 5
Proximal penile urethra 223
Pubectomy, inferior 358
Pulse
  energy 207
  energy, use of 204
Pulsed laser 199
P-value 400*f*
Pyelolithotomy, laparoscopic 249
Pyeloplasty 367

Q

Quasi-bipolar 39

R

Rack and pinion system 29
Radiation therapy, complications after 374
Radical cystectomy 305, 372
  complications 373
Radical inguinal orchiectomy 380*f*
Radical nephrectomy 366
  indications 366

Radical orchiectomy 380
    complications 382
Radical penectomy 310, 311, 313
    specimen 310f
Radical prostatectomy 321, 369, 373
    complications 371, 372
    specimen 321, 321f
    surgical technique 370
Radiofrequency 122
    ablation 133
    energy 162
Radiopacity, differential diagnosis of 247
Randomization 431
    types of 431t
Randomized controlled trials 426, 427fc
    advantages of 428
    disadvantages of 428
    types of 428, 428f
Rectal injury 371, 373
Red rubber catheter 145
Re-entry catheter 150, 150f
Reflux
    disease 230
    primary 234
    secondary 234
Regression analysis 413
    types of 414t
Renal angiography 261
Renal calculi, bilateral 237
Renal cell carcinoma 175, 264, 336
    adjuvant therapy for 336
    metastatic 336
Renal dysfunction 366
Renal exploration 278
Renal imaging 250
Renal injury 276
Renal mass 256, 258, 258f
    right 257f
Renal oncocytoma 319
Renal reconstructive surgery 278
Renal trauma 274f, 275f, 278
    classification of 276
    indications for
        nephrectomy in 279
        surgery in 277
    management in 277
    postoperative complications of 279
    radiological investigations for 276
    role of angioembolization in 277
    severity of 276
Renal tubular acidosis 244
    types 244
Renal tumors, differential diagnoses in 302
Renal vein thrombus 264f
Renovascular injuries 279
Resectoscope 25, 27, 27f, 191
    electrodes 193f
    external end of 28, 28f
    obturator 29f
    parts of 25
    sheath 25
        parts of 28
Retracting instruments 91
Retrocaval ureter 279, 279f, 280
    types of 280
Retrograde endopyelotomy, instruments used in 79
Retrograde intrarenal surgery 393, 440f
Retrograde urethrogram 215, 215f, 217f, 219f, 220f, 222f-224f
Retroperitoneal approach, instruments used for 104
Retroperitoneal hematoma 277
Retroperitoneal lymph node 175
    dissection 382, 384f, 385f
        preoperative planning 382
        steps 382
        types 382
Retropulsion devices 150, 152
    types of 151f
Retrospective cohort study 425
    design of 425f
Reusable flexible ureteroscopes 85t
Reusable trocars 104
Richard wolf ureteroscopes 78
Rigid biopsy forceps 19, 19f
Rigid neonatal cystourethroscope 186
Ring retractor 176, 176f
Road traffic accident 273
Robinson catheter 145
Robotic
    devices 118
    drapes 119
    instrumentation 119
    instruments 91
    surgery 117, 123, 370

systems 120, 121
trocars 119
working instruments 119
Rod-lens system 11, 12f
Roizen criteria 375

S

Sachse's optical urethrotome 21, 21f, 23
Saline, transurethral resection in 39
Satinsky forceps, laparoscopic 114
Satinsky vascular clamp 92, 177, 178f
Scardino spiral flap 368
Scatter graph 419f
Scintigraphy, dynamic 311
Scissors
  parts of 108
  types of 212
Screw dilators 50, 51, 52f
Scrotal skin lymphatic drainage 314
Self-retaining catheters 145
Seminal vesicles 323
Seminoma 341
Semirigid ureteroscope, parts of 76f
Semirigid ureteroscopy 74
  classification 75
Sensor wire 142
Sepsis 233
Serial teflon ureteral dilator 153, 154f, 218
Shah superperc sheaths 65f
Shapiro–Wilk normality test 396
Sheldon staging system 305
ShockPulse and lithoclast master 70t
ShockPulse lithotripter 70f
  mechanism of action of 71f
ShockPulse, shockwaves of 71f
Shockpulse-SE™ lithotripter 69
Silicone 143
  Foley catheters 146
  stent 143
Siliconized latex Foley catheters 146
Simple rubber catheter 145
Single-use flexible ureteroscopes 86t, 87
Sinusoidal obstructive syndrome 349
SIOP staging system 303
Skewness 399
Small renal mass 260, 261
Small testicular carcinoma 314f
Snodgrass repair 350
Sober ureterostomy 231

Solid state lasers 200
Spatula blade 130
Spermatocytic tumor 316
Spiral tip ureteral access catheter 140
Splenic injury 365
Squamous cell carcinoma 305, 312
  chemotherapy in 340
Stacked bar chart 418f
Staghorn stone 238, 241
  common composition of 241
Stainless steel core guidewire 140
Stapler
  laparoscopic 113
  parts of 113f
Statistical test 406fc, 410t
  paired data 406fc
  unpaired data 405fc
Steam sterilization 161
Stents
  length of 144f
  removal forceps 19, 19f
  types of 143
Sterilization 160, 161, 165, 170, 171
  different methods of 161
  methods 173t
  steps of 167
Stethoscopes 164
Stone 240, 244
  basket 17
  burden 241
  catcher 66f
  clinic effect 238
  crushing forceps 43
  holding forceps 114, 179
  management, laser for 199
  score 242t
  score, types of 241
Storz and Wolf instrument 106f
Storz camera hub 93f
Storz miniperc dilator 58f
Storz nephroscope 59f
Storz new minimally invasive
    percutaneous nephrolithotomy
    system 63
Storz pediatric cystourethroscope 187
Straight distending obturator 28
Stricture disease 215
Stripping fiber 206
Study design, types of 394fc
Study subjects, selection of 425
Substitution urethroplasty 356

Suction cannula 157, 157f
Suction irrigation
　apparatus 92
　cannula 92
Sulfhydryl enzymes, alkylation of 164
Sunitinib 336, 337
Super hi-vision system 95
Suprapubic catheter 220
Suprapubic cystolithotomy 180
Suprapubic cystolithotripsy 46
Surgery 122
　laparoscopic 122, 123
Survival analysis Kaplan–Meier curves 421, 421f
Swiss lithoclast master 67, 68
　shockwaves of 69f
Symphysis pubis, umbilicus to 372

T

T test 408
Telescope 3, 11, 92
　basic structure of 13
　channel 9
　laparoscopic 91
　parts of 13
　sterilization of 172
Telescopic metal dilators 50
Temsirolimus 339
Teratoma syndrome 317
Testicular
　cancers, chemotherapy in 341
　mass 314
　tumor 314
　　types of 315
Testis, carcinoma of 316, 380
Thiersch-Duplay technique 352
Thompson walker suprapubic cystolithotomy forceps 179, 181f
Three dimensional video technology 96f
Three-incision technique 211
Three-way
　catheters with color codes 148f
　Foley hematuria catheters 147
　hemostatic catheters 146, 147
Thromboembolism, venous 374
Thrombus, venous 259
Thudicum 183, 184f
Thulium fiber laser 200, 203, 203f, 204, 211, 212
　advantages of 204

Thulium:yttrium aluminum garnet laser 200, 203, 212
Tiemann catheter 148, 149f
Tissue ischemia 353
Titanium alloy 143
Toomey syringe 36f, 37
Toothed grasper 92
Torqueable tip ureteral access catheter 139f, 140
Toxicity 343, 344, 346
Tract dilators 50
Transitional cell carcinoma 133, 263, 264
Transurethral cystolithotripsy 46
Transurethral resection syndrome 39
Transverse preputial island flap 351
Trauma, abdominal 277
Trocars 91, 92, 99
　classification 99f
Tumor
　benign 263
　in ureter, types of 262
　malignant 263
　metastatic 317
　origin of 310
　paratesticular 315
　stages of 302
　T stage of 257
　thrombus 259
　triphasic nature of 301
　type of 313
Turkey's test 409
Turner Warwick 185f
　needle holder 185
　retractor set 176
Two-tailed test 402

U

Ultramini percutaneous nephrolithotomy 60, 62f
Ultrasonic
　devices 131
　dissectors 129, 130
　generator 129, 129f
　hook 130
Ultrasonography 171
Ultrasound
　instruments 164
　physics of 129
Ultrathin ureteroscope 79

Unpaired T test 408
Upper urinary tract 74
Urachal carcinoma, stages of 305
Ureter
  bilateral 373
  pathology 304
Ureteral balloon dilator 153
Ureteric catheter 137, 138f
  types of 137, 145
Ureteric dilator 153
Ureteric injury 371
Ureteric mass, lower 262
Ureteric stone
  bilateral 244
  right 245f
Ureterocalycostomy 368
Ureterocele 196
Ureteropelvic junction, abnormal 367
Ureteroresectoscope 79
Ureteroscopes 78, 172
  evolution of 74
  semicritical item, sterilization of 171
Ureteroscopy 154f
Urethra
  posterior 220f, 222, 223
  prostatic 304
  supracorporal rerouting of 359
  tubularization of 352
Urethral balloon dilators 153
Urethral catheters 145
Urethral diverticulum 354
Urethral length gain 359
Urethral stricture 354, 356
  anterior 216, 355
Urethral surgery, instruments used in 181
Urethral tumor 310, 311
  treatment 311
Urethral valve
  anterior 223
  posterior 233
Urethrectomy, indications of 306
Urethroplasty 218
Urethrotome knifes 191f
Urethrotomy 23f, 219
Urinary catheter 145
Urinary tract
  infection 196, 222
  symptoms 227
Urine leak 365, 374

Urinoma, drainage of 368
Urolithiasis 237
Urologic laparoscopy, armamentarium
    required for 91
Urological malignancies, chemotherapy
    in 327
Urology 199
  lasers in 199
Uroradiology 213
Urothelial bladder cancer 332
Urticaria 345

V

Vaginal repair 360, 361
Valves, types of 233
Vancouver and Harvard style of
    referencing, differences between
    442t
Vapor pulse coagulation 127
Vascular instruments 177
  use of 179
Vena cava
  inferior 175, 258
  thrombectomy, inferior 387
Veno-occlusive disease 349
Ventilators 164
Veress needle 92, 97, 98, 100f
  mode 96
  parts of 98f
Vesical end knob 9
Vesicoureteric junction 142, 306
Vesicoureteric reflux, causes of 369
Vesicovaginal fistula repair 360
Video monitor 91
Video output 94, 94f
Video resolution and pixels 94, 94t
Video-imaging armamentarium 91
Vinblastine 345
Visiport 101, 102f
Visual internal urethrotomy 21, 218
  blades, types of 22f
Voiding dysfunction 196

W

Waveform 124f
Weiss criteria 319
Whistle tip catheter 138
Whitish infiltrative growth 310f

Wilms' tumor 300, 302
   chemotherapy for 347, 348, 348*t*
   origin of 301
   types of 301
Windsock sign 233
Wolf and Storz nephroscopes, major
   differences in 56
Wolf miniature compact fiber
   cystourethroscope 186
Wolf miniperc
   dilators and sheath 59*f*
   nephroscope 60*f*
Wolf pediatric
   optical urethrotome 190
   ureterorenoscope 194, 194*f*

Wound
   infection 354
   separation 354

X

X-ray pelvis anteroposterior 221*f*

Y

Yttrium aluminum garnet 199
Y-V plasty 367

Z

Zebra guidewire 142

EU GSPR Authorised Reprsentative
Logos Europe, 9 rue Nicolas Poussin
1700, La Rochelle, France
Phone: +33 (0) 6 67 93 73 78
E-mail: contact@logoseurope.eu

www.ingramcontent.com/pod-product-compliance
Ingram Content Group UK Ltd.
Pitfield, Milton Keynes, MK11 3LW, UK
UKHW050427150426
5217IPUK00019B/1279